Evidence-based Clinical Chinese Medicine

Volume 27

Overweight and Obesity in Adults

Evidence-based Clinical Chinese Medicine

Print ISSN: 2529-7562
Online ISSN: 2529-7554

Series Co Editors-in-Chief

Charlie Changli Xue *(RMIT University, Australia)*
Chuanjian Lu *(Guangdong Provincial Hospital of Chinese Medicine, China)*

Published

More information on this series can also be found at https://www.worldscientific.com/series/ebccm

(Continued at end of book)

Evidence-based Clinical Chinese Medicine

Co Editors-in-Chief

Charlie Changli Xue
RMIT University, Australia

Chuanjian Lu
Guangdong Provincial Hospital of Chinese Medicine, China

Volume 27
Overweight and Obesity in Adults

Lead Authors

Johannah Shergis
RMIT University, Australia

Jiaxin Chen
Guangdong Provincial Hospital of Chinese Medicine, China

World Scientific

NEW JERSEY · LONDON · SINGAPORE · BEIJING · SHANGHAI · HONG KONG · TAIPEI · CHENNAI · TOKYO

Published by

World Scientific Publishing Co. Pte. Ltd.

5 Toh Tuck Link, Singapore 596224

USA office: 27 Warren Street, Suite 401-402, Hackensack, NJ 07601

UK office: 57 Shelton Street, Covent Garden, London WC2H 9HE

Library of Congress Cataloging-in-Publication Data

Names: Xue, Charlie Changli, author. | Lu, Chuan-jian, 1964–   author.

Title: Evidence-based clinical Chinese medicine / Charlie Changli Xue, Chuanjian Lu.

Description: New Jersey : World Scientific, 2016. | Includes bibliographical references and index.

Identifiers: LCCN 2015030389| ISBN 9789814723084 (v. 1 : hardcover : alk. paper) |
   ISBN 9789814723091 (v. 1 : paperback : alk. paper) |
   ISBN 9789814723121 (v. 2 : hardcover : alk. paper) |
   ISBN 9789814723138 (v. 2 : paperback : alk. paper) |
   ISBN 9789814759045 (v. 3 : hardcover : alk. paper) |
   ISBN 9789814759052 (v. 3 : paperback : alk. paper)

Subjects: | MESH: Medicine, Chinese Traditional--methods. | Clinical Medicine--methods. |
   Evidence-Based Medicine--methods. | Psoriasis. | Pulmonary Disease, Chronic Obstructive.

Classification: LCC RC81 | NLM WB 55.C4 | DDC 616--dc23

LC record available at http://lccn.loc.gov/2015030389

Volume 27: Overweight and Obesity in Adults

ISBN 978-981-126-039-1 (hardcover)

ISBN 978-981-126-040-7 (ebook for institutions)

ISBN 978-981-126-041-4 (ebook for individuals)

British Library Cataloguing-in-Publication Data

A catalogue record for this book is available from the British Library.

For any available supplementary material, please visit
https://www.worldscientific.com/worldscibooks/10.1142/12967#t=suppl

Disclaimer

The information in this monograph is based on systematic analyses of the best available evidence for Chinese medicine interventions, both historical and contemporary. Every effort has been made to ensure the accuracy and completeness of the data in this publication. This book is intended for clinicians, researchers and educators. The practice of evidence-based medicine considers the best available evidence, practitioners' clinical experience and judgement, and patients' preference. Not all interventions are acceptable in all countries. It is important to note that some of the substances mentioned in this book may no longer be in use, toxic, prohibited, or restricted under the provisions of the Convention on International Trade in Endangered Species of Wild Fauna and Flora (CITES). Practitioners, researchers and educators are advised to comply with the relevant regulations in their country and with the restrictions on the trade of the species included in CITES appendices I, II and III. This book is not intended as a guide for self-medication. Patients should seek professional advice from qualified Chinese medicine practitioners.

Foreword

Since the late 20th century, Chinese medicine, including acupuncture and herbal medicine, has been increasingly used throughout the world. The parallel development and spread of evidence-based medicine has provided challenges and opportunities for Chinese medicine.

The opportunities have been evidence-based medicine's emphasis on the effective use of the best available clinical evidence, incorporating the clinicians' clinical experience, subject to patients' preference. Such practices have a patient focus that reflects the historical nature of Chinese medicine practice. However, the challenges are also significant due to the fact that, despite the long-term development and very rich literature accumulated over 2,000 years, there is an overall lack of high-level clinical evidence for many of the interventions used in Chinese medicine.

To address this knowledge gap, we need to generate clinical evidence through high-quality clinical studies and evaluate evidence to enable the effective use of such available evidence to promote evidence-based Chinese medicine practice.

Modern Chinese medicine is rooted in its classical literature and the legacies of ancient doctors, grounded in the practice of expert clinicians and increasingly informed by clinical and experimental research efforts. In recognition of the unique features of Chinese medicine, for each of the conditions in this series, a 'whole-evidence' approach is used to provide a synthesis of different types and levels of evidence to enable practitioners to make clinical decisions informed by the current best evidence.

There are four main components of this 'whole-evidence' approach. Firstly, we present the current approaches to the diagnosis, differentiation and treatment of each condition based on expert consensus in published textbooks and clinical guidelines. This provides an overview of how the condition is currently managed. The second section provides an analysis of the condition in a historical context based on systematic searches of the *Zhong Hua Yi Dian* 中华医典, which includes the full texts of more than 1,000 classical medical books. These analyses provide objective views on how the condition has been treated over two millennia, reveal continuities and discontinuities between traditional and modern practice, and suggest avenues for future research.

The third component is the assessment of evidence derived from modern clinical studies of Chinese medicine interventions. The methods established by the Cochrane Collaboration are used as the basis for conducting systematic reviews and undertaking meta-analyses of outcome data for randomised controlled trials (RCTs). In addition, the clinical relevance of meta-analysis data is enhanced by examining the herbal formulae, individual herbs, and acupuncture treatments that were assessed in the RCTs and the evidence base is broadened by the inclusion of data from controlled clinical trials and non-controlled studies. The fourth component is to determine how the herbal medicine interventions may achieve the effects indicated by the clinical trials. Thus, for each of the most frequently used herbs, we provide reviews of their effects in pre-clinical models and their likely mechanisms of action.

For each condition, this 'whole-evidence' approach links clinical expertise, historical precedent, clinical research data, and experimental research to provide the reader with assessments of the current state of the evidence for the efficacy, effectiveness and safety of Chinese medicine interventions using herbal medicines, acupuncture and moxibustion, and other health care practices, such as *tai chi* 太极.

Since these books are available in Chinese and English, they can benefit patients, practitioners and educators internationally and enable practitioners to make clinical decisions informed by the current best evidence.

These publications represent a major milestone in the development of Chinese medicine and make a significant contribution to the development of evidence-based Chinese medicine globally.

Co-Editors-In-Chief

Distinguished Professor Charlie Changli Xue,
RMIT University, Australia

Professor Chuanjian Lu, Guangdong Provincial Hospital of
Chinese Medicine, China

Purpose of the Monograph

This book is intended for clinicians, researchers and educators. It can be used to inform tertiary education and clinical practice by providing systematic, multi-dimensional assessments of the best available evidence for using Chinese medicine to manage each common clinical condition.

How to Use this Monograph

Some Definitions

A glossary is included, containing terms and definitions that frequently appear in the book. It also describes the definitions of statistical tests, methodological terms, evaluation tools, and interventions. For example, in this book, Integrative Medicine refers to the combined use of a Chinese medicine treatment with conventional medical management, and Combination Therapies refer to two or more Chinese medicines from different therapy groups (Chinese herbal medicine, acupuncture or other Chinese medicine therapies) administered together. The terminology used throughout the monograph is based on the World Health Organization's *Standard Terminologies on Traditional Medicine in the Western Pacific Region* (2007), where possible or from the cited reference.

Data Analysis and Interpretation of Results

In order to synthesise the clinical evidence, a range of statistical analysis approaches are used. In general, the effect size for dichotomous data is reported as a risk ratio (RR) with a 95% confidence interval (CI), and for continuous data, they are reported as mean difference (MD) with 95% CI. Statistically significant effects are indicated with an asterisk. Readers should note that being statistical significant does not necessarily correspond with a clinically important effect. Interpretation of results should take into consideration of the clinical significance, quality of studies (expressed as "high", "low" or "unclear" risk of bias in this book), and heterogeneity amongst the studies. Tests for heterogeneity are conducted using the I^2 statistic. An I^2 score greater than 50% may indicate substantial heterogeneity.

Use of Evidence in Practice

The Grading of Recommendations Assessment, Development and Evaluation (GRADE) approach was used to summarise the results and the certainty of the evidence for critical and important comparisons and outcomes. Due to the diverse nature of Chinese medicine practice, treatment recommendations are not included with the summary of findings tables. Therefore readers will need to interpret the evidence with reference to the local practice environment.

Limitations

Readers should note some of the methodological limitations of the classical literature and the clinical evidence.

- Search terms used to search the *Zhong Hua Yi Dian* 中华医典 database may not include all terms that have been used for the condition, which may alter the findings.
- The Chinese language has changed over time. Citations have been interpreted for analysis, and such interpretations may be subject to disagreement.
- The Chinese medicine theory has evolved over time. As such, concepts described in classical Chinese medical literature may no longer be found in contemporary works.

- Symptoms described in citations may be common to many conditions, and a judgement was required to determine the likelihood of the citation being related to the condition. This may have introduced some bias due to the subjective nature of the judgement.
- The vast majority of the clinical evidence for Chinese medicine treatments has come from China. The applicability of the findings to other populations and countries requires further assessment.
- Many studies included participants with varying disease severity. Where possible, subgroup analyses were undertaken to examine the effects in different sub-populations. As this was not always possible, the findings may be limited to the population included and not to sub-populations.
- The potential risk of bias found in many included studies suggested methodological limitations. The findings for GRADE assessments based on studies of very low to moderate quality evidence should be interpreted accordingly.
- Nine major English and Chinese language databases were searched to identify clinical studies, in addition to clinical trial registers. Other studies may exist that were not identified through searches and which may alter the findings.
- The calculation of the frequency of herbal formula use was based on formula names. It is possible that studies evaluated herbal treatments with the same or similar herb ingredients but were given different formula names. Due to the complexity of herbal formulas, it was considered not appropriate to make a judgement as to the similarity of the formulas for analysis. As such, the frequency of the formulas reported in Chap. 5 may be underestimated.
- The most frequently utilised herbs that may have contributed to the treatment effect have been described in Chap. 5. These herbs may provide leads for further exploration. Calculation of the herbs with potential effects is based on the frequency of formulae reported in the studies and does not take into consideration the clinical implications and functions of every herb in a formula.

Authors and Contributors

CO-EDITORS-IN-CHIEF
Distinguished Prof. Charlie Changli Xue (*RMIT University, Australia*)
Prof. Chuanjian Lu (*Guangdong Provincial Hospital of Chinese Medicine, China*)

CO-DEPUTY EDITORS-IN-CHIEF
Prof. Anthony Lin Zhang (*RMIT University, Australia*)
Dr. Brian H May (*RMIT University, Australia*)
Prof. Xinfeng Guo (*Guangdong Provincial Hospital of Chinese Medicine, China*)
Prof. Zehuai Wen (*Guangdong Provincial Hospital of Chinese Medicine, China*)

LEAD AUTHORS
Dr Johannah Shergis (*RMIT University*)
Dr Jiaxin Chen (*Guangdong Provincial Hospital of Chinese Medicine, China*)

CO-AUTHORS:
RMIT University (Australia):
Prof. Anthony Lin Zhang
Distinguished Prof. Charlie Changli Xue

Guangdong Provincial Hospital of Chinese Medicine (China):
Prof. Changcai Xie
Prof. Wenbin Fu
Prof. Xinfeng Guo

Members of Advisory Committee and Panel

CO-CHAIRS OF PROJECT PLANNING COMMITTEE
Prof. Peter J Coloe (*RMIT University, Australia*)
Prof. Yubo Lyu (*Guangdong Provincial Hospital of Chinese Medicine, China*)
Prof. Dacan Chen (*Guangdong Provincial Hospital of Chinese Medicine, China*)

CENTRE ADVISORY COMMITTEE (ALPHABETICAL ORDER)
Prof. Keji Chen (*The Chinese Academy of Sciences, China*)
Prof. Aiping Lu (*Hong Kong Baptist University, China*)
Prof. Caroline Smith (*Western Sydney University, Australia*)
Prof. David F Story (*RMIT University, Australia*)

METHODOLOGY EXPERT ADVISORY PANEL (ALPHABETICAL ORDER)
Prof. Zhaoxiang Bian (*Hong Kong Baptist University, China*)
The Late Prof. George Lewith (*University of Southampton, United Kingdom*)
Prof. Lixing Lao (*The University of Hong Kong, China*)
Prof. Jianping Liu (*Beijing University of Chinese Medicine, China*)
Prof. Frank Thien (*Monash University, Australia*)
Prof. Jialiang Wang (*Sichuan University, China*)

CONTENT EXPERT ADVISORY PANEL (ALPHABETICAL ORDER)
Prof. Bin Xu (*Nanjing University of Chinese Medicine, China*)
Prof. Li Yan (*Peking Union Medical College Hospital, China*)

Distinguished Professor Charlie Changli Xue, PhD

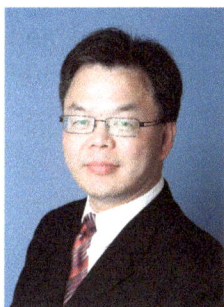

Distinguished Professor Charlie Changli Xue holds a Bachelor of Medicine (majoring in Chinese Medicine) from the Guangzhou University of Chinese Medicine, China (1987) and a PhD from RMIT University, Australia (2000). He has been an academic, researcher, regulator, and practitioner for over three decades. Distinguished Professor Xue has made significant contributions to evidence-based educational development, clinical research, regulatory framework and policy development, and provision of high-quality clinical care to the community. Distinguished Professor Xue is recognised internationally as an expert in evidence-based traditional medicine and integrative healthcare.

Distinguished Professor Xue is the Inaugural National Chair of the Chinese Medicine Board of Australia appointed by the Australian Health Workforce Ministerial Council (in 2011), and he was reappointed for a second term in 2014. Since 2007, he has been a Member of the World Health Organization (WHO) Expert Advisory Panel for Traditional and Complementary Medicine, Geneva. Professor Xue is also Honorary Senior Principal Research Fellow at the Guangdong Provincial Academy of Chinese Medical Sciences, China.

At RMIT, Distinguished Professor Xue is an Associate Deputy Vice-Chancellor (International). He is also Director of the World Health Organization (WHO) Collaborating Centre for Traditional Medicine.

Between 1995 and 2010, Professor Xue was Discipline Head of Chinese Medicine at RMIT University. He leads the development of five successful undergraduate and postgraduate degree programs in Chinese Medicine at RMIT University, which is now a global leader in Chinese medicine education and research.

Professor Xue's research has been supported by over AU$15 million worth of research grants, including six project grants from the Australian Government's National Health & Medical Research Council (NHMRC) and two Australian Research Council (ARC) grants. He has contributed over 200 publications and has been frequently invited as a keynote speaker for numerous national and international conferences. Professor Xue has contributed to over 300 media interviews on issues related to complementary medicine education, research, regulation and practice.

Professor Chuanjian Lu, MD

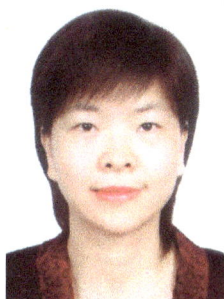

Professor Chuanjian Lu is Doctor of Medicine. She is the vice president of the Guangdong Provincial Hospital of Chinese Medicine (Guangdong Provincial Academy of Chinese Medical Sciences, Second Clinical Medical College of Guangzhou University of Chinese Medicine). She also is the chair of the Guangdong Traditional Chinese Medicine (TCM) Standardization Technical Committee and the vice-chair of the Immunity Specialty Committee of the World Federation of Chinese Medicine Societies (WFCMS).

Professor Lu has engaged in scientific research into TCM, clinical practice, and teaching for some 25 years. Her research has been devoted to integrated traditional and western medicine. She has edited and published 12 monographs and 120 academic research articles as the first author and corresponding author, with over 30 articles being included in SCI journals.

She has received widespread recognition for her achievements, with awards for Excellent Teacher of South China, National Outstanding Women TCM Doctor, and National Outstanding Young Doctor of TCM. She also received The Science and Technology Star of the Association of Chinese Medicine, the National Excellent Science and Technology Workers of China Award, and the Five-Continent Women's Scientific Awards of China Medical Women's Association.

Professor Lu has won the Award of Science and Technology Progress over 10 times from the Guangdong Provincial Government, China Association of Chinese Medicine, and Chinese Hospital Association.

Acknowledgements

The authors and contributors would like to acknowledge the valuable contributions of the following people who assisted with database searches, data extraction, data screening, data assessment, translation of documents, editing, and/or administrative tasks: Kevin Wang, Iris Zhou, Dr Mary Zhang, Edward Caruso, Hanlin Wang, Jieling Lin, and Shiya Huang.

Contents

Contents

Contents

List of Figures

List of Tables

1

Introduction to Overweight and Obesity

OVERVIEW

Overweight and obesity is recognised as one of the world's leading health concerns. It is a result of many interacting factors, including genes and the environment, with an energy imbalance due to a sedentary lifestyle, excessive calorie intake, or both. It has significant effects on morbidity, quality of life, mortality and health expenditure. It is associated with many complications and chronic illnesses, including diabetes mellitus, cardiovascular disease, hypertension, stroke and some cancers.

Definition of Overweight and Obesity

Overweight and obesity are physical states as well as chronic diseases. Specifically, they are conditions in which weight gain is caused by an increase in the volume of body fat and/or the number of adipose cells, or an abnormally high percentage of body fat, usually with excessive fat deposits in some local areas. It is increasing in prevalence and is associated with a significant risk of metabolic disorders, cardiovascular disease, cancer, mental health disease, as well as physical and social effects. Overweight and obesity are classified using the body mass index (BMI), calculated by dividing weight (kilograms [kg]) by height squared (metres^2). A person with a BMI of 25–29.9 kg/m^2 is classified as overweight and obesity is classified as a BMI greater than or equal to 30 kg/m^2.

Clinical Presentation

People will appear overweight and have excess fat on the abdomen, upper arms, legs, face, etc. They are most likely overeating relative to their energy expenditure and are often unable to manage their food intake and physical activity. As well as ongoing and routine monitoring of BMI, screening and managing comorbidities, assessing other health risks is important for this group of people. Obesity contributes to cardiovascular risk factors, including hypertension, impaired fasting glucose, and dyslipidaemia. It is also associated with many comorbidities including type 2 diabetes mellitus, cardiovascular disease, sleep apnoea and certain cancers.[1] Therefore, proper assessment, ongoing monitoring and treatment are required. People often make multiple attempts to lose weight, and this may assist in understanding the underlying factors and developing an appropriate treatment plan.

Epidemiology

Obesity is increasing in most regions of the world. In developed countries, the number of people who are overweight and obese is reaching epidemic proportions, and those with morbid obesity is also on the rise.[2,3] It is estimated that more than 1.9 billion adults (39%) are overweight, and the proportion is projected to be 60% in 2030.[4] Occupation-related physical activity, as well as household management energy expenditure, has declined over the last 50 years.[5,6] As developed and developing countries move towards service-based or technology-enhanced occupations without the need for physical activity, coupled with people spending more time doing sedentary activities, such as watching TV, the number of people with obesity has continued to rise.

The global age-standardised mean BMI increased from 21.7 kg/m² (95% confidence interval [CI] 21.3 to 22.1) in 1975 to 24.2 kg/m² (95% CI 24.0 to 24.4) in 2014 in men, and from 22.1 kg/m² (95% CI 21.7 to 22.5) in 1975 to 24.4 kg/m² (95% CI 24.2 to 24.6) in 2014 in women. Age-standardised prevalence of obesity increased from 3.2% (95% CI 2.4 to 4.1) in 1975 to 10.8% (95% CI 9.7 to 12.0) in 2014 in men, and from 6.4% (95% CI 5.1 to 7.8) to 14.9% (95% CI 13.6 to 16.1) in women. Men account for 2.3% (95% CI 2.0 to 2.7) and women 5.0% (95% CI 4.4 to 5.6) of severely obese people in 2014 (i.e., have a BMI $\geq$ 35 kg/m^2).[7]

The prevalence of obesity in the United States (US) is one of the highest in the world. It has significantly increased over the last 20 years and is currently estimated at almost 40% of adults.[8] Obesity prevalence among men and women follows a similar pattern by age, with a slight increase as people get older. Men and women aged 40–59 account for the highest proportion (40.8% and 44.7%, respectively).[8] In other regions of the world, the prevalence of obesity is lower but still significant. Most countries, such as Canada, China, Europe, Australia, Latin America, Southern and Northern African countries and the Middle East, report that about 20–30% of their adult population are obese. However, these data are for obesity only, and the prevalence of people who are overweight is much higher at about 60%. In Western and Central African countries and many Asian countries, the number is much lower at about 2–10%.[9,10]

Burden

Despite many government agencies and health organisations developing guidelines for managing people with overweight and obesity, there has been no substantial effect in reducing overweight and obesity rates. Overweight and obesity is the cause of about four million deaths per year, 3.9% of years of life lost and 3.8% of disability-adjusted life-years (DALYs) worldwide.[9] It is also associated with other serious health risks[11] and increases the risk of cardiovascular disease and all-cause mortality.[12] Health burden aside, it represents a significant economic burden, including direct and indirect health care costs. In the US, the annual costs relating to obesity are US$1.4 trillion[13] and medical costs alone are US$147 billion per year, US$1,429 higher than those of people with normal weight.[14]

Risk Factors

People can become overweight and obese at any age, and there are many modifiable contributing factors (and some unmodifiable factors). Starting in gestation, nutrition in early life is thought to have an effect on metabolic states and future obesity. For example, a higher BMI and greater gestational weight gain in mothers are associated with a higher BMI in their children.[15] Furthermore, children whose mothers have type 2 diabetes are more likely to be overweight.[16] Lifestyle factors during childhood and adolescence can have an effect on future obesity. Obesity in childhood typically persists during adolescence and into adulthood, especially in children with an obese parent. However, in most overweight and obese people, the problem starts in adulthood due to lifestyle factors (secondary causes are uncommon but still need to be ruled out).

Lifestyle

The primary risk factors include lifestyle choices, such as reduced physical activity and maintaining a high-energy (food) intake. This is particularly problematic as occupational physical and household activities are rapidly declining, and sedentary time, including watching TV, is rapidly increasing, leading to reduced energy expenditure.[17]

Genetic

There is a genetic component, and heritability is high. Generally, genes do not directly cause obesity, but they can predispose certain people to become obese and make them susceptible to obesogenic environmental factors.[18] Some research has shown that genetic mutations in leptin pathways can cause obesity, but this is very rare, and only a handful of people worldwide have been diagnosed with genetically based leptin deficiency.[19]

Gender

Gender and hormones also play a role in obesity in terms of food intake, sensitivity to insulin and leptin and body fat distribution. For example, males tend to have more visceral fat, whereas females have more subcutaneous fat deposits.[20] Women have certain periods in their lives when the risk of becoming overweight and obese is higher, such as during pregnancy and postpartum. Menopause is also a significant risk for weight gain in women, with a shift to more abdominal fat distribution with increased associated health risks.[21] In men, as in women, ageing is a significant risk for weight gain. A decline in physical activity as well as hormonal changes, including oestrogen and testosterone, lead to increased fat mass.

Socioeconomic and Ethnic Factors

There is a higher prevalence of obesity in lower socioeconomic groups, possibly due to a lack of nutrition education or access to affordable healthy foods or the local environment.[22] In addition, ethnicity influences the risk of obesity, with white men, Black women and Hispanics being at higher risk than other groups.[23]

Medical

Medical disorders can also lead to overweight and obesity, such as hypothyroidism, due to slowing metabolic activity, an injury to brain centres that regulate the hypothalamus,[24] polycystic ovarian syndrome and growth hormone deficiencies.

Behavioural

Other factors that may lead to obesity (or prevent successful weight loss) include sleep deprivation, which is thought to increase appetite. Smoking cessation can also be a factor, and most people gain weight while trying to quit.[25] Furthermore, people who smoke and are over-weight have at a greater risk of obesity morbidity and mortality.

Medications

Some antipsychotic medications, tricyclic antidepressants, antiepi-leptics and insulin are associated with weight gain,[26] as are glucocorticoids, which in some cases lead to Cushing's Syndrome.

Pathological Processes

A decline in physical activity accompanied by energy-dense food intake leads to increased deposition of fat and subsequently causes people to become overweight and obese. There are complex feed-back control systems involving the hormonal and neural mechanisms that maintain energy balance, body weight and fat stores. Nutrients are a fundamental and ongoing need for life and the biological mechanisms that strongly drive food-seeking behaviours. The central nervous system receives afferent signals about ingested and stored nutrients and triggers behavioural, autonomic and endocrine out-put. There is a highly complex homeostatic system whereby the body is resistant to losing weight. It involves the hypothalamus, caudal brainstem, as well as areas in the cortex and limbic system that com-plicate food, reward and emotions.[27] Leptin is one of the most potent hormones in the feedback system, and its production is closely related to body fat mass. It can reduce food intake and increase the activity of the sympathetic nervous system, whereas ghrelin, another important gut hormone, can increase food intake. After weight loss, ghrelin increases, thereby stimulating appetite and making the diet-induced weight loss difficult to maintain.

Obesity has many adverse effects on hemodynamics and cardio-vascular structure and function,[1] leading to an increased risk of weight-related comorbidities. There is increased cardiac output and cardiac work, potentially leading to cardiomyopathy and heart fail-ure. In terms of hemodynamics, obesity increases blood volume, stroke volume and arterial pressure and contributes to increased left ventricular wall stress and pulmonary artery hypertension. It negatively effects the cardiac structure by causing left ventricular remodelling, left atrial enlargement and ventricular hypertrophy, leading to increased heart weight and wall thickness. Inflammation, including increased C-reactive protein and the overexpression of tumour necrosis factor, is common.[28] Furthermore, obesity is associated with changes in lipid metabolism, leading to high concentrations of cholesterol and triglycerides.

In terms of diabetes risk, obesity is associated with metabolic syndrome and type 2 diabetes, including insulin resistance and hyperinsulinemia, leptin insensitivity and hyperleptinemia, reduced adiponectin, sympathetic nervous system, renin-angiotensin-aldosterone system activation, etc.[28] People with obesity and metabolic syndrome are also at an increased risk of heart failure and stroke compared to the general population.[29]

Diagnosis

The BMI is widely accepted as the measure to determine if a person is at a healthy weight. The BMI is calculated as weight in kilograms divided by height in metres squared (kg/m^2), and it is classified into four categories. However, the categories are different for Europids and Asian populations, as the latter have increased risks with a lower BMI (Table 1.1).[30] People with a BMI of between 25 and 29.9 kg/m^2 are classified as overweight, and those with a BMI greater than or equal to 30 kg/m^2 are classified as obese.[23]

Waist circumference should also be measured to classify and monitor changes over time. It can help to assess the risk of obesity-related complications and is a recommended measurement in clinical practice guidelines to predict cardiovascular disease and diabetes.[31] Furthermore, it is useful in certain groups, including the elderly or people with high muscle mass, such as bodybuilders. In these groups, the BMI may overestimate or underestimate weight categorisation. Waist circumference may not be necessary for people

Table 1.1. Classification of Weight by Body Mass Index in Adults

Classification	BMI kg/m²*	BMI kg/m² (Asian Populations)†	Risk of Comorbidities
Underweight	Below 18.5 kg/m²	Below 18.5 kg/m²	Low
Healthy weight	18.5 to 24.9 kg/m²	18.5 and 22.9 kg/m²	Average
Overweight	25 to 29.9 kg/m²	23 to 24.9 kg/m²	Increased
Obese	30 or greater kg/m²	25 or greater kg/m²	Moderate/severe

Abbreviations: BMI, body mass index; kg, kilograms; m², metres squared.
* General Body Mass Index classifications.
† BMI classifications based on Asian individuals.
Table adapted from NIH and WHO guidelines.[11,30,33,34]

with a BMI greater than 35. A waist circumference greater than or equal to 40 inches (102 cm) in men and greater than or equal to 35 inches (88 cm) in women indicates an increased cardiometabolic risk.[32]

Obesity-related health risks should also be investigated, including diabetes mellitus, cardiovascular disease (hypertension, dyslipidemia, impaired fasting glucose), heart disease, sleep apnoea, non-alcoholic fatty liver disease, osteoarthritis, polycystic ovarian syndrome, etc. These conditions are strongly associated with obesity. Together, they put people at a higher risk of mortality.

Management

A multi-component approach is better than single interventions (Table 1.2). It primarily includes reduced energy intake, increased physical activity and behavioural change. The choice of management will depend on how much weight the person needs to lose, comorbidities and preference. In addition to weight loss, goals of treatment should include the prevention and reversal of complications and improved quality of life. Most countries have clinical practice guidelines for overweight and obesity, and most contain similar advice in terms of screening, management and treatment.[35] A reduction of at least 5% of one's body weight is beneficial. Generally, a weight loss

Table 1.2.   Chapter Summary

Definition of overweight and obesity	• Overweight: body mass index (BMI) of 25–29.9 kg/m² • Obesity: BMI ≥ 30 kg/m²
Risk factors	• Lifestyle behaviours, including reduced physical activity and energy-rich foods • Genetic factors — interacting with environmental factors • Gender • Socioeconomic and ethnic factors • Medical conditions (e.g., polycystic ovarian syndrome) • Medications
Management	• Diet (calorie reduction) • Increased physical activity • Behavioural change • Pharmacological (e.g., orlistat) • Non-pharmacological (e.g., surgery, complementary and alternative therapies)

Abbreviations: BMI, body mass index; kg, kilograms; m², metres squared.

of 10 to 15% is a good result, whereas anything exceeding 15% is an excellent result.[32]

People who are overweight with a BMI between 25 and 29.9 kg/m² and risk factors for cardiovascular disease are encouraged to lose weight. A multi-component intervention is required, including a healthy diet and regular exercise to create an energy deficit, as well as behavioural counselling to prevent further weight gain. People with a BMI of 30 kg/m² or more are advised to adopt a healthy lifestyle in addition to requiring more intense weight loss interventions and weight loss programs. These may include a very low-energy diet, weight loss medications and/or bariatric surgery.

Before a management plan is implemented, it is important to assess a person's willingness to make lifestyle and behavioural changes. This may include understanding their motivations, confidence to make the changes, identifying possible barriers and their support network. People should also be encouraged to self-manage their weight loss alongside ongoing monitoring.

Generally, management should focus on gradual weight loss and then weight maintenance. Small amounts of weight loss over time can improve health and well-being[35] by lowering cardiovascular risk, preventing or delaying the progression, improving control of type 2 diabetes and improving other health conditions. It can also improve one's quality of life and self-esteem and reduce depression.[35] Weight gain is largely triggered by behavioural, medical and socioeconomic factors, so prevention and early management are important.

Lifestyle Interventions

Multi-component lifestyle interventions, including increased physical activity and diet adjustment, are needed to induce an energy deficit. In addition, behavioural changes are needed for (and to maintain) weight loss.[32,35]

Diet

Calorie restriction below expenditure should produce initial weight loss (usually a calorie deficit of 500 to 1,000 kcal/day).[32] Many types of diets can produce weight loss, and there is no global recommendation. Rather, energy intake and diet adherence are the key factors. Common diets include low-calorie, low-fat, low-carbohydrate, high-protein and Mediterranean diets.[36] It is important that patients are referred to the appropriate services, such as a dietitian to assist with making diet changes to ensure they have balanced nutrition, especially for those on a very low–energy diet. The gut microbiome also plays a key role in digestion and can influence obesity as well as the body's ability to lose weight through dietary interventions. Therefore, a varied diet rich in fibre may be beneficial. In many countries, there are national dietary guidelines that can advise on nutrition, and a diet of 800 to 1,200 kcal/day will induce weight loss. However, the rate of weight loss is not always predictable. This may be due to one's diet adherence, body composition and energy expenditure, as well as metabolic adaptations that lead to a less than expected weight loss.

Gender and age may also play a role in how much weight is lost through diet.[37] For example, men generally lose more than women as they have higher energy expenditure, as do younger individuals because metabolic rate declines as people get older.[38]

Physical Activity

Physical activity and energy expenditure is an important element for weight loss in the short and long term in conjunction with diet modifications, as exercise alone only produces modest weight loss.[39] Most energy is expended through resting metabolic processes, including maintaining one's body temperature, cardiac and respiratory function, muscle function and gastrointestinal processes. However, for weight loss, physical activity through movement and exercise is essential. The total energy expenditure of both active and resting forms plays a significant role in weight loss or weight gain. In addition to the former, exercise has other physiologic benefits, such as fat mass reduction. In terms of physical activity, there is no consensus on an ideal or optimal activity, but a combination of aerobic and resistance exercise might be the most beneficial.[40] Exercise should be of moderate intensity for at least 30 minutes each time on most days of the week.[41]

Behaviour

Behavioural changes are important to ensure weight loss success and weight maintenance, especially in the long term. When people do not undergo behaviour therapy, they often return to baseline weight. Eating behaviours may need to be modified, and ongoing monitoring of food intake is important. People will benefit from understanding their food habits, including stimuli and triggers, especially in people who overeat, night-eat or binge-eat. Group programs and/or psychologist support may be beneficial for some people that have difficulty achieving their weight goals. People with mental health comorbidities, such as depression, may also benefit from psychologist support early in their weight loss care.

Pharmacological

For individuals with obesity and a BMI of greater than or equal to 30 kg/m^2 (or greater than or equal to 27 kg/m^2 with obesity-related comorbidities) who are unable to achieve their weight loss goals with lifestyle interventions, pharmacologic therapies may be indicated. Medications include orlistat (a lipase inhibitor), lorcaserin (appetite suppressant), liraglutide (acts on insulin and glucagon) and phentermine-topiramate (reduces hunger). These medications are prescribed as an adjunct to lifestyle interventions.[35] Metformin is also used, particularly in people at risk of type 2 diabetes.[42]

Surgery

Bariatric surgery may improve weight loss in people with a BMI of greater than 40 kg/m^2 (or greater than 30 kg/m^2 with obesity-related comorbidities). This requires a multi-disciplinary team and continued follow-up to ensure proper nutrition, as well as management of overall mental health and physical health.

Complementary and Alternative Therapies

Complementary and alternative therapies are often used by people wanting to lose weight, similar to that of the general population.[43] There are many products on the market, but the results vary. Acupuncture has been studied for the treatment of obesity and it appears to have a modest benefit for weight loss. In the following chapters, the evidence for and use of Chinese medicine therapies, including acupuncture, have been comprehensively reviewed.

Prognosis

Many factors contribute to overweight and obesity; however, the most impactful are one's lifestyle, physical activity and diet. With appropriate lifestyle and behavioural adjustments, most people can successfully lose weight and improve their physical and mental health. Even a weight loss of 5% of one's body weight can improve many health aspects, and an additional weight loss of greater than 5% can reduce cardiovascular risk factors.[44] Due to the body's strong homeostatic drive to maintain body weight and a set point of fat tissue, people will experience plateaus and may regain weight. After a period of low-calorie intake, there can be rebound weight gain, and appetite-stimulating mediators and hormones that favour weight gain are increased.[45] Therefore, weight maintenance needs ongoing monitoring and support.

References

1. Lavie CJ, McAuley PA, Church TS, *et al.* (2014) Obesity and cardiovascular diseases: Implications regarding fitness, fatness, and severity in the obesity paradox. *J Am Coll Cardiol* **63(14):** 1345–1354.
2. World Health Organization. (2018) Obesity and overweight. WHO, Geneva. https://www.who.int/news-room/fact-sheets/detail/obesity-and-overweight
3. Sturm R. (2007) Increases in morbid obesity in the USA: 2000–2005. *Public Health* **121(7):** 492–496.
4. Kelly T, Yang W, Chen CS, *et al.* (2008) Global burden of obesity in 2005 and projections to 2030. *Int J Obes.* **32(9):** 1431–1437.
5. Archer E, Shook RP, Thomas DM, *et al.* (2013) 45-Year trends in women's use of time and household management energy expenditure. *PLoS One* **8(2):** e56620.
6. Church TS, Thomas DM, Tudor-Locke C, *et al.* (2011) Trends over 5 decades in U.S. occupation-related physical activity and their associations with obesity. *PLoS One* **6(5):** e19657.
7. NCD Risk Factor Collaboration (NCD-RisC). (2016) Trends in adult body-mass index in 200 countries from 1975 to 2014: A pooled analysis of 1698 population-based measurement studies with 19.2 million participants. *Lancet* **387(10026):** 1377–1396.
8. Hales CM, Carroll MD, Fryar CD, *et al.* (2017) Prevalence of obesity among adults and youth: United States, 2015–2016. NCHS Data Brief, No 288. National Center for Health Statistics, Hyattsville, MD.
9. Ng M, Fleming T, Robinson M, *et al.* (2014) Global, regional, and national prevalence of overweight and obesity in children and adults

during 1980–2013: A systematic analysis for the Global Burden of Disease Study 2013. *Lancet* **384(9945):** 766–781.

10. Wu YF, Ma GS, Hu YH, *et al.* (2005) [The current prevalence status of body overweight and obesity in China: Data from the China National Nutrition and Health Survey]. *Zhonghua Yu Fang Yi Xue Za Zhi* **39(5):** 316–320.

11. National Institutes of Health, National Heart Lung and Blood Institute. (1998) Clinical guidelines on the identification, evaluation, and treatment of overweight and obesity in adults. The evidence report. *Obes Res* **6(Suppl 2):** 51S–209S.

12. Flegal KM, Kit BK, Orpana H, *et al.* (2013) Association of all-cause mortality with overweight and obesity using standard body mass index categories: A systematic review and meta-analysis. *JAMA.* **309(1):** 71–82.

13. Waters H, DeVol D. (2016) Weighing down America: The health and economic impact of obesity. Milken Institute. https://milkeninstitute.org/report/weighing-down-america-health-and-economic-impact-obesity

14. Finkelstein EA, Trogdon JG, Cohen JW, *et al.* (2009) Annual medical spending attributable to obesity: Payer-and service-specific estimates. *Health Aff* **28(5):** w822–831.

15. Oken E, Taveras EM, Kleinman KP, *et al.* (2007) Gestational weight gain and child adiposity at age 3 years. *Am J Obstet Gynecol* **196(4):** 322. e1–e3228.

16. Baptiste-Roberts K, Nicholson WK, Wang NY, *et al.* (2012) Gestational diabetes and subsequent growth patterns of offspring: The National Collaborative Perinatal Project. *Matern Child Health J* **16(1):** 125–132.

17. Katzmarzyk PT, Church TS, Craig CL, *et al.* (2009) Sitting time and mortality from all causes, cardiovascular disease, and cancer. *Med Sci Sports Exerc* **41(5):** 998–1005.

18. Ramachandrappa S, Farooqi IS. (2011) Genetic approaches to understanding human obesity. *J Clin Invest* **121(6):** 2080–2086.

19. Licinio J, Caglayan S, Ozata M, *et al.* (2004) Phenotypic effects of leptin replacement on morbid obesity, diabetes mellitus, hypogonadism, and behavior in leptin-deficient adults. *Proc Natl Acad Sci USA* **101(13):** 4531–4536.

20. Clegg DJ, Brown LM, Woods SC, *et al.* (2006) Gonadal hormones determine sensitivity to central leptin and insulin. *Diabetes* **55(4):** 978–987.

21. Lovejoy JC. (2003) The menopause and obesity. *Prim Care* **30(2):** 317–325.
22. Drewnowski A. (2012) The economics of food choice behavior: Why poverty and obesity are linked. *Nestle Nutr Inst Workshop Ser* **73:** 95–112.
23. NHLBI Obesity Education Initiative Expert Panel on the Identification Evaluation and Treatment of Obesity in Adults (US). (1998) Clinical guidelines on the identification, evaluation, and treatment of overweight and obesity in adults: The evidence report. https://www.ncbi.nlm.nih.gov/books/NBK2003/
24. Hochberg I, Hochberg Z. (2010) Expanding the definition of hypothalamic obesity. *Obes Rev* **11(10):** 709–721.
25. Filozof C, Fernandez Pinilla MC, Fernandez-Cruz A. (2004) Smoking cessation and weight gain. *Obes Rev* **5(2):** 95–103.
26. Leslie WS, Hankey CR, Lean ME. (2007) Weight gain as an adverse effect of some commonly prescribed drugs: A systematic review. *QJM* **100(7):** 395–404.
27. Berthoud HR, Morrison C. (2008) The brain, appetite, and obesity. *Ann Rev Psychol* **59:** 55–92.
28. Lavie CJ, Alpert MA, Arena R, *et al.* (2013) Impact of obesity and the obesity paradox on prevalence and prognosis in heart failure. *JACC Heart Fail* **1(2):** 93–102.
29. Isomaa B, Almgren P, Tuomi T, *et al.* (2001) Cardiovascular morbidity and mortality associated with the metabolic syndrome. *Diabetes Care.* **24(4):** 683–689.
30. World Health Organization. Regional Office for the Western Pacific. (2000) The Asia-Pacific perspective: Redefining obesity and its treatment. http://iris.wpro.who.int/handle/10665.1/5379
31. Gelber RP, Gaziano JM, Orav EJ, *et al.* (2008) Measures of obesity and cardiovascular risk among men and women. *JACC* **52(8):** 605–615.
32. Jensen MD, Ryan DH, Apovian CM, *et al.* (2014) 2013 AHA/ACC/TOS guideline for the management of overweight and obesity in adults: A report of the American College of Cardiology/American Heart Association Task Force on Practice Guidelines and The Obesity Society. *Circulation.* **129(25 Suppl 2):** S102–S138.
33. World Health Organization Expert Consultation. (2004) Appropriate body-mass index for Asian populations and its implications for policy and intervention strategies. *Lancet* **363(9403):** 157–163.

34. World Health Organization. (2000) Obesity: Preventing and managing the global epidemic. Report of a WHO Consultation (WHO Technical Report Series 894).

35. National Health and Medical Research Council. (2013) Clinical practice guidelines for the management of overweight and obesity in adults, adolescents and children in Australia. National Health and Medical Research Council, Melbourne.

36. Dansinger ML, Gleason JA, Griffith JL, *et al.* (2005) Comparison of the Atkins, Ornish, Weight Watchers, and Zone diets for weight loss and heart disease risk reduction: A randomized trial. *JAMA* **293(1):** 43–53.

37. Heymsfield SB, Harp JB, Reitman ML, *et al.* (2007) Why do obese patients not lose more weight when treated with low-calorie diets? A mechanistic perspective. *Am J Clin Nutr* **85(2):** 346–354.

38. Roberts SB, Rosenberg I. (2006) Nutrition and aging: Changes in the regulation of energy metabolism with aging. *Physiol Rev* **86(2):** 651–667.

39. Shaw K, Gennat H, O'Rourke P, *et al.* (2006) Exercise for overweight or obesity. *Cochrane Database Syst Rev* **(4):** Cd003817.

40. Villareal DT, Aguirre L, Gurney AB, *et al.* (2017) Aerobic or resistance exercise, or both, in dieting obese older adults. *N Engl J Med* **376(20):** 1943–1955.

41. Donnelly JE, Blair SN, Jakicic JM, *et al.* (2009) American College of Sports Medicine Position Stand. Appropriate physical activity intervention strategies for weight loss and prevention of weight regain for adults. *Med Sci Sports Exerc* **41(2):** 459–471.

42. Knowler WC, Barrett-Connor E, Fowler SE, *et al.* (2002) Reduction in the incidence of type 2 diabetes with lifestyle intervention or metformin. *N Engl J Med* **346(6):** 393–403.

43. Bertisch SM, Wee CC, McCarthy EP. (2008) Use of complementary and alternative therapies by overweight and obese adults. *Obesity* **16(7):** 1610–1615.

44. Douketis JD, Macie C, Thabane L, *et al.* (2005) Systematic review of long-term weight loss studies in obese adults: Clinical significance and applicability to clinical practice. *Int J Obes* **29(10):** 1153–1167.

45. Sumithran P, Prendergast LA, Delbridge E, *et al.* (2011) Long-term persistence of hormonal adaptations to weight loss. *N Engl J Med* **365(17):** 1597–1604.

2

Overweight and Obesity in Chinese Medicine

OVERVIEW

In Chinese medicine (CM), overweight and obesity is called *Fei ren* 肥人 or *Fei man* 肥满. It relates to the Spleen and Stomach but also includes the dysfunction of the Kidney, Liver, Heart and Lung. Deficiency and excess patterns are common, and treatment often involves *qi* promotion and water draining. This chapter introduces the main aetiologies, pathogenesis and syndromes of overweight and obesity in CM. Treatments are described based on CM textbooks and clinical practice principles and guidelines, including Chinese herbal medicine, acupuncture, massage and diet therapy.

Introduction

Records of diagnosis and treatment of overweight and obesity can be found in classic Chinese medicine (CM). Being overweight relates to various factors such as the body's constitution, an unhealthy diet, insufficient exercise and age. The location of the condition is primarily in the Spleen, Stomach and muscles, with a close relationship with Kidney deficiency. It is also related to the Heart and Lung, as well as Liver failing in the free flow of *qi*. The excess is mainly caused by Stomach heat or phlegm-dampness, and deficiency patterns include deficient Spleen *qi*, *yang* deficiency in the Spleen and Kidney, *qi* deficiency in the Heart and Lungs, or Liver–Gallbladder failing in free flow *qi*. Combined deficiency and excess patterns are also common.

In clinical practice, it is important to identify the *Ben xu* 本虚 (Root) and *Biao shi* 标实 (Branch) and deficiency/excess, as well as the location of the condition. According to the principle of reinforcing deficiency and reducing excess, deficiency conditions need to be treated by tonifying the Spleen and Kidney, and excesses treated by reducing heat, dispelling dampness or resolving phlegm, together with *qi* promotion, water draining, bowel regulation, resolving stasis and eliminating accumulated undigested food.

This chapter introduces the CM understanding of overweight and obesity in terms of terminology, aetiology and pathogenesis. It also includes syndrome differentiation, common herbal medicine and acupuncture treatments, as well as prevention strategies recommended in CM.

Definition

Obesity is identified under the CM terms for 'fatness', 'portliness' and 'phlegm-dampness'. There is no special diagnosis or treatment of obesity mentioned in classical CM literature; however, obesity was recorded as early as the Warring States in the *Ling Shu Wei Qi Shi Chang Pian* (灵枢·卫气失常篇).[1] It says that 'there are three body types: people with quite a lot of muscle/fat and firm skin (called *Zhi*), not much muscle/fat with loose skin (called *Gao*), or tight skin and muscle/fat (*Rou*)'. Obesity was divided into these three types: *Zhi*, *Gao* and *Rou*, and the related body size and features were described, such as cold and heat, and *qi* and Blood. For example, the *Gao* type was described as a 'wide body with a large amount of fat on the belly'. In *Ling Shu Yin Yang Er Shi Wu Ren* (灵枢·阴阳二十五人),[1] obesity was regarded as a constitution with 'excessive *qi*' and related to many diseases, such as diabetes (*xiao ke* 消渴), stroke, hemiplegia and flaccidity. For example, *Su Wen Tong Ping Xu Shi Lun* (素问·通评虚实论)[2] says excessive *qi*, due to overeating, is related to *xiao dan* 消瘅 (diabetes), syncope, hemiplegia, weakness, the fullness of *qi* and the dysfunction of *qi* flow.

Aetiology and Pathogenesis

According to the theory of CM, the pathogenesis of overweight and obesity is related to various factors, such as the body's constitution, an unhealthy diet, insufficient exercise or old age.[3-4] Spleen, Stomach and muscles are primarily affected, with a close relationship with Kidney deficiency and Liver failing in the free flow of *qi*, as well as Heart and Lung impairment. Deficiency or excess, or both, are involved. Excess patterns are mainly caused by Stomach heat or phlegm-dampness, and Stomach heat is normally the cause of the accumulation of fat and then phlegm-dampness. Phlegm-dampness often combines with *qi* and Blood stagnation or water-dampness, leading to an obstruction of phlegm and Blood stasis, binding of phlegm and *qi*, or phlegm-fluid retention. Deficiency patterns are usually due to a lack of Spleen *qi*, causing the failure of the Spleen to transform and distribute food and drink to all parts of the body, in turn storing fat water-dampness. Other patterns may include Spleen and Kidney *yang* deficiency, *qi* deficiency in the Heart and Lungs, or Liver–Gallbladder failing to free flow *qi*, resulting in deficiency patterns. In addition, people may also present with a combination of deficiency in *Ben* and excess in *Biao*. This combination, regardless of which one is more dominant, will lead to an accumulation of fat tissues and eventually cause obesity.

Pathological processes can transform during the development of obesity. There are three common clinical circumstances:

1. Overweight and obesity patterns can change and often fluctuate between excess and deficiency, as well as being influenced by pathological factors. For example, excessive eating will cause dampness-turbidity to aggregate in the body and convert to fat. When dampness-turbidity transforms into heat, Stomach heat will stagnate in the Spleen and contribute to weight gain. Unhealthy diets and eating habits will further damage the Spleen and Stomach function, and they will fail to transport and transform food. Spleen diseases can affect the Kidney and cause dual

deficiency of the Spleen and Kidney, leading to excessive pathogenic *qi*, causing a deficiency of healthy *qi*. In the later stage of disease, deficiency syndromes may be converted to an excess or a deficiency–excess complex syndrome, including:

- Chronic Spleen deficiency engendering dampness-turbidity, causing fat accumulation.
- Dual diseases of *Wood* and *Earth* — original disease of the Spleen leads to Liver dysfunction, Blood stasis, and *qi* stagnation.
- Spleen dysfunction leading to Kidney *yang* deficiency — this will then fail in its function to move water and generate *qi*, causing water-dampness retention in the meridians and skin, worsening obesity.

2. Over a long period of time, phlegm-dampness retention will block the flow of *qi* and Blood and cause *qi* stagnation or Blood stagnation. Long-term *qi* stagnation and Blood stagnation will convert to heat and form accumulated-heat, phlegm-heat, dampness-heat or stasis-heat.

3. People with obesity are likely to develop other diseases. The *Huang Di Nei Jing* mentions that obesity has a relationship to other diseases, such as *xiao dan* 消瘅 (diabetes). Being overweight for long periods will usually develop into complications such as wasting and thirsting (diabetes), headaches, dizziness, chest pain/oppression, stroke, gallbladder distention and impediment symptoms.*

Syndrome Differentiation and Treatments

The treatment principles for obesity are to tonify deficiency and reduce excess. Deficiency conditions can be treated by boosting healthy *qi* and fortifying the Spleen. If the Kidney is affected, then it

---

*A group of diseases caused by the invasion of wind, cold, dampness or heat pathogen in the meridian/channel, involving muscles, sinews, bones and joints, manifesting as local pain, soreness, heaviness or hotness, and even articular swelling, stiffness and deformities, also called wind impediment.

should be replenished (*qi*) and tonified. Excess conditions can be treated by clearing the Stomach and down-bearing turbidity or by dispelling dampness and phlegm, in combination with enhancing bowel movements to eliminate accumulated undigested food, regulate *qi* to disperse stagnation, clear phlegm and Blood stasis, and eventually to reduce the excess factors and resolve obesity. In sum, the deficiency–excess complex conditions should be treated with both reinforcement and elimination methods (Table 2.1).[4–6]

Table 2.1. Summary of Chinese Medicine Syndromes and Herbal Treatments

Syndromes	Treatment Principle	Herbal Medicine	
		Formula	Patent Herbal Medicine
Stomach heat with dampness obstruction	Clear Stomach heat, drain dampness and resolve turbidity, promote digestion and remove food stagnation	*Xiao cheng qi tang* plus *Bao he wan* (modified)	*Bao he wan, Fang feng tong sheng wan, Jiu zhi da huang wan*
Spleen deficiency with dampness encumbrance	Fortify the Spleen and replenish *qi*, drain water-dampness	*Shen ling bai zhu san* (modified) combined with *Fang ji huang qi tang*	—
Spleen and Kidney *yang* deficiency	Tonify the Spleen and Kidney, warm *yang* to form *qi*	*Zhen wu tang* (modified) combined with *Ling gui zhu gan tang*	*Ji sheng shen qi wan*
Liver depression and *qi* stagnation	Sooth the Liver *qi*, move *qi* to resolve phlegm	*Xiao yao san* (modified) combined with *Dao tan tang*	—

Stomach Heat with Dampness Obstruction 胃热湿阻

Clinical manifestations: Strong body constitution, an excessive amount of body fat, overeating, swift digestion with rapid hunger, excessive sweating; distending headache and dizziness, abdominal distention and fullness; incomplete bowel motions or hard stools; dark urine, red tongue body with thick and sticky tongue coat; yellow tongue coat; a rapid and slippery pulse or a rapid and wiry pulse.

Treatment principle: Clear Stomach heat, drain dampness and resolve turbidity, promote digestion and remove food stagnation.

Formula: *Xiao cheng qi tang* 小承气汤 combined with *Bao he wan* 保和丸 (with modifications).

Formula ingredients: *Da huang* 大黄, *zhi shi* 枳实, *hou pou* 厚朴, *lian qiao* 连翘, *huang lian* 黄连, *shan zha* 山楂, *shen qu* 神曲, *lai fu zi* 莱菔子, *chen pi* 陈皮, *ban xia* 半夏 and *fu ling* 茯苓.

Modifications: For patients with the syndrome of heat binding in the Stomach and intestines, dry stools or constipation, red tongue body with thick and yellow coating, add fried *lai fu zi* 炒莱菔子, scorched *bin lang* 焦槟榔 and *yuan ming* powder 元明粉 (mix power with water), or mix with *fan xie ye* 番泻叶 decoction to clear heat and regulate the bowels. For patients with an internal accumulation of damp-heat, abdominal distention and fullness, sticky and incomplete stools and a red tongue with sticky and yellow coating, add *cang zhu* 苍术, *sheng yi yi ren* 生薏苡仁, *hu zhang* 虎杖, *yin chen* 茵陈, and *jin qian cao* 金钱草 to clear heat and drain dampness. For patients with exuberant heat damaging *qi*, lassitude or a lack of strength, add *tai zi shen* 太子参 to tonify *qi*, or *xi yang shen* 西洋参. For patients with rapid digestion and hunger with a bitter taste in the mouth or gastric upset, add *huang lian* 黄连 to discharge fire with its bitter-cold properties. If there is dry mouth and thirst, add *tian hua fen* 天花粉 and *ge gen* 葛根 to clear heat and engender fluid. If there is dizziness or distending headache, add *ye ju hua* 野菊花.

Patent herbal medicine: *Bao he wan* 保和丸.

Spleen Deficiency with Dampness 脾虚湿阻

Clinical manifestations: Being overweight with excessive body fat, heavy sensation of the limbs, lassitude of spirit, lack of strength, shortness of breath, a reluctance to speak, excessive sleepiness during the night and day, a dry mouth but with no desire to drink, poor appetite, abdominal stuffiness and fullness and sloppy stools; an enlarged and pale tongue with teeth-marks and a white sticky coating or with white and slippery coating; a soggy and relaxed pulse or a fine and slippery pulse.

Treatment principle: Fortify the Spleen and replenish *qi*, drain water-dampness.

Formula: *Shen ling bai zhu san* 参苓白术散 combined with *Fang ji huang qi tang* 防己黄芪汤 (with modifications).

Formula ingredients: *Dang shen* 党参, *fu ling* 茯苓, *bai zhu* 白术, *da zao* 大枣, *jie geng* 桔梗, *shan yao* 山药, *bian dou* 扁豆, *yi yi ren* 薏苡仁, *lian zi rou* 莲子肉, *chen pi* 陈皮, *sha ren* 砂仁, *fang ji* 防己, *huang qi* 黄芪, *zhu ling* 猪苓, *ze xie* 泽泻 and *che qian zi* 车前子.

Modifications: For patients with a heavy sensation of the limbs, add *pei lan* 佩兰 and *huo xiang* 藿香 to enliven the Spleen with aroma; add *ban xia* 半夏 to alleviate stuffiness or add *ping wei san* 平胃散 to soothe the middle and relieve stuffiness. For patients with abdominal fullness and sloppy stools, add *hou pou* 厚朴, *chen pi* 陈皮 and *guang mu xiang* 广木香 to regulate *qi* and resolve distention. For patients with swollen limbs, add *ze xie* 泽泻, *zhu ling* 猪苓 or *wu pi yin* 五皮饮 to drain the dampness.

Spleen and Kidney *Yang* Deficiency 脾肾阳虚

Clinical manifestations: Being overweight, a swollen face, a lack of vitality and strength, spontaneous sweating with rapid and difficult breathing that worsens with movement; a fear of the cold, cold extremities, and soreness and weakness of the lumbar region and knees; cold and fullness in the lower abdomen, or swollen limbs and body, clear and abundant urine, frequent urination at night, a lack of copulative power in males or menstrual irregularities or amenorrhea in females; a pale and enlarged tongue body with white and thin coating and a fine and sunken pulse.

Treatment principle: Tonify the Spleen and Kidney, warm *yang* to form *qi*.

Formula: *Zhen wu tang* 真武汤 combined with *Lin gui zhu gan tang* 苓桂术甘汤 (with modifications).

Formula ingredients: *Fu zi* 附子, *gui zhi* 桂枝, *fu ling* 茯苓, *bai zhu* 白术, *bai shao* 白芍, *sheng jiang* 生姜, and *gan cao* 甘草.

Modifications: For severe *qi* deficiency and symptoms of shortness of breath and spontaneous sweating, add *ren shen* 人参 and *huang qi* 黄芪. For patients with obvious water retention and symptoms such as swelling with decreased urine output, add *wu ling san* 五苓散, *ze xie* 泽泻, *zhu ling* 猪苓 or *da fu pi* 大腹皮. For patients with a preference for hot food and aversion to cold food, add *pao jiang* 炮姜 to warm the Spleen and dissipate cold. For patients with soreness and weakness of the lumbar region and knees, add *niu xi* 牛膝, *rou cong rong* 肉苁蓉 or *du zhong* 杜仲. For patients with a fear of the cold and with cold extremities, add *bu gu zhi* 补骨脂, *xian mao* 仙茅, *xian ling pi* 仙灵脾, *yi zhi ren* 益智仁 and a high dose of *rou gui* 肉桂 and *fu zi* 附子 to warm the Kidneys to dissipate the cold.

Patent herbal medicine: *Ji sheng shen qi wan* 济生肾气丸.

Liver Depression and *Qi* Stagnation 肝郁气滞证

Clinical manifestations: Being overweight, depressed, having fullness in the chest, hypochondrium and abdomen, excessive belching and hiccups, menstrual irregularities or amenorrhoea in females, insomnia and dream-disturbed sleep and irregular stools; a light red or slightly dark tongue body with a white or thin and sticky coat, a string-like pulse or a string-like and slippery pulse.

Treatment principle: Soothe Liver *qi* stagnation, move *qi* to resolve phlegm.

Formula: *Xiao yao san* 逍遥散 combined with *Dao tan tang* 导痰汤 (with modifications).

Formula ingredients: *Chai hu* 柴胡, *zhi shi* 枳实, *bai shao* 白芍, *chen pi* 陈皮, *ban xia* 半夏, *fu ling* 茯苓, *dan nan xing* 胆南星, *bai zhu* 白术, *dang gui* 当归, *gan cao* 甘草, *bo he* 薄荷 and *sheng jiang* 生姜.

Modifications: For patients with hypochondriac pain, add *chuan lian zi* 川楝子 and *chuan xiong* 川芎. If there is chronic Liver *qi* depression and stagnant *qi* transforming into heat, symptoms will include a bitter taste in the mouth and a dry throat, dizziness, blurred vision and vexation, and a red tongue with yellow coating — add *mu dan pi* 丹皮, *zhi zi* 栀子, *huang qin* 黄芩, *yin chen* 茵陈, *lian qiao* 连翘, *xia ku cao* 夏枯草 and *jue ming zi* 决明子 to clear heat and relieve depression. If there is internal harassment of *qi* stagnation and phlegm-heat, a patient will have symptoms such as vexation or oppression in the chest, insomnia and a dream-disturbed sleep, a red tongue with yellow coat, and a slippery, rapid and string-like pulse — add *huang lian* 黄连, *huang qin* 黄芩, *gua lou* 瓜蒌, *suan zao ren* 酸枣仁 or *yuan zhi* 炙远志 to tranquilise the Heart heat and resolve phlegm.

Chinese Herbal Medicine Commercial Products

The herbal products in this section are referenced to three key books, including the *Chinese Internal Medicine National Teaching Materials of the 11th Five-year Plan for Higher Education* (中医内科学; 普通高等教育 '十一五' 国家级规划教材, 2007),[3] the *Chinese Internal Medicine National Teaching Materials of the 12th Five-year Plan for TCM Higher Education, 9th edition* (中医内科学; 全国中医药行业高等教育 '十二五' 规划教材; 第九版, 2012),[4] and the *Pharmacopoeia of the People's Republic of China* (中华人民共和国药典, 2015).[7]

1. *Bao he wan* 保和丸
   Herbs: *Ban xia* 半夏, *chen pi* 陈皮, *fu ling* 茯苓, *lai fu zi* 莱菔子, *lian qiao* 连翘, *shen qu* 神曲, *mai ya* 麦芽 and *shan zha* 山楂.

Functions: Promotes digestion and removes food stagnation; suitable for patients with food accumulation in the Stomach causing disharmony of Stomach *qi*.

2. *Fang feng tong sheng wan* 防风通圣丸

   Herbs: *Fang feng* 防风, *chuan xiong* 川芎, *dang gui* 当归, *shao yao* 芍药, *da huang* 大黄, *bo he* 薄荷, *ma huang* 麻黄, *lian qiao* 连翘, *mang xiao* 芒硝, *sheng shi gao* 生石膏, *huang qin* 黄芩, *jie geng* 桔梗, *hua shi* 滑石, *gan cao* 甘草, *jing jie* 荆芥, *bai zhu* 白术 and *zhi zi* 栀子.

   Functions: For patients who have wind-fire in the Stomach and intestines, and dual excess of the exterior and interior.

3. *Jiu zhi da huang pian* 九制大黄片

   Herbs: *Da huang* 大黄.

   Functions: Clears heat and drains dampness, purges fire and relaxes the bowels; can reduce body fat and contribute to weight control; suitable for people with obesity and constipation.

4. *Ji sheng shen qi wan* 济生肾气丸

   Herbs: *Shu di huang* 熟地黄, *shan zhu yu* 山茱萸, *mu dan pi* 牡丹皮, *shan yao* 山药, *fu ling* 茯苓, *ze xie* 泽泻, *rou gui* 肉桂, *zhi fu zi* 制附子, *niu xi* 牛膝 and *che qian zi* 车前子.

   Functions: Suitable for obesity with Spleen and Kidney *yang* deficiency pattern, with obvious oedema, inhibited urination or pain and soreness of the lumbar region and knees. Note that some herbs such as *ma huang* and *fu zi* may be restricted in some countries.

Acupuncture and Relevant Therapies

1. Filiform needle therapy/electroacupuncture (Table 2.2).[8]

   Treatment principle: Resolve phlegm and relieve bowels to regulate meridians, select points mainly on the Conception Vessel, Spleen and Stomach meridians.

   Main points: CV12 *Zhongwan* 中脘, ST25 *Tianshu* 天枢, ST28 *Shuidao* 水道, LI11 *Quchi* 曲池, ST37 *Shangjuxu* 上巨虚 and SP6 *Sanyinjiao* 三阴交.

Table 2.2. Summary of Acupuncture and Other Treatments

Treatments	Treatment Principles	Treatment Details
Filiform needle therapy/ electroacupuncture	Resolve phlegm, relieve bowels and regulate meridians.	CV12 *Zhongwan* 中脘, ST25 *Tianshu* 天枢, ST28 *Shuidao* 水道, LI11 *Quchi* 曲池, ST37 *Shangjuxu* 上巨虚, SP6 *Sanyinjiao* 三阴交
Ear acupuncture	Regulate *Zang-fu* function, especially the Spleen and Stomach, dredge meridians.	Mouth 口 (CO1), Stomach 胃 (CO4), Endocrine 内分泌 (CO18), *San Jiao* 三焦 (CO17), Spleen 脾 (CO13), Hunger 饥点, Subcortex 皮质下(AT4)
Diet therapy	Tonify the Spleen, clear dampness, resolve phlegm and lower lipids.	Various
Cupping therapy	Regulate meridians, resolve phlegm and reduce body fat.	CV12 *Zhongwan* 中脘, ST25 *Tianshu* 天枢, CV14 *Juque* 巨阙, SP15 *Daheng* 大横, SP14 *Fujie* 腹结
Tuina	Regulate meridians, resolve phlegm and reduce body fat.	Pushing, rubbing, kneading, grasping, tapping manipulation on abdominal region/points, etc.
Qigong	Boost healthy *qi*, regulate *Zang-fu* function and fortify the Spleen.	*Tai chi quan* 太极拳 and *Wu qin xi* 五禽戏

Analysis: Obesity is usually related to the disorder of the Spleen, Stomach and intestines; the abdomen is where the corresponding points for the Stomach and intestines are located. CV12 is the Front-*mu* point of the Stomach and Influential point of *fu* organs, LI11 is the sea point of the Large Intestine meridian, ST25 is the Stomach point corresponding to the Large Intestine, ST37 is the lower sea point of the Large Intestine; use these four points to regulate the bowels. ST28 can separate the clear and turbid, SP6 fortifies the Spleen, induces diuresis and clears phlegm turbidity; needle the above points to fortify the Spleen and Stomach, regulate the bowels and resolve phlegm.

Other points: Add ST44 *Neiting* 内庭 for intestinal and bowel heat. Add PC6 *Neiguan* 内关 and ST36 *Zusanli* 足三里 for phlegm-dampness obstruction. Add CV6 *Qihai* 气海, BL23 *Shenshu* 肾俞, BL20 *Pishu* 脾俞 and ST36 for Spleen and Kidney *yang* deficiency pattern. Add LR14 *Qimen* 期门 and LR3 *Taichong* 太冲 for Liver depression and *qi* stagnation.

Needle manipulation: Filiform needling, according to the principle of treat deficiency by tonification and treat the excess by purgation; moxibustion can be applied on Back-*shu* points.

2. Ear acupuncture

Main points: Select 3–5 points, including Mouth 口 (CO1), Stomach 胃 (CO4), Endocrine 内分泌 (CO18), *San Jiao* 三焦 (CO17), Spleen 脾 (CO13), Hunger 饥点 and Subcortex 皮质下 (AT4). Filiform needles or seeds can be used on the points.

Other Therapies

Therapies described in this section are taken from *Diagnosis and Treatment of Obesity and Related Diseases in Chinese and Western Medicine* (肥胖及相关疾病中西医诊疗, 2010)[9] and the *Evidence-based Clinical Practice Guidelines of Chinese Medicine — Chinese Internal Medicine* (中医循证临床实践指南 — 中医内科, 2011).[10]

Diet Therapy

1. *Yin er* and green bean porridge (银耳绿豆粥): *Yin er* (Tremella mushroom) (20 g), sliced white radish (50 g) and green beans (20 g). Boil for 30 minutes. Add some rice when eating.
2. Cucumber soup with *Yu mi xu* (金丝黄瓜汤): *Yu mi xu* (corn silk) (20 g), cucumber (50 g) and vinegar (600 mL). Cook corn silk and cucumber until it boils, then add vinegar for 5 minutes.

3. White gourd, bamboo shoot and *Kun bu* soup (冬瓜笋丝海带汤): *Kun bu* (kelp) (50 g), sliced bamboo shoots (30 g), white gourd (50 g), *chen pi* 陈皮 (20 g) and *da zao* 大枣 (10 pieces); with onions, ginger, garlic, salt and corn flour. Vegetable oil, vinegar and *kun bu* are essential foods for weight loss. Small amounts of daily consumption can be beneficial.
   Method: Add onions, ginger and garlic into heated vegetable oil, then add *kun bu* and bamboo shoots and stir-fry. Add water to boil, then add white gourd, *chen pi* and *da zao*. Add corn flour to thicken the soup, and then some salt and vinegar, as required. This soup can clear phlegm and reduce body fat, as well as promote urination and regulate the Spleen and Stomach.
4. *Yin Yu Ping Shen* tea (银菊平身茶): *Huai hua* 槐花 (10 g), *ju hua* 菊花 (10 g) and *yin er* 银耳 (6 g). Boil the three ingredients and drink daily. It can clear the Heart and improve vision, nourish the Liver and engender fluid, and reduce body fat and dispel heat.
5. *Hai Dai Yu Mi Geng Sui* (海带玉米梗碎): Corn kernels (30 g), boil with water for 10 minutes, then add *kun bu* (30 g), *hu tao ren* (walnuts) (10 g) and *tao ren* (6 g). Boil until the *kun bu* is soft. This formula will detoxify and nourish the skin, reduce body fat, fortify the Spleen and engender fluids, clear phlegm and free the vessels. It can be used as a diet therapy for daily intake.
6. *Shan Zha Jue Ming* tea (山楂决明茶): *Shan zha* 山楂 (10 g), *jue ming zi* 决明子 (10 g), white radish (20 g) and green beans (20 g). Boil *shan zha* and *jue ming zi* for 10 minutes, then add other ingredients until the green beans are soft. Drink as a tea. It can pacify the Liver and dissipate stasis, promote urination and purge fire to clear toxins and reduce body fat.

Cupping Therapy

Cupping can be applied to acupuncture points. Select 4–5 points: CV12 *Zhongwan* 中脘, ST25 *Tianshu* 天枢, CV14 *Juque* 巨阙, SP15 *Daheng* 大横 and SP14 *Fujie* 腹结. A large or medium-sized cup may be used. Keep the cups on the points for 10 to 15 minutes, once per day — 15 times is one treatment course.

Tuina

1. Massage on the abdomen; 30 minutes for each treatment, 3 times per week. ① Rubbing manipulation: use finger tips or the palm to rub, in a gentle, rhythmic manner, the abdomen, clockwise from the top right to the bottom left for 2–3 minutes. Apply evenly to make the local area warm. ② Pushing manipulation: push with the fingers or palms forward, apart or spirally, to regulate *yin* and *yang,* for 2–3 minutes. ③ Kneading manipulation: press and move to and fro or circularly on an affected area with the flat of the thumb, the thenar eminence or the root of the palm, with force, for 5 minutes. ④ Grasping manipulation: lifting and squeezing the affected areas with the fingers, a relaxed wrist, gradually with force and then back to gentle manipulation for 5–8 minutes. ⑤ Tapping points technique: apply around the umbilicus for 5 minutes, repeat once. ⑥ Tapping points according to syndrome differentiation: select points based on the four syndromes (Stomach heat with dampness obstruction, Spleen deficiency with dampness, Spleen and Kidney *yang* deficiency, or Liver depression and *qi* stagnation); three months is one treatment course.

2. Massage along the five meridians on the abdomen (Conception Vessel, Kidney meridian, Stomach meridian, Spleen meridian and Liver meridian) for 2–3 minutes, rubbing around the umbilicus. Warm the hands before covering the umbilicus and start rubbing from the middle to the edge of the abdomen, clockwise with force for 2–3 minutes then 2–3 minutes anticlockwise. Pinching manipulation: hold and lift the soft tissue around CV12 and BL24, lift quickly and put it down gently, repeat 20–30 times. Pushing manipulation: push with force from the hypochondrium area to the abdomen with two palms until the affected skin becomes warm. Grasping manipulation on hypochondrium: lift with force and squeeze the muscles on the hypochondrium, manipulate from the upper to lower hypochondrium, repeat 20–30 times. Push upwards to the right and left sides to regulate *yin* and *yang.* Place all fingertips just under the xiphoid process, then move along the

last rib from the xiphoid process to both sides of the body, repeat 20–30 times. Pressing manipulation on acupoints: use one fingertip and press CV13, CV12, CV8, CV6, CV4 and ST25 for 30 seconds on each point. Apply one treatment per day for the first five days, then once every second day; 20 days as one treatment course. Rest for five days before the second course; two treatment courses are recommended.

Qigong Therapies

Tai chi quan 太极拳 and *Wu qin xi* 五禽戏 may assist in weight loss. *Tai chi quan* can be strenuous and is more beneficial when used with breath regulation. The simplified *tai chi quan* is easier to master but is less strenuous than the traditional style. People can repeat the simplified form several times in a row to achieve the level of exercise required for weight loss. *Wu qin xi* is a type of physical exercise created by Huatuo according to the movement characteristics of a tiger, deer, bear, ape and bird. Regular *wu qin xi* exercise can make people energetic, quick, agile, fit and healthy.

Prevention and Care of Obesity

The prevention of obesity can start as early as childhood. Since obesity is difficult to treat, prevention at an early stage is extremely important. Weight control is a long-term commitment, and close monitoring and proper treatments will prevent rebound weight gain.[3-4]

1. Eat a healthy diet, avoid heavy food and alcohol, have plenty of vegetables and fruits rich in fibre and vitamins. Take in enough proteins and reduce the consumption of sugar, fat and salt. Avoid excessive food intake and snacks. In certain circumstances, it might also be beneficial to add herbal medicines into the diet.
2. Calorie-burning activities, such as walking or brisk walking, jogging, bike riding, climbing stairs or boxing, are important.

Housework and other physical activities will be helpful as well. There is no need to be too vigorous while exercising, as consistency is very important to prevent weight gain.

3. Gradual weight loss is recommended; it will not damage the healthy *qi* and will eventually achieve long-term weight loss success.

References

1. 佚名. (2018) 黄帝内经·灵枢. 北京: 中国医药科技出版社.
2. 佚名. (2018) 黄帝内经·素问. 中国医药科技出版社, 北京.
3. 周仲瑛. (2007) 中医内科学 (普通高等教育 '十一五' 国家级规划教材). 中国中医药出版社, 北京.
4. 吴勉华, 王新月. (2012) 中医内科学 (全国中医药行业高等教育 '十二五' 规划教材 (第九版)). 中国中医药出版社, 北京.
5. 危北海, 贾葆鹏. (1998) 单纯性肥胖病的诊断及疗效评定标准. *中国中西医结合杂志*. **5:** 317–319.
6. 魏子孝. (2000) 中西医结合内分泌代谢疾病诊疗手册. 人民军医出版社, 北京.
7. 国家药典委员会. (2015) 中华人民共和国药典. 中国医药科技出版社, 北京.
8. 许能贵, 符文彬. (2016) 临床针灸学 (广州中医药大学特色教材). 科学出版社, 北京.
9. 仝小林, 毕桂芝, 李敏. (2010) 肥胖及相关疾病中西医诊疗. 人民军医出版社, 北京.
10. 中国中医科学院. (2011) 中医循证临床实践指南-中医内科. 中国中医药出版社, 北京.

3

Classical Chinese Medicine Literature

OVERVIEW

Classical Chinese medicine literature has contributed valuable experience for the prevention and management of various health conditions and diseases. As an important component of the 'whole evidence' approach, this chapter systematically summarises and evaluates the evidence obtained from classical Chinese medicine literature for obesity. This literature was derived from the *Zhong Hua Yi Dian* 中华医典, which is one of the most comprehensive digital collections of Chinese medicine books. A total of 306 citations contained details of Chinese herbal medicine management for overweight and obesity. The aetiology and pathogenesis, as well as formulae and herbs, were analysed and summarised.

Introduction

The earliest written records of Chinese medicine (CM) history date back to the periods of Spring and Autumn (770–476 BCE) and Warring States (474–221 BCE). Texts from these periods describe concepts such as *yin* and *yang*, as well as herbal decoctions, acupuncture and moxibustion as ways to treat health complaints.[1] Some of the experience from the classical literature continues to inform contemporary understanding and the management of overweight and obesity.

Obesity in classical literature was commonly described using the terms *fei gui ren* 肥贵人, *zun rong ren* 尊荣人, *fei pang* 肥胖 and *fei ren* 肥人. The first known classical literature citation describing obesity was from the *Huang Di Nei Jing Su Wen* 黄帝内经素问 (before CE 618). The passage described different types of obesity based on the theory of body constitution and noted that excessive eating could be one of the factors leading to obesity. Over centuries, the knowledge, understanding and management of obesity have gradually developed.

In order to systematically evaluate and synthesise the evidence of the classical and pre-modern medical literature, a search of the *Zhong Hua Yi Dian* (ZHYD) 中华医典 was undertaken. The ZHYD 'Encyclopaedia of Traditional Chinese Medicine' is an electronic record of more than 1,000 medical books.[2] This collection is the largest currently available and is representative of other large collections of classical and pre-modern CM literature.[3–4]

Search Terms

To identify the possible citations of obesity in the classical literature, contemporary CM textbooks,[5–7] monographs,[8–26] journal articles[27–30] and CM specialists and experts were consulted for possible search terms. A list of 36 search terms was developed (Table 3.1).

Table 3.1. Terms Used to Identify Classical Literature Citations

Search Terms of Obesity in Pinyin	Search Terms of Obesity in Chinese	English Translation
Fei ren	肥人	Obese people
Pang ren	胖人	Obese people
Zhi ren	脂人	Fat people
Gao ren	膏人	Fat people
Rou ren	肉人	Muscular people
Sheng ren	盛人	Strong people
Fei pang	肥胖	Obesity
Fei sheng	肥盛	Fat and strong
Ti sheng	体盛	Strong body
Ti fei	体肥	Fat body

Table 3.1. *(Continued)*

Search Terms of Obesity in Pinyin	Search Terms of Obesity in Chinese	English Translation
Duo shi	多湿	Dampness
Duo tan	多痰	Phlegmatic
Tan shi	痰湿	Phlegm-dampness
Tan yin	痰饮	Phlegm and retained fluid
Ti pang	体胖	Fat body
Fei gui	肥贵	Fat and rich
Gao liang	膏粱	Rich food
Ren zhi	人脂	Body fat
Xiao zhi	消脂	Reduce lipid
Ling ren shou	令人瘦	Make people slim
Xiao fei	消肥	Reduce fat
Xiao shou	消瘦	Slim down
Fei shuo	肥硕	Stout
Fei man	肥满	Fat and plump
Tan zheng	痰证	Phlegm syndrome
Pi shi	脾湿	Spleen dampness
Shui zhong	水肿	Edema
Yu zhang	瘀胀	Stasis and distention
Gao zhi	膏脂	Fat
Zun rong ren	尊荣人	Honored and glorious people
Ren gao	人膏	Fat
Jiang zhi	降脂	Reduce lipid
Qu zhi	祛脂	Reduce lipid
Shou shen	瘦身	Slimming
Jian fei	减肥	Lose weight
Qing shen	轻身	Light body weight

- Terms relating to obese people included *fei ren* 肥人 (obese people), *pang ren* 胖人 (obese people), *zhi ren* 脂人 (fat people), *gao ren* 膏人 (fat people), *rou ren* 肉人 (muscular people), *sheng ren* 盛人 (strong people), *fei gui* 肥贵 (fat and rich) and *zun rong ren* 尊荣人 (honoured and glorious people).

- Symptom terms relating to obesity included *fei pang* 肥胖 (obesity), *fei sheng* 肥盛 (fat and strong), *ti sheng* 体盛 (strong body), *ti fei* 体肥 (fat body), *ti pang* 体胖 (fat body), *fei shuo* 肥硕 (stout), *fei man* 肥满 (fat and plump) and *shui zhong* 水肿 (oedema).
- Syndrome terms included *duo shi* 多湿 (dampness), *duo tan* 多痰 (phlegmatic), *tan shi* 痰湿 (phlegm-dampness), *tan yin* 痰饮 (phlegm and retained fluid), *tan zheng* 痰证 (phlegm syndrome), *pi shi* 脾湿 (Spleen dampness) and *yu zhang* 瘀胀 (stasis and distention).
- Chinese medicine function terms related to the management for obesity, such as *xiao zhi* 消脂 (reduce lipid), *ling ren shou* 令人瘦 (make people slim), *xiao fei* 消肥 (reduce fat), *xiao shou* 消瘦 (slim down), *jiang zhi* 降脂 (reduce lipid), *qu zhi* 祛脂 (reduce lipid), *shou shen* 瘦身 (slimming), *jian fei* 减肥 (lose weight) and *qing shen* 轻身 (light weight body).
- Other terms related to obesity included *gao liang* 膏粱 (rich food), *ren zhi* 人脂 (body fat), *gao zhi* 膏脂 (fat) and *ren gao* 人膏 (fat).

Procedures for Search

Search terms were entered into both the heading and text search fields of the ZHYD, and the search results were downloaded into spreadsheets. Duplicate citations found by multiple search terms were excluded. A 'citation' was defined as a distinct passage of text referring to one or more of the search terms. Codes were allocated for the types of citations, books and the dynasties in which they were written, according to the procedures described by May and colleagues.[4] Books published after 1949 (the end of the Minguo/Republic of China) were excluded. The process for searching, sorting and analysing information from classical literature is illustrated in Fig. 3.1.

Data Coding and Data Analysis Procedure

After removing the duplicates, the citations were reviewed to identify the symptoms relevant to obesity. Inclusion and exclusion criteria

Search	*Zhong Hua Yi Dian* 中华医典, which contains over 1,000 books .
Collect	Collect citations that mention any of the search terms (Table 3.1).
Sort	Sort citations and remove those that are not relevant.
Analyse	Formulae and herbs
	Total treatment citations = 306

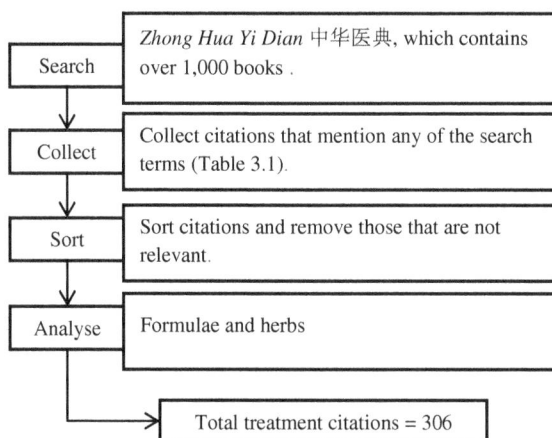

Fig. 3.1. Classical literature citations.

were applied to judge the eligibility of each citation in terms of their likelihood of describing obesity. Citations that mentioned children, adolescents or pregnant women as patients were excluded. Citations that met any of the following criteria were included:

- Describing symptoms and CM treatment for obesity.
- Describing symptoms, aetiology or pathogenesis for obesity.
- Describing 'losing weight' as the main function of any CM management.
- Describing obesity-related complications or comorbidities.

Citations were separated for analysis if they contained multiple treatments. Where herbal ingredients for Chinese herbal medicine (CHM) formulae were not detailed in a citation, the herbs were sought from other descriptions of the formula within the same book. If herb ingredients were not able to be identified from the same book, the ingredients were then sourced from the *Zhong Yi Fang Ji Da Ci Dian* 中医方剂大辞典, which is one of the most comprehensive collections of CHM formulae. Descriptive statistics methods were used to analyse the most frequently mentioned CHM formulae and herbal ingredients in the classical literature.

Search Results

A total of 27,273 hits (instances) in the ZHYD were obtained by the 36 search terms (Table 3.2). Not surprisingly, terms such as *tan zheng* 痰证 (6,721 hits, 24.64%) and *shui zhong* 水肿 (5,215 hits, 19.12%) produced the largest number of hits. This is because they were the general terms describing the syndrome of phlegm and oedema, respectively. Other search terms that yielded more than 5% of hits included *qing shen* 轻身 (light body weight, 4,800 hits, 17.6%), *xiao shou* 消瘦 (slim down, 2,260 hits, 8.29%) and *gao liang* 膏粱 (rich food, 1,760 hits, 6.45%). The term *qu zhi* 祛脂 did not yield any results.

Table 3.2. Hit Frequency by Search Term

Pinyin	Chinese Characters	Total Hit Frequency (n, %)
Tan zheng	痰证	6,721 (24.6%)
Shui zhong	水肿	5,215 (19.1%)
Qing shen	轻身	4,800 (17.6%)
Xiao shou	消瘦	2,260 (8.3%)
Gao liang	膏粱	1,760 (6.5%)
Duo tan	多痰	1,353 (5.0%)
Fei ren	肥人	1,149 (4.2%)
Pi shi	脾湿	1,146 (4.2%)
Tan shi	痰湿	842 (3.1%)
Duo shi	多湿	441 (1.6%)
Ti fei	体肥	275 (1.0%)
Tan yin	痰饮	275 (1.0%)
Fei sheng	肥盛	179 (0.7%)
Fei pang	肥胖	156 (0.6%)
Ling ren shou	令人瘦	103 (0.4%)
Gao zhi	膏脂	84 (0.3%)
Fei gui	肥贵	68 (0.3%)
Fei man	肥满	59 (0.2%)
Ren zhi	人脂	55 (0.2%)

Table 3.2. (*Continued*)

Pinyin	Chinese Characters	Total Hit Frequency (n, %)
Ti sheng	体盛	51 (0.2%)
Sheng ren	盛人	34 (0.1%)
Rou ren	肉人	33 (0.1%)
Ren gao	人膏	33 (0.1%)
Zun rong ren	尊荣人	30 (0.1%)
Shou shen	瘦身	27 (0.1%)
Ti pang	体胖	24 (0.1%)
Pang ren	胖人	20 (0.1%)
Xiao zhi	消脂	15 (0.05%)
Gao ren	膏人	14 (0.05%)
Fei shuo	肥硕	14 (0.05%)
Jian fei	减肥	13 (0.05%)
Zhi ren	脂人	9 (0.03%)
Yu zhang	瘀胀	8 (0.03%)
Jiang zhi	降脂	4 (0.01%)
Xiao fei	消肥	3 (0.01%)
Qu zhi	祛脂	0
Total		27,273

Citations Related to Obesity

A total of 430 citations met the criteria and were preliminarily included. After splitting citations for aetiology and pathogenesis and multiple CM treatments, 466 citations were pooled for further confirmation of eligibility. After the final eligibility assessment process, 437 citations met the inclusion criteria, of which 306 citations mentioned CM treatments and 131 citations described the aetiology, pathogenesis and other discussions related to obesity. The treatments described in the included citations were all identified as herbal medicines, and the details were extracted, coded and further analysed.

Descriptions of Obesity

Typical clinical manifestations of obesity were mentioned in many classical literature citations. *Zhen Jiu Jia Yi Jing* 针灸甲乙经 (c. 282) differentiated three types of obese people: *zhi ren* 脂人 (fat people), *rou ren* 肉人 (muscular people) and *gao ren* 膏人 (fat people). *Zhi ren* are obese people with stiff muscles and skin full of fat. In contrast, *gao ren* refers to obese people with soft muscles and skin. *Rou ren* are obese people with skin and muscle that do not separate from each other (曰: 人有脂, 有膏, 有肉. 曰: 别此奈何? 曰: 肉坚, 皮满者, 脂; 肉不坚, 皮缓者, 膏; 皮肉不相离者, 肉). The *qi* and Blood status of these three groups of people are also different, resulting in different manifestations:

- *Zhi ren* usually have less *qi* when compared to *Gao ren* and less Blood when compared to *Rou ren*, so the body size is not as large as other types (脂者, 其血清, 气滑少, 故不能大).
- *Rou ren* commonly have excessive Blood, which could induce the body to be plump and strong (肉者多血, 多血者则形充, 形充者则平也). As a result, the body size of *rou ren* is usually large (肉者, 身体容大).
- *Gao ren* commonly have excessive *qi*, which induces heat inside the body, so *gao ren* are usually cold-resistant (曰: 膏者多气, 多气者热, 热者耐寒也). The excessive *qi* also can cause the skin to sag, and abdominal fat could be present (膏者, 多气而皮纵缓, 故能纵腹垂腴).

Descriptions of the Aetiology of Obesity

The earliest description of obesity aetiology was from the *Huang Di Nei Jing* 黄帝内经. Improper diet was considered to be the main factor inducing obesity. In *Su Wen, Yi Fa Fang Yi Lun* section 素问 · 异法方宜论, the authors noted that overeating could induce people to gain weight and become obese (其民华食而脂肥). A similar discussion was also seen in another section of *Su Wen, Qi Bing Lun* 素问 ·

奇病论, stating that obese people frequently overeat sweet food in their daily life (此人必数食甘美而多肥也).

Apart from an improper diet, *qi* deficiency, dampness and phlegm were commonly mentioned causes of obesity. In *Gu Jin Yi Tong Da Quan* 古今医统大全 (c. 1556), Dr Xu Chun Pu indicated that '*Qi* deficiency with phlegm can cause obesity, thus the treatment method is to eliminate phlegm and tonify *qi*' (肥人气虚有痰, 宜豁痰而补气).

In *Dan Xi Xin Fa* 丹溪心法 (c. 1481), Dr Zhu Dan Xi indicated that 'dampness and heat can cause people to be obese and feel tired and lazy, and the patient could be treated by *cang zhu* 苍术, *fu ling* 茯苓 and *hua shi* 滑石' (凡肥人沉困怠惰, 是湿热, 宜苍术, 茯苓, 滑石); *qi* deficiency can induce people to become overweight, have white colour skin, feel fatigued, and this can be managed by *cang zhu* 苍术, *ren shen* 人参, *ban xia* 半夏, *cao guo* 草果, *hou po* 厚朴 and *shao yao* 芍药 (凡肥白之人, 沉困怠惰是气虚, 宜二术, 人参, 半夏、草果、厚朴, 芍药).

Dr Zhu Shi Jing, in his book *Yi Jian Neng Yi* 一见能医 (published in the Qing dynasty), held a similar view: '*Qi* deficiency and Blood excess can cause obesity' (血实气虚, 则体易肥).

Dr Chen Shi Duo, in his book *Shi Shi Mi Lu* 石室秘录 (c. 1687), discussed the relationship between *qi* deficiency and phlegm in the pathogenic process of obesity. The author indicated that the treatment method for obesity with phlegm syndrome is to tonify *qi* and nourish the Spleen, Stomach Earth and *Ming men* (life gate) fire (则治痰焉可仅治痰哉, 必须补其气, 而后带消其痰为得耳。然而气之补法, 又不可纯补脾胃之土, 而当兼补其命门之火, 盖火能生土, 而土自生气, 气足而痰自消, 不治痰, 正所以治痰也).

In the book *Yin Hai Zhi Nan* 银海指南 (c.1807), Dr Gu Xi further noted that when deficiency of the middle *qi* occurs, the Spleen fails to transport and transform food and drink, and phlegm is produced. In these obese people, phlegm syndrome is the cause, which is commonly produced by a dysfunction of the middle *qi* in transporting the essence of food and drink (盖痰涎之化, 本由中气衰弱, 水谷入胃, 不能尽化, 留而为痰...故肥人多痰者, 因中气不能健运所致).

Descriptions of Chinese Medicine Syndrome Differentiation of Obesity

Few citations stated the CM syndrome differentiation of obesity in classical literature citations. However, there were some descriptions.

In *Shi Shi Mi Lu* 石室秘录 (c. 1687), Dr Chen Shi Duo stated that the 'phlegm syndrome is commonly seen in obese people, and this is actually induced by *qi* deficiency; if the body is weak, the *qi* flow stops and generates phlegm' (肥人多痰, 乃气虚也, 虚则气不能营运, 故痰生之). This indicates that *qi* deficiency and phlegm obstruction may be one of the syndromes of obesity. A similar opinion was documented in *Gu Jin Yi Tong Da Quan* 古今医统大全 (c. 1556), in which Dr Xu Chun Pu described that '*qi* deficiency with phlegm can cause obesity, thus the treatment method is to eliminate phlegm and tonify *qi*' (肥人气虚有痰, 宜豁痰而补气).

Dr Ye Gui, in his book *Ye Tian Shi Cao Ren Bo He Yuan Yi An* 叶天士曹仁伯何元长医案 (c.1821), indicated that Spleen deficiency with dampness and phlegm (or Spleen deficiency with phlegm-heat) were common in obese people. He noted that 'dampness in obese people was mainly caused by the Spleen deficiency. There was no way out for dampness, thus it gradually transformed into phlegm and then phlegm generates heat' (肥人之湿多起于脾, 脾主湿, 又主土, 土气不旺, 湿邪无路可出, 则变而为痰, 化而为热, 所谓湿生痰、痰生热是也).

Chinese Herbal Medicine

The 306 CHM treatment citations were identified from 134 books. *Ji Yang Gang Mu* 济阳纲目 (c. 1626) was the book that produced the largest number of citations (*n* = 30). Other books with a high number of citations included *Ji Yin Gang Mu* 济阴纲目 (c. 1620) (*n* = 9), *Zhang Shi Yi Tong* 张氏医通 (c. 1695) (*n* = 8), *Dan Xi Zhi Fa Xin Yao*

丹溪治法心要 (c. 1368) (*n* = 7), and *Luo Shi Hui Yue Yi Jing* 罗氏会约医镜 (c. 1789) (*n* = 7). All the treatments obtained from the included citations were administered orally.

Frequency of Treatment Citations by Dynasty

The included CHM citations were obtained from the classical literature published from the Song and Jin Dynasties (c. 961–1271) to Minguo/Republic of China (1912–1949). Most citations (94%) were published in the Ming dynasty (c. 1369–1644) and the Qing dynasty (c. 1645–1911) (Table 3.3). This high number of citations may be due to advancing printing techniques and more books being published during these periods.

The earliest citation of CHM use was obtained from *Xue Shi Ji Yin Wan Jin Shu* 薛氏济阴万金书 (c. 1265). The author noted that *Dao tan tang* 导痰汤 plus *huang lian* 黄连 and *chuan xiong* 川芎 could be used to manage obese people with phlegm syndrome and amenorrhea when phlegm is hiding in the sea of Blood. The formulation should avoid the herb *sheng di* 生地 because of its sweetness, which may diminish the function of the middle energiser. (乃若肥人脂满多痰, 而痰或潜住血海, 亦主经闭, 法当用导痰汤加黄连, 川芎, 不可用生地, 恐其性腻膈). The most recent citation was a case report from *Quan Guo Ming Yi Yan An Lei Bian* 全国名医验案类编 (c. 1929). The author reported an obese man with cold *Bi* disease 寒痹证. After taking CHM formulae with the function of dispelling dampness and activating Blood, the symptoms were resolved.

Table 3.3   Dynastic Distribution of Treatment Citations

Dynasty	No. of Citations
Song and Jin Dynasties (961–1271)	4
Yuan Dynasty (1272–1368)	6
Ming Dynasty (1369–1644)	144
Qing Dynasty (1645–1911)	144
Minguo/Republic of China (1912–1949)	8
Total	306

Treatment with Chinese Herbal Medicine

A total of 281 formulae and 25 *materia medica* entries were obtained from the 306 CHM treatment citations. Of the 281 formulae, 83 were named (29.5%), and the others only included herbal ingredients but did not provide a formula name. Most formulae contained multiple herbal ingredients (*n* = 258, 91.8%), while 23 were identified as single herb formulae. Formulae with different names were pooled together for frequency analysis if they originated from the same basic formula and shared similar ingredients.

Most Frequent Formulae in Possible Obesity Citations

The 281 formulae were sorted into the following categories based on the description of the condition:

- Described obesity as an individual symptom (12 citations).
- Described obesity as a symptom of a disease consistent with polycystic ovarian syndrome (PCOS) (84 citations).
- Described obesity as a complication of a stroke (65 citations).
- Described obesity as a complication of diabetes (8 citations).
- Described obesity as a complication of hypertension (7 citations).
- Described obesity as a complication of other diseases (105 citations).

Note: The 105 citations describing obesity as a complication of other diseases, such as *han bi* 寒痹, *pi zheng* 痞症, etc., were not analysed in this chapter.

Obesity as an Individual Symptom

A total of 12 formulae were used for managing obesity as an individual symptom, including six named and six unnamed formulae. They all had a similar function: to tonify Spleen *qi* and/or expel phlegm. This is consistent with the contemporary understanding from

CM textbooks and guidelines that *qi* deficiency and phlegm are the two main causes of obesity (see Chapter 2).

The functions of these formulae were categorised as follows:

- Tonify Spleen *qi* to expel phlegm: *Liu jun zi tang* 六君子汤, *Bai zhu tang* 白术汤, *Huo tu liang pei dan* 火土两培丹, *Bu qi xiao tan yin* 补气消痰饮, *Yi qi hua tan wan* 益气化痰丸, *Si jun er chen he yi wei tang* 四君二陈合益胃汤 and three unnamed formulae.
- Expel Phlegm: Two unnamed formulae.
- Clear Heart and tonify *qi* to expel Phlegm: one unnamed formula.

> *Representative citation (Yang Sheng Si Yao* 养生四要, *c. 1549):*
> Phlegm syndrome in people with obesity is likely generated by excessive eating and an unhealthy lifestyle. The fat blocks meridians all over the body and slows down the transportation of *ying qi* 营气 (nutrient *qi*) and *wei qi* 卫气 (defensive *qi*). This could induce the dysfunction of transporting the essence of food and water and generating phlegm. As a result, the treatment principle for obesity should be to nourish the Spleen and tonify *qi*. *Yi qi hua tan wan* 益气化痰丸 could be considered as a treatment. (肥人痰者, 奉养太厚, 躯脂塞壅, 故营卫之行少缓, 水谷之化不齐, 所以多痰; 故治肥人者, 补脾益气为主, 宜用: 益气化痰丸).

Obesity and Polycystic Ovarian Syndrome

In past eras, there was no specific term for PCOS. Typical symptoms of PCOS were described as *bu yun* 不孕 (infertility), *bi jing* 闭经 (amenorrhea), *jing hou bu tiao* 经候不调 (abnormal period) and obesity terms. In reviewing the total treatment pool, 84 citations mentioned obesity and symptoms possibly related to PCOS (abnormal period, amenorrhea and infertility) and were pooled for analysis. A total of 70 named and 14 unnamed formulae were obtained from the included citations. Of the 70 named formulae, nine were mentioned in multiple citations and are presented in Table 3.4.

Table 3.4.   Most Frequent Formulae in Possible Obesity and Polycystic Ovarian Syndrome Citations

Formula Name	Herb Ingredients	No. of Citations (*n*)
Dao tan tang 导痰汤	*Chen pi* 陈皮, *ban xia* 半夏, *fu ling* 茯苓, *gan cao* 甘草, *zhi shi* 枳实, *tian nan xing* 天南星 (from *Ren Zhai Zhi Zhi Fang Lun* 仁斋直指方论, c. 1264)	28
Er chen tang 二陈汤	*Chen pi* 陈皮, *ban xia* 半夏, *fu ling* 茯苓, *gan cao* 甘草 (from *Dan Xi Shou Jing* 丹溪手镜, c. 1621)	7
Bu zhong yi qi tang 补中益气汤	*Ren shen* 人参, *huang qi* 黄芪, *chai hu* 柴胡, *gan cao* 甘草, *dang gui* 当归, *bai zhu* 白术, *sheng ma* 升麻, *chen pi* 陈皮 (from *Bian Zheng Lu* 辨证录, c. 1687)	5
Qi gong wan 启宫丸	*Chuan xiong* 川芎, *bai zhu* 白术, *ban xia* 半夏, *xiang fu* 香附, *fu ling* 茯苓, *shen qu* 神曲, *chen pi* 陈皮, *gan cao* 甘草 (from *Feng Shi Jing Nang Mi Lu* 冯氏锦囊秘录, c.1694)	5
Er chen tang he si wu tang 二陈汤合四物汤	*Chen pi* 陈皮, *ban xia* 半夏, *fu ling* 茯苓, *gan cao* 甘草, *sheng jiang* 生姜, *wu mei* 乌梅, *dang gui* 当归, *chuan xiong* 川芎, *bai shao* 白芍, *shu di huang* 熟地黄 (from *Nv Ke Jing Lun* 女科经纶, c. 1684)	4
Cang fu dao tan wan 苍附导痰丸	*Cang zhu* 苍术, *xiang fu* 香附, *cheng pi* 陈皮, *tian nan xing* 天南星, *zhi ke* 枳壳, *ban xia* 半夏, *chuan xiong* 川芎, *hua shi* 滑石, *fu ling* 茯苓, *shen qu* 神曲 (from *Guang Si Ji Yao* 广嗣纪要, c. 1549)	2
Ji yin dao tan tang 济阴导痰汤	*Ban xia* 半夏, *tian nan xing* 天南星, *chen pi* 陈皮, *zhi ke* 枳壳, *fu ling* 茯苓, *hua shi* 滑石, *chuan xiong* 川芎, *fang feng* 防风, *qiang huo* 羌活, *che qian zi* 车前子, *sheng jiang* 生姜 (from *Ji Yin Gang Mu* 济阴纲目, c. 1620)	2
Miao ying wan 妙应丸	*Cang zhu* 苍术, *ren shen* 人参, *huang qi* 黄芪, *bai zhu* 白术, *di huang* 地黄, *chen pi* 陈皮, *ban xia* 半夏, *dang gui* 当归, *fu ling* 茯苓, *hua shi* 滑石, *zhi gan cao* 炙甘草 (from *Gu Jin Yi Tong Da Quan* 古今医统大全, c. 1556)	2

Table 3.4. (*Continued*)

Formula Name	Herb Ingredients	No. of Citations (*n*)
Ren shen ban xiao wan 人参半夏丸	*Ren shen* 人参, *ban xia* 半夏, *tian nan xing* 天南星, *fu ling* 茯苓, *bo he* 薄荷, *ming fan* 明矾, *ge fen* 蛤粉, *huo xiang* 藿香, *han shui shi* 寒水石 (fom *Nu Ke Qie Yao* 女科切要, c. 1773)	2

The use of some herbs/ingredients may be restricted in some countries. Readers are advised to comply with relevant regulations.

Dao tan tang 导痰汤 was the most frequently cited formula to treat obesity and PCOS. The earliest citation mentioned *Dao tan tang* was from *Ren Zhai Zhi Zhi Fang Lun* 仁斋直指方论 (c. 1264). Herbal ingredients can dry dampness and expel phlegm, regulate *qi* and resolve stuffiness. Most of the other frequently cited formulae have a similar function. The functions of the most frequent formulae can be categorised into three groups:

- Dry dampness, regulate *qi* and expel phlegm: *Dao tan tang* 导痰汤, *Er chen tang* 二陈汤, *Cang fu dao tan wan* 苍附导痰丸 and *Ji yin dao tan tang* 济阴导痰汤.
- Nourish the Spleen, tonify and regulate *qi* to expel phlegm: *Bu zhong yi qi tang* 补中益气汤, *Er chen tang he si wu tang* 二陈汤合四物汤, *Miao ying wan* 妙应丸 and *Ren shen ban xia wan* 人参半夏丸.
- Dry dampness, regulate *qi*, expel phlegm and activate Blood: *Qi gong wan* 启宫丸.

In contemporary CM textbooks of gynaecology,[29] *Dao tan tang* and *Cang fu dao tan wan* are both recommended for managing PCOS, with dampness and phlegm blocking the meridians. This highlights their importance for managing obesity in PCOS.

Representative citation (Fu Qing Zhu Nv Ke Ge Kuo 傅青主女科歌括, *c. 1827):*
Female patients suffering from obesity, sputum and infertility suffer from excessive dampness rather than *qi* deficiency (妇人有身

体肥胖，痰涎甚多，不能受孕者，人以为气虚之故，谁知是湿盛之故乎). The dampness pathogen causing obesity is not an external pathogen but is induced by an internal disease of Spleen Earth. The excessive dampness can induce obesity, *qi* deficiency, phlegm and sputum, and finally internal deficiency, though the patient may look strong in appearance. *Qi* and internal deficiency occur, and the circulation of water is interrupted, causing dampness to be retained in the Spleen and Stomach. As a result, the water cannot be transferred into essence but becomes sputum and phlegm (不知湿盛者，多肥胖；肥胖者，多气虚；气虚者，多痰涎，外似健壮而内实虚损也. 内虚则气必衰，气衰则不能行水，而湿停于肠胃之间，不能化精而化涎矣). The exuberant phlegm aggravates the Spleen's dampness, and it is not able to receive heat, thus causing the dampness to flow into the uterus. Exuberant dampness and body fat can cause dysfunction of the uterus and infertility. *Jia wei bu zhong yi qi tang* 加味补中益气汤 can be selected for managing this disease (夫脾本湿土，又因痰多愈加其湿，脾不能受热，必津润于胞胎，日积月累，则胞胎竟变为汪洋之水窟矣. 且肥胖之妇，内肉必满，遮隔子宫，不能受精，此必然之势也. 方用加味补中益气汤).

Obesity and Stroke

The classical literature citations indicated that stroke patients can present with obesity. One possible explanation is that both stroke and obesity have a similar pathological factor in CM, that is, an improper diet with excessive eating and drinking. The over-indulgence of food and wine can induce dysfunction of the Spleen and Stomach, generating internal phlegm and heat and causing internal wind. The phlegm, heat and wind harass the head and can induce a stroke. A total of 65 citations mentioned obesity and disease/symptom terms, possibly related to strokes, including *zhong feng* 中风 (sudden wind attack), *qi tuo cu dao* 气脱卒倒 (suddenly falling due to *qi* collapse), and *si zhi bu ju* 四肢不举 (paralysis). Most of the formulae obtained from the citations were named (*n* = 51, 78.5%). Ten formulae were mentioned in multiple citations (Table 3.5).

Table 3.5.   Most Frequent Formulae in Possible Obesity and Stroke Citations

Formula Name	Herb Ingredients	No. of Citations (*n*)
Liu jun zi tang 六君子汤	*Chen pi* 陈皮, *ban xia* 半夏, *ren shen* 人参, *bai zhu* 白术, *fu ling* 茯苓, *gan cao* 甘草 (from *Ming Yi Za Zhu* 明医杂著, c. 1502)	10
Huo xiang zheng qi san he xing xiang san 藿香正气散合星香散	*Da fu pi* 大腹皮, *bai zhi* 白芷, *zi su* 紫苏, *fu ling* 茯苓, *ban xia* 半夏, *bai zhu* 白术, *chen pi* 陈皮, *hou po* 厚朴, *jie geng* 桔梗, *huo xiang* 藿香, *gan cao* 甘草, *tian nan xing* 天南星, *mu xiang* 木香, *sheng jiang* 生姜 (from *Dan Xi Xin Fa* 丹溪心法, c. 1481)	5
Bei mu gua lou san 贝母瓜蒌散	*Bei mu* 贝母, *tian nan xing* 天南星, *jing jie* 荆芥, *fang feng* 防风, *qiang huo* 羌活, *huang bo* 黄柏, *huang qin* 黄芩, *huang lian* 黄连, *bai zhu* 白术, *chen pi* 陈皮, *ban xia* 半夏, *bo he* 薄荷, *gan cao* 甘草, *wei ling xian* 威灵仙, *tian hua fen* 天花粉 (from *Yi Fang Xuan Yao* 医方选要, c. 1495)	3
Bu zhong yi qi tang 补中益气汤	*Huang qi* 黄芪, *bai zhu* 白术, *chen pi* 陈皮, *ren shen* 人参, *chai hu* 柴胡, *sheng ma* 升麻, *dang gui* 当归, *gan cao* 甘草 (from *Dan Xi Zhi Fa Xin Yao* 丹溪治法心要, c. 1543)	3
Da xu ming tang 大续命汤	*Ma huang* 麻黄, *gui zhi* 桂枝, *dang gui* 当归, *shi gao* 石膏, *gan jiang* 干姜, *gan cao* 甘草, *chuan xiong* 川芎, *xing ren* 杏仁, *huang qin* 黄芩, *zhu li* 竹沥 (from *Zhang Shi Yi Tong* 张氏医通, c. 1695)	3
San hua tang 三化汤	*Hou po* 厚朴, *da huang* 大黄, *zhi shi* 枳实, *qiang huo* 羌活 (from *Dan Xi Xin Fa* 丹溪心法, c. 1481)	3
Shi quan da bu tang 十全大补汤	*Ren shen* 人参, *bai zhu* 白术, *fu ling* 茯苓, *gan cao* 甘草, *dang gui* 当归, *chuan xiong* 川芎, *jiu bai shao* 酒白芍, *shu di huang* 熟地黄, *huang qi* 黄芪, *rou gui* 肉桂 (from *Jing Yue Quan Shu* 景岳全书, c. 1624)	3
Si jun zi tang 四君子汤	*Ren shen* 人参, *bai zhu* 白术, *fu ling* 茯苓, *gan cao* 甘草 (from *Jing Yue Quan Shu* 景岳全书c. 1624)	3

(Continued)

Table 3.5.   (*Continued*)

Formula Name	Herb Ingredients	No. of Citations (*n*)
Er chen tang 二陈汤	*Chen pi* 陈皮, *ban xia* 半夏, *fu ling* 茯苓, *gan cao* 甘草, (from *Gu Jin Yi An An* 古今医案 按, c.1778)	2
Xing xiang san 星香散	*Tian nan xing* 天南星, *mu xiang* 木香, *sheng jiang* 生姜 (from *Ming Yi Zhi Zhang* 明医指掌, c. 1579)	2

The use of some herbs/ingredients may be restricted in some countries. Readers are advised to comply with relevant regulations.

Liu jun zi tang 六君子汤 was the most frequently cited formulae (*n* = 10). The earliest citation was from *Ming Yi Za Zhu* 明医杂著 (c. 1502). Herbs were formulated to tonify *qi* and promote *yang*, remove dampness and expel phlegm. Other frequently mentioned formulae were from three main categories, targeting different syndromes of a stroke and obesity:

- Tonify *qi* and promote *yang*, remove dampness and expel phlegm: *Liu jun zi tang* 六君子汤, *Bu zhong yi qi tang* 补中益气汤, *Shi quan da bu tang* 十全大补汤 and *Si jun zi tang* 四君子汤.
- Regulate *qi*, dry dampness and expel phlegm: *Huo xiang zheng qi san he xing xiang san* 藿香正气散合星香散, *Bei mu gua lou san* 贝母瓜蒌散, *Er chen tang* 二陈汤 and *Xing xiang san* 星香散.
- Regulate *qi*, activate Blood and unblock the meridians: *San hua tang* 三化汤 and *Da xu ming tang* 大续命汤.

Representative citation (Ming Yi Za Zhu 明医杂著, *c. 1502):*
There was an obese patient living an alcoholic life. One day, he suddenly felt his tongue stiffen, and he could not speak normally. He also had symptoms of facial paralysis, coughing sputum and weak limbs. This obese patient caught a pathogen, which appeared externally and induced internal deficiency. In addition to this, the heat and dampness due to excessive drinking aggravated the symptoms. He should be treated by *Liu jun zi tang* 六君子汤 plus *ge gen* 葛根,

shen qu 神曲 and *ren shen* 人参 (有形体肥胖, 平素善饮, 忽舌本强硬, 语言不清, 口眼㖞斜, 痰气上涌, 肢体不遂, 此肥人多中气, 以盛于外而歉于内, 兼之酒饮湿热, 症乃成矣。须用六君子, 加煨葛根神曲, 多用人参以挽之).

Obesity and Diabetes

A total of eight citations mentioned obesity as a complication under the disease term '*xiao ke* 消渴' (emaciation and polydipsia disease), which is an umbrella term possibly referring to diabetes in classical literature. This is consistent with the contemporary understanding of clinical medicine that obesity is one of the risk factors for type 2 diabetes.[31] Of these eight citations, seven named formulae were obtained. Consistent with contemporary CHM management for diabetes, three cited formulae, *Liu wei di huang wan* 六味地黄丸, *Tiao wei cheng qi tang* 调胃承气汤 and *Bai hu jia ren shen tang* 白虎加人参汤, were also recommended in contemporary CM guidelines and textbooks.[32,33] These formulae are proposed to treat different CM syndromes of diabetes, including Kidney *yin* deficiency, excessive heat in the Stomach and *yin* deficiency with excessive heat, respectively. The clinical functions of the other formulae include clearing excessive heat in the Stomach (*San huang wan* 三黄丸) and dry dampness, regulating *qi* and expelling phlegm (*Dao tan tang* 导痰汤, *Liu jun zi tang he zuo jin zhi shi tang* 六君子汤合左金枳实汤 and *Qian shi bai zhu san* 钱氏白术散).

   Representative citation (San Xiao Lun 三消论, *c. 1884):*
   Huang Di Nei Jing 黄帝内经 says, 'Obese patients overindulge in greasy and sweet food. The greasy food causes internal heat, while sweet foods cause abdominal distention. Consequently, excessive *qi* overflows upwards and causes emaciation and polydipsia.' (经曰: 此肥美之所发也, 此人必数食甘美而多肥也. 肥者令人内热, 甘者令人中满, 故其气上溢, 转而为消渴).

Obesity and Hypertension

Seven citations described headache and/or dizziness in obese patients, which was considered possibly hypertension disease. The aetiology and pathogenesis are similar between obesity and hypertension, including an improper diet and the harassment of internal phlegm and wind. A total of four named and one unnamed formula were obtained from the included citations. Most of them tonify *qi* and expel phlegm, including *Si jun zi tang* 四君子汤, *Er chen tang* 二陈汤 and *Liu jun zi tang* 六君子汤.

Representative citation (*Ji Yang Gang Mu* 济阳纲目, *c. 1626*):

Jia wei liu jun zi tang 加味六君子汤 can be used for managing obese patients with *qi* deficiency, excessive phlegm and wind pathogen manifesting as dizziness (加味六君子汤, 治肥人气虚痰盛, 兼挟风邪, 眩晕不休).

Most Frequent Herbs from Obesity Citations

All of the 306 CHM treatment citations were further analysed for herb frequency. Forty-five citations were found to be single herb formulae or *materia medica* entries, and they were analysed as a sub-set. Multiple herbs were included in 261 citations, and they were split into two sub-sets for analysis based on their characteristics, including:

1. Citations that mentioned the CHM management was for obesity only, or described the add-on herb for obesity when managing other conditions; and
2. Citations that mentioned CHM management were for other conditions, including obesity as a complication.

A total of 64 citations mentioned CHM management for simple obesity or described the add-on herbs for obesity when managing other diseases. In total, 51 herbs were obtained from these citations. The clinical functions of the most frequently cited herbs were grouped into nine categories:

1. Dry dampness to expel phlegm: *ban xia* 半夏, *tian nan xing* 天南星 and *hou po* 厚朴.

2. Nourish Spleen, drain dampness to expel phlegm: *cang zhu* 苍术, *bai zhu* 白术 and *fu ling* 茯苓.
3. Tonify *qi* and nourish Spleen: *ren shen* 人参.
4. Regulate *qi* and nourish Spleen to dry dampness and expel phlegm: *chen pi* 陈皮, *gan cao* 甘草 and *sha ren* 砂仁.
5. Clear heat and expel phlegm: *zhu li* 竹沥.
6. Promote urination and remove dampness: *hua shi* 滑石.
7. Activate Blood and move *qi*, expel wind and alleviate pain: *chuan xiong* 川芎.
8. Promote digestion and harmonise the Stomach: *shen qu* 神曲.
9. Release the exterior and expel the cold, and warm the middle energiser: *sheng jiang* 生姜.

Most of the commonly cited herbs have the function to expel dampness and phlegm, tonify *qi* and nourish Spleen, which is consistent with the aetiology of obesity, according to contemporary knowledge. There were two herbs, *sheng jiang* 生姜 and *chuan xiong* 川芎, that have functions unrelated to the aetiology of obesity. They may have been used for managing other symptoms in the formulation.

The most frequently cited herbs included *ban xia* 半夏 (*n* = 39), *cang zhu* 苍术 (*n* = 31), *bai zhu* 白术 (*n* = 22) and *fu ling* 茯苓 (*n* = 17) (Table 3.6). *Ban xia* 半夏 has the therapeutic function of draining dampness and expelling phlegm. *Ban xia* manifests its therapeutic action on the Spleen and Stomach meridians, and it can dry dampness and phlegm accumulating in the middle energiser. This can be beneficial for obesity syndromes related to phlegm and dampness retention in the Spleen and Stomach. In the formulation of the widely used phlegm-dispelling formula *Er chen tang* 二陈汤, *ban xia* acts as the sovereign herb. *Gu Jin Yi Tong Da Quan* 古今医统大全 (c. 1556) states that '*Ban xia*, *chen pi*, *ren shen* and *bai zhu* can be used for treating obese patients with *qi* deficiency and phlegm syndrome' (肥人气虚有痰, 宜二陈, 参, 术).

Cang zhu 苍术 and *bai zhu* 白术, the second and third most frequently cited ingredients, are sourced from the same species of

Table 3.6.   Most Frequent Herbs in Possible Obesity Citations

Herb Name	Scientific Name	No. of Citations (*n*)
Ban xia 半夏	*Pinellia ternata* (Thunb.) Breit.	39
Cang zhu 苍术	*Atractylodes lancea* (Thunb.) DC. var. *chinensis* (DC.) Koidz.	31
Bai zhu 白术	*Atractylodes macrocephala* Koidz.	22
Fu ling 茯苓	*Poria cocos* (Schw.) Wolf.	17
Ren shen 人参	*Panax ginseng* C. A. Mey.	14
Sheng jiang 生姜	*Zingiber officinale* Rosc.	14
Chen pi 陈皮	*Citrus reticulata* Blanco	14
Tian nan xing 天南星	1. *Arisaema* spp.	9
Zhu li 竹沥	1. *Phyllostachysnigra* (Lodd. ex Lindl.) 2. *Munrovar henonis* (Mitf.) StapfetRendle	8
Hua shi 滑石	Talcum	7
Gan cao 甘草	1. *Glycyrrhiza* spp.	7
Sha ren 砂仁	1. *Amomum villosum* Lour. var. *xanthioides* T. L. Wu et Senjen 2. *Amomum longiligulare* T. L. Wu	5
Chuan xiong 川芎	*Ligusticum chuanxiong* Hort.	4
Liu shen qu 六神曲	Fermented combination of herbs (dried mass)	3
Hou po 厚朴	*Magnolia officinalis* Rehd. et Wils. var. *biloba* Rehd. et Wils.	3

The use of some herbs/ingredients may be restricted in some countries. Readers are advised to comply with relevant regulations.

Atractylodes. They have a similar clinical function of drying dampness to fortify the Spleen by encumbering the Spleen *yang*. These two herbs are commonly seen in dampness draining and tonifying, and replenishing formulae. They can be beneficial for managing the obesity generated by the Spleen *qi* deficiency and dampness obstruction in the middle energiser. For example, in *Yang Sheng Si Yao* 养生四要 (c. 1549), both *cang zhu* and *bai zhu* were mentioned in the formulation of *Yi qi hua tan wan* 益气化痰丸 for the management of obese people with the phlegm syndrome, caused by overeating and fat blocking the movement of *qi* in the meridians (肥人痰者, 奉养太厚, 躯脂塞壅, 故营卫之行少缓, 水谷之化不齐, 所以多痰. 故治肥人者, 补脾益气为主, 宜用: 益气化痰丸).

Fu ling 茯苓, mentioned in 17 formulae, was the fourth most frequently cited herb. Similar to *cang zhu* and *bai zhu*, *fu ling* nourishes the Spleen *qi* and drains dampness. *Fu ling* can also reduce excessive dampness by promoting urination. It can be helpful for expelling dampness and phlegm in obese people, combined with other dampness-draining medicinals (*Jian Ming Yi Gou* 简明医觳, c. 1629, 肥人湿痰, 半夏, 茯苓, 苍术, 滑石).

Most Frequent Herbs for Obesity as a Complication of Other Conditions

A total of 197 citations mentioned CHM treatment for other conditions with obesity as a complication (e.g., PCOS, stroke, hypertension, etc.). In total, 199 herbal ingredients were obtained from these citations, and the most frequently cited herbs are listed in Table 3.7. Although these citations did not mention that herbal management was especially for obesity, many of these herbs are known to be used

Table 3.7. Most Frequent Herbs in Citations with Obesity and Accompanied Complications

Herb Name	Scientific Name	No. of Citations (*n*)
Ban xia 半夏	*Pinellia ternata* (Thunb.) Breit.	139
Gan cao 甘草	*Glycyrrhiza* spp.	132
Fu ling 茯苓	*Poria cocos* (Schw.) Wolf.	125
Chen pi 陈皮	*Citrus reticulata* Blanco	125
Tian nan xing 天南星	*Arisaema* spp.	84
Bai zhu 白术	*Atractylodes macrocephala* Koidz.	84
Chuan xiong 川芎	*Ligusticum chuanxiong* Hort.	74
Sheng jiang 生姜	*Zingiber officinale* Rosc.	64

(Continued)

Table 3.7. (*Continued*)

Herb Name	Scientific Name	No. of Citations (*n*)
Dang gui 当归	*Angelica sinensis (Oliv.)* Diels	52
Cang zhu 苍术	*Atractylodes lancea* (Thunb.) DC. var. *chinensis* (DC.) Koidz.	52
Ren shen 人参	*Panax ginseng* C. A. Mey.	48
Xiang fu 香附	*Cyperus rotundus* L.	48
Zhi shi 枳实	*Citrus aurantium* L. var. *sinensis* Osbeck	45
Huang lian 黄连	*Coptis* spp.	33
Wu mei 乌梅	*Prunus mume* (Sieb.) Sieb. et Zucc.	24
Zhu li 竹沥	1. *Phyllostachysnigra* (Lodd. ex Lindl.) 2. *Munrovar henonis* (Mitf.) StapfetRendle	21
Huang qin 黄芩	*Scutellaria baicalensis* Georgi	20
Huang qi 黄芪	*Astragalus membranaceus* (Fisch.) Bge. var. *mongholicus* (Bge.) Hsiao	20
Hua shi 滑石	Talcum	19
Mu xiang 木香	*Aucklandia lappa* Decne.	17

The use of some herbs/ingredients may be restricted in some countries. Readers are advised to comply with relevant regulations.

for obesity. There were seven new herbs identified in the obesity as a complication of other conditions citations, including herbs that:

- Regulate *qi*, soothe the Liver and expel phlegm: *xiang fu* 香附 and *mu xiang* 木香.
- Remove food retention and expel phlegm: *zhi shi* 枳实.
- Clear heat: *huang lian* 黄连 and *huang qin* 黄芩.
- Nourish Spleen and tonify *qi*: *huang qi* 黄芪.
- Nourish *yin* and promote *jin*: *wu mei* 乌梅.

The functions of these seven herbs are consistent with contemporary CM textbooks in managing different syndromes of obesity.

Table 3.8   Most Frequent Single Herb Formula and *Materia Medica* Herbs

Herb Name	Scientific Name	No. of Citations (*n*)
Cha 茶	*Camellia sinensis* O. Ktze	26
He ye 荷叶	*Nelumbo nucifera* Gaertn.	5
Kun bu 昆布	1. *Laminaria japonica* Aresch. 2. *Ecklonia kurome* Okam.	4
Hai zao 海藻	*Sargassum fusiforme* (Harv.) Setch. var. *pallidum* (Turn.) C. Ag.	3
Dong gua 冬瓜	*Benincasa hispida* (Thunb.) Cogn.	2
Shan zha 山楂	*Crataegus pinnatifida* Bge. var. *major* N. E. Br.	2
Chi xiao dou 赤小豆	*Phaseolus calcaratus* Roxb.	2

The use of some herbs/ingredients may be restricted in some countries. Readers are advised to comply with relevant regulations.

Single Herb Formulae and Meteria Medica

Eleven herbs were obtained from single herb formula or *materia medica* entries. Seven herbs were identified in multiple citations (Table 3.8).

Cha 茶 (tea) was the most frequently mentioned single herb formula. The earliest citation was from the book *Zheng Lei Ben Cao* 证类本草 (c. 1108). The author Tang Shen Wei described the function of *cha* was to 'make people slim, reduce body fat, and help people remain awake' (久食令人瘦, 去人脂, 使不睡). Although many citations in later eras mentioned that *cha* could make people slim and reduce body fat, this was actually regarded as a side effect when drinking it in large amounts, according to the citation records. Nevertheless, it was cited for its usefulness for obesity by expelling phlegm, regulating *qi* and promoting digestion. For the other most frequently mentioned single herb formulae/*materia medica* entries, *he ye* 荷叶, *kun bu* 昆布, *hai zao* 海藻 and *dong gua* 冬瓜 have the function to expel phlegm or drain dampness and thus reduce body fat; *shan zha* 山楂 promotes digestion, regulates *qi* and reduces fat; and *chi xiao dou* 赤小豆 promotes urination and reduces oedema.

Classical Literature in Perspective

In past eras, obesity was commonly described in many classical literature citations. It could appear as an individual symptom or a complication alongside another health condition. Over a long period of exploration and documentation, comprehensive understanding and knowledge have been developed in terms of the aetiology, pathogenesis and treatments for obesity in CM theory.

The aetiology and pathogenesis of obesity had been discussed in several classical literature books. As early as the Spring and Autumn periods and the Warring States, the ancient CM practitioners found that overindulgence in food and wine could be one of the main factors inducing obesity. Consistent with contemporary CM understanding of obesity, *qi* deficiency, dampness and phlegm were commonly mentioned pathogens generating the dysfunction of the Spleen and Stomach, further leading to obesity.

The citations including CHM treatments were mostly obtained from the books published in the Ming dynasty (c. 1369–1644) and the Qing dynasty (c. 1645–1911). The first citation describing CHM management was from *Xue Shi Ji Yin Wan Jin Shu* 薛氏济阴万金书 (c. 1265); however, classical evidence for CHM managing obesity as an individual symptom (without complications) is limited. General functions of the herbal formulae included tonifying Spleen *qi* and expelling phlegm. Formulae cited for obesity as a complication of other conditions differed. However, some formulae and treatment principles for these conditions are similar to current CM guidelines and textbooks. Herbs commonly mentioned for managing obesity were aligned with the aetiology and pathogenesis of obesity. The general functions included expelling dampness and phlegm, nourishing the Spleen and tonifying *qi*.

The review of the evidence of classical CM literature showed that the aetiology, pathogenesis and treatment methods of obesity have been documented in depth in past eras, and the precious CM knowledge documented in this classical literature continues to inform and guide the management of obesity in CM clinical practice today.

References

1. Needham J, Lu G, Sivin N. (2000) Science and civilisation in China. Vol 5, Part VI: Medicine. Cambridge University Press, Cambridge, UK.
2. Hu R. (2000) *Encyclopedia of Traditional Chinese Medicine*. Hunan Electronic and Audio-Visual Publishing House, Changsha.
3. May B, Lu C, Xue C. (2012) Collections of traditional Chinese medical litearture as resources for systematic searches. *J Altern Complement Med* **18(12):** 1101–1107.
4. May B, Lu Y, Lu C, *et al.* (2013) Systematic assessment of the representativeness of published collections of the traditional literature on Chinese medicine. *J Altern Complement Med* **19(5):** 403–409.
5. 刘亦选, 陈镜合. (1998) 中医内科学. 人民卫生出版社, 北京.
6. 吴勉华, 王新月. (2012) 中医内科学. 中国中医药出版社, 北京.
7. 周仲瑛. (2007) 中医内科学. 中国中医药出版社, 北京.
8. 李经纬, 邓铁涛. (1995) 中医大辞典. 人民卫生出版社, 北京.
9. 朱文锋. (1999) 国家标准应用中医内科疾病诊疗常规. 湖南科学技术出版, 长沙.
10. 魏子孝. (2000) 中西医结合内分泌代谢疾病诊疗手册. 人民军医出版社, 北京.
11. 冯建华. (2001) 内分泌与代谢病的中医治疗. 人民卫生出版社, 北京.
12. 吕光荣. (2001) 中医内科证治学. 人民卫生出版社, 北京.
13. 吴承玉. (2001) 现代中医内科诊断治疗学. 人民卫生出版社, 北京.
14. 林昭庚. (2002) 中西医病名对照大辞典. 人民卫生出版社, 北京.
15. 张洪义, 陆小左. (2002) 中医临床诊断. 天津科学技术出版社, 天津.
16. 郑筱萸. (2002) 中药新药临床研究指导原则. 中国医药科技出版社, 北京.
17. 赵进喜. (2004) 内分泌代谢病中西医诊治. 辽宁科学技术出版社, 辽宁.
18. 姜喆. (2006) 内分泌代谢病临床诊治. 科学技术文献出版社, 北京.
19. 吴绪平. (2006) 现代针灸治疗大成. 中国医药科技出版社, 北京.
20. 雷磊. (2007) 内分泌与代谢病 · 名家医案 · 妙方解析. 人民军医出版社, 北京.
21. 罗云坚, 孙塑伦. (2007) 中医临床治疗特色与优势指南. 人民卫生出版社, 北京.
22. 夏征农, 陈至立. (2009) 辞海. 上海辞书出版社, 上海.
23. 施红. (2011) 中西医结合内分泌与代谢性疾病. 科学出版社, 北京.
24. 范冠杰, 邓兆智. (2013) 专科专病中医临床诊治丛书 · 内分泌科专病与风湿病中医临床诊治. 人民卫生出版社, 北京.

25. 倪青. (2016) 内分泌代谢病中医循证治疗学. 科学技术文献出版社, 北京.
26. 刘学兰. (2017) 中医内分泌代谢病学. 科学出版社, 北京.
27. 龚海洋, 张惠敏, 王睿林, *et al.* (2004) 古代医家对肥胖的认识. *北京中医*. **(06):** 336–338.
28. 周正, 郭洁, 刘培枝. (2018) 基于古代文献探讨肥胖与疾病相关性. *中国民族民间医药*. **27(03):** 26–27.
29. 王姬. (2017) 中医对肥胖认识研究的发展概况. *中国中医药现代远程教育*. **15(11):** 152–154.
30. 黎健明. (2013) 成年单纯性肥胖的中医证治文献研究: 广州中医药大学.
31. American Diabetes Association. (2019) Classification and diagnosis of diabetes: Standards of medical care in diabetes. *Diabetes Care.* **42(Suppl 1):** S13.
32. 张伯礼, 吴勉华, 林子强. (2017) 中医内科学. 中国中医药出版社, 北京.
33. 中华中医药学会. (2011) 糖尿病中医药防治指南. *中国中医药现代远程教育*. **9(4):** 148–151.

4

Methods for Evaluating Clinical Evidence

OVERVIEW

This chapter describes the methods used to identify and evaluate a range of Chinese medicine (CM) interventions for overweight and obesity in clinical studies. Studies identified through a comprehensive search were assessed against eligibility criteria. A review of the methodological quality of the studies was undertaken using standardised methods. Results from included studies were evaluated to provide an estimate of the effects of a range of CM therapies.

Introduction

The use of Chinese medicine (CM) for overweight and obesity has been well described in contemporary literature and classical CM literature. Several systematic reviews have been conducted to evaluate the efficacy and safety of Chinese medicine treatment for overweight and obesity. These have included three reviews of Chinese herbal medicines and six reviews of acupuncture. Systematic reviews have been summarised in the relevant chapters.

This chapter includes the methods of examining the CM interventions for overweight and obesity in clinical studies. Efficacy and safety will be examined in controlled clinical trials. Interventions have been categorised as follows:

- Chinese herbal medicine (CHM) (Chapter 5).
- Acupuncture and related therapies (Chapter 7).

- Other CM therapies (Chapter 8).
- Combination CM therapies (Chapter 9).

References to clinical trials were obtained and assessed by an expert group. Randomised controlled trials (RCTs), non-randomised controlled clinical trials (CCTs) and non-controlled studies were evaluated in detail. Controlled trials were evaluated using the same approach as RCTs and have been described separately. Evidence from non-controlled studies is more difficult to evaluate; therefore the approach was taken to describe the characteristics of the studies, details of the intervention and any adverse events. References to included studies are denoted by a letter and then a number. Studies of CHM are indicated by 'H' (e.g., H1), studies of acupuncture and related therapies are indicated by 'A' (e.g., A1), studies of other CM therapies are indicated by 'O' (e.g., O1), and studies of combinations of CM therapies are indicated by 'C' (e.g., C1).

Search Strategy

Evidence was searched for in English-language and Chinese-language databases, and the methods followed the *Cochrane Handbook of Systematic Reviews*.[1] English-language databases included PubMed, Excerpta Medica Database (Embase), Cumulative Index of Nursing and Allied Health Literature (CINAHL), Cochrane Central Register of Controlled Trials (CENTRAL), including the Cochrane Library, and Allied and Complementary Medicine Database (AMED). Chinese-language databases included China BioMedical Literature (CBM), China National Knowledge Infrastructure (CNKI), Chongqing VIP (CQVIP) and Wanfang. Databases were searched from the dates of inception to November 2018. No restrictions were applied. Search terms were mapped to controlled vocabulary (where applicable), in addition to being searched as keywords.

To conduct a comprehensive search of the literature, searches were run according to the study design (reviews, controlled trials, non-controlled studies). This was done for each of the three intervention types (CHM, acupuncture and related therapies, and other CM therapies), resulting in nine searches in each of the nine databases:

1. CHM reviews.
2. CHM controlled trials (randomised and non-randomised).
3. CHM non-controlled studies.
4. Acupuncture and related therapies reviews.
5. Acupuncture and related therapies controlled trials (randomised and non-randomised).
6. Acupuncture and related therapies non-controlled studies.
7. Other CM therapies reviews.
8. Other CM therapies controlled trials (randomised and non-randomised).
9. Other CM therapies non-controlled studies.

Studies of combination CM therapies were identified through the above searches. In addition to electronic databases, reference lists of systematic reviews and included studies were searched for additional publications. Clinical trials registries were searched to identify clinical trials that were ongoing or completed, and where required, trial investigators were contacted to obtain data. The searched trial registries were the Australian New Zealand Clinical Trial Registry (ANZCTR), the Chinese Clinical Trial Registry (ChiCTR), the European Union Clinical Trials Register (EU-CTR), and the United States National Institutes of Health's register (ClinicalTrials.gov).

If required, trial investigators were contacted to obtain further information. Trial investigators were contacted by email or telephone and were followed up after two weeks if no reply was received. Where no response was received after one month, any unknown information was marked as not available.

Inclusion Criteria

*   Study type: Controlled prospective studies with or without randomisation and uncontrolled studies (cohort, case series and case studies).
*   Participants: Adults aged 18 years and older with a body mass index (BMI) of greater than 24 kg/m^2 (Table 4.1).[2-3] People with overweight and obesity with weight-related complications that are either caused or exacerbated by excess adiposity were also

Table 4.1.   Inclusion and Exclusion Criteria

	Inclusion	Exclusion

Study type	1. Controlled prospective studies
	  – Randomised
	  – Quasi-randomised
	2. Uncontrolled studies
	  – Cohort
	  – Case series
	  – Case studies
		1. Epidemiological studies
		2. Retrospective studies
		3. Duplicated studies

Population	1. Adults (18 years of age and older)
	2. Overweight: BMI of 25 to 29.9 kg/m²*
	3. Obese: BMI of 30 kg/m² or more
	  – If Chinese studies, overweight: BMI of 24 to 27.9 kg/m², and obese: BMI of 28 kg/m² or greater
	  – Overweight/obesity with complications (based on 2016 AACE/ACE Guidelines)[†]
		1. People less than 18 years of age
		2. Obesity secondary to other diseases (e.g., anterior pituitary hypofunction, hypothyroidism, hypercortisolism)
		3. Obesity related to taking medications
		4. Gestational obesity

Intervention	1. Intervention administered for at least four weeks (28 days) 2. Chinese medicine therapies alone or in combination with other Chinese medicine therapies or guideline-recommended therapies	1. Non-Chinese medicine therapies 2. Western herbal medicine 3. Tea (*Camellia sinensis*) alone 4. Herbal medicine given intravenously

Comparison	1. Dietary measures
	  – Reduced-calorie, healthy meal plan
	  – Individualised diet
	  – Meal replacement
	  – Other dietary interventions
	2. Physical activities
	  – Aerobic physical activity
	  – Resistance exercise
	  – Individualised program
	  – Other exercise interventions
	3. Behavioural/lifestyle counselling
	4. Pharmacotherapy (recommended in guidelines)[‡]
	  – Orlistat
		1. Pharmacotherapies not recommended in guidelines
		2. Bariatric surgery or other surgery
		3. Chinese medicine
		4. If integrative medicine study, control group is different to intervention group

Table 4.1. (*Continued*)

Inclusion	Exclusion
– Naltrexone/bupropion – Liraglutide – Lorcaserin – Phentermine/topiramate – Metformin 5. Placebo 6. Cognitive behavioural therapy or psychotherapy 7. No treatment 8. Treatment for weight-related complications such as lipid-lowering treatments and hypoglycaemics	

Abbreviations: BMI, body mass index; kg, kilograms; m^2, metres squared.

* Body Mass Index (BMI): Underweight: BMI less than 18.5 kg/m^2, normal weight: BMI of 18.5 to 24.9 kg/m^2, overweight: BMI of 25 to 29.9 kg/m^2, obese: BMI of 30 kg/m^2 or more.

Note that BMI values may vary depending on the definition of overweight and obese in each country. For example, the overweight classification in China is lower. Therefore, studies published in China on the Chinese population showed that overweight was classified as 24 to 27.9 kg/m^2, and obesity was greater than or equal to 28 kg/m^2.[2,3] In Chinese studies that followed the WHO Guidelines published in 2000, overweight was classified as being 23 to 24.9 kg/m^2, and obesity, 25 kg/m^2 or greater.[5]

† Complications from the 2016 AACE/ACE Guidelines[4]: Pre-diabetes (including impaired fasting glucose and impaired glucose tolerance), metabolic syndrome, type 2 diabetes, dyslipidaemia, hypertension, cardiovascular disease and cardiovascular disease mortality, non-alcoholic fatty liver disease/non-alcoholic steatohepatitis, polycystic ovarian syndrome (PCOS), female infertility, male hypogonadism, obstructive sleep apnoea, asthma/reactive airway disease, osteoarthritis, urinary stress incontinence, gastroesophageal reflux disease and depression.

‡ Obesity guidelines include:

- 2016 AACE/ACE Guidelines: American Association of Clinical Endocrinologists and American College of Endocrinology comprehensive clinical practice guidelines for medical care of patients with obesity.[4]
- 2015 European guidelines for obesity management in adults.[6]
- 2011 Chinese expert consensus for obesity prevention and treatment in adults.[2] (In Chinese: 2011 年中国成人肥胖症防治专家共识.)
- 2003 Chinese Guidelines for the Prevention and control of overweight and obesity in Chinese adults.[7] (In Chinese: 2003 年中国成人超重和肥胖症预防控制指南 (试行.))
- 2000 WHO Guidelines: The Asia-Pacific perspective: redefining obesity and its treatment.[5]
- 1998 Chinese Guidelines: Standard for diagnosis and efficacy evaluation of simple obesity.[8] (In Chinese: 1998 年单纯性肥胖病的诊断及疗效评定标准.)

included, based on the complications listed in the 2016 AACE/ACE Guidelines, such as pre-diabetes, metabolic syndrome, type 2 diabetes, dyslipidaemia, hypertension and polycystic ovarian syndrome.[4]

- Interventions: CHM, acupuncture and related therapies, or other CM therapies, alone or in combination with other CM therapies or with pharmacotherapy/routine care or with lifestyle interventions, such as diet restriction and exercise. Studies combining CM therapies with pharmacotherapy/routine care/lifestyle interventions were required to use the same therapies in both the intervention and comparator groups. Studies must have administered the interventions for at least four weeks (28 days).

  Comparators: Placebo, no treatment or waiting list, pharmacotherapies recommended in clinical practice guidelines, such as orlistat; lifestyle interventions, such as diet modification, physical activities, behavioural/lifestyle counselling or other routine care therapies for studies that recruited participants with complications, such as diabetes.

- Outcome measures: Studies reported at least one of the pre-specified body composition outcome measures (Table 4.2).

Exclusion Criteria

- Study type: Epidemiological studies and retrospective studies. Duplicated studies reporting the same results (those published at the later date were excluded).
- Participants: Obesity secondary to other diseases (e.g., anterior pituitary hypofunction, hypothyroidism, hypercortisolism); people aged under 18 years; obesity related to taking medications; gestational obesity.
- Intervention: Chinese medicine interventions that are not commonly practiced worldwide, such as catgut embedding; Western herbal medicine; tea (*Camellia sinensis*) used alone.
- Comparators: Drugs not recommended in guidelines; bariatric surgery or other surgery; Chinese medicine therapies; in an

Table 4.2.   Pre-specified Outcomes

Outcome Categories	Outcome Measures
Body composition	1. Weight
	2. Body mass index
	3. Waist circumference
	4. Waist–hip ratio
	5. Fat mass
Cardiovascular risk factors	− Serum glucose − Serum lipids − Blood pressure − HbA1c − Fasting insulin − Other.
Effective rate	Effective rate according to a recognised standard such as the 1998 *Chinese guidelines: Standard for diagnosis and efficacy evaluation of simple obesity*[8] and the 1995 *Guidelines for the clinical research of Chinese medicine new drugs.*[9]
Health-related quality of life	Any validated instrument that measures quality of life.
Adverse events	Number and type of adverse events.

integrative medicine study, control is different to the intervention group.

- Outcomes: Effective rate measures that do not provide an acknowledged reference to the rating scale.

Outcomes

Pre-specified outcomes were separated into two main categories: body composition, including changes in body weight or body mass, and indices of cardiovascular risk factors. Changes in body weight and BMI are important measures used to evaluate interventions for overweight and obesity and were the primary outcomes for the assessment of the clinical trials. The waist circumference and waist–hip ratio were secondary outcomes used as a more practical clinical estimate of abdominal/visceral adipose tissue. Changes in body composition, including fat mass, were also evaluated. A reduction in fat mass was an indication of a favourable effect of an intervention, separate from weight reduction. Indices of related complications and cardiovascular risk factors, such as blood pressure, serum glucose, lipids, etc., were also assessed as secondary outcome measures. The outcomes and measurements are included in Table 4.2.

Other outcomes included the effective rate and quality of life measurements. The effective rate is a popular outcome measure in clinical trials in China. Effective rate measures were only included if they were in accordance with recognised standards, such as the 1998 *Chinese guidelines: Standard for diagnosis and efficacy evaluation of simple obesity*[8] and the 1995 *Guidelines for the clinical research of Chinese medicine new drugs.*[9] Being clinically effective usually includes more than 3 kg of weight reduction (or more than 2 kg/m^2 of BMI reduction) or more than 3% of fat mass reduction after three months of treatment according to these standards. The assessment of the quality of life measurements was planned; however, few of the included studies used these types of measures. Adverse events, including the number and type of events, were also assessed.

Risk of Bias Assessment

The risk of bias was assessed for randomised controlled trials using the Cochrane Collaboration's tool.[1] In clinical trials, bias can be categorised as selection bias, performance bias, detection bias, attrition bias and reporting bias. Each domain is assessed to determine whether the bias is at a low, high or unclear risk. Low risk of bias indicates that bias is unlikely, high risk indicates plausible bias that seriously weakens confidence in the results and unclear bias indicates a lack of information or uncertainty over potential bias and raises some doubt about the results. The risk of bias assessment is verified by two people and disagreements are resolved by discussion or consultation with a third person.

Risk of bias is categorised using the following six domains:

- Sequence generation: The method used to generate the allocation sequence is given in sufficient detail to allow an assessment of whether it should produce comparable groups. Low risk of bias refers to a random number table or computer random generator. High risk of bias includes studies that describe a non-random sequence generation, such as an odd or even date of birth or date of admission.
- Allocation concealment: The method used to conceal the allocation sequence is given in enough detail to determine whether intervention allocations could have been foreseen before or during enrolment. Low risk of bias includes central randomisation or sealed envelopes, and high risk of bias includes open random sequence, etc.
- Blinding of participants and personnel: Measures used to describe whether the study participants and personnel are blind to the intervention received. In addition, information relating to whether the blinding was effective is also assessed. Studies that ensure blinding of participants and personnel are at low risk of bias. If the study is not blind or incompletely blind, it is at high risk of bias.
- Blinding of outcome assessors: Measures used to describe if the outcome assessors are blind to knowing which intervention a participant received. In addition, information relating to whether the blinding was effective is also assessed. Studies that ensure the blinding of outcome assessors are at low risk of bias. If the study is not blind or incompletely blind, it is at high risk of bias.
- Incomplete outcome data: Completeness of outcome data for each main outcome, including dropouts, exclusions from the analysis with numbers missing in each group, and reasons for dropping out or exclusions. Studies with low risk of bias would include all outcome data. If there is missing data, it is unlikely to relate to the true

outcome or is balanced between groups. Studies at high risk of bias would have unexplained missing data.

- Selective reporting: The study protocol is available, and the pre-specified outcomes are included in the report. Studies with a published protocol that include all pre-specified outcomes in their report would be at low risk of bias. Studies at high risk of bias would not include all pre-specified outcomes or the outcome data may be reported incompletely.

Statistical Analyses

The frequency of CM syndromes, CHM formulae, herbs and acupuncture points reported in included studies are presented using descriptive statistics. CM syndromes reported in two or more studies are presented. The 10 most frequently reported CHM formulae and 20 most frequently reported herbs are presented where used in at least two studies, although for CHM formulae, this was not always possible. The top 10 acupuncture points used in two or more studies are presented or as available. Where data were limited, reports of single CM syndromes or acupuncture points were provided as a guide for the reader.

Definitions of statistical tests and results are described in the glossary. Dichotomous data are reported as a risk ratio (RR) with 95% confidence intervals (CI), and continuous data are reported as the mean difference (MD) or standardised mean difference (SMD) with 95% CI. For dichotomous data, when the RR is greater than one and the upper and lower values of the 95% CI are both greater than one, this indicates we can be 95% certain that there is a difference between the groups and that the true effect lies within these CIs. The same is true for values less than one. In such cases, we say there is a 'significant difference' between the groups. For continuous data, when the MD is greater than zero and both the upper and lower values of the 95% CI are greater than zero, we say there is a 'significant difference' between the groups. The same is true on the negative side of the scale.[1] For all analyses, RR or MD and 95% CI were reported, together with a formal test for heterogeneity using the I^2 statistic. An I^2 score greater than 50% was considered to indicate substantial heterogeneity.[1] Where possible and appropriate, planned subgroup analyses included the CM formula and complications of overweight and obesity, such as studies that assessed participants with diabetes, PCOS, hypertension, etc. Available case analysis with a random effects model was used in all analyses. The random effects model was used to take into account the clinical heterogeneity likely to be encountered within and between included studies and the variation in treatment effects between included studies.

Assessment Using Grading of Recommendations Assessment, Development and Evaluation

The Grading of Recommendations Assessment, Development and Evaluation (GRADE) approach was used.[10–11] The GRADE approach summarises and rates the strength and quality ('certainty') of evidence in systematic reviews using a structured process for presenting evidence summaries. The results are presented in a summary of findings tables. The results provide an important overview for overweight and obesity outcomes.

A panel of experts was established to evaluate the certainty of evidence. The panel included the systematic review team, Chinese medicine practitioners, integrative medicine experts, research methodologists and conventional medicine physicians. The experts were asked to rate the clinical importance of key interventions from CHM and acupuncture therapies as well as comparators and outcomes. Results were collated and, based on the rating scores and subsequent discussion, a consensus on the content for the summary of findings tables was achieved.

The certainty of the evidence for each outcome was rated according to the five factors outlined in the GRADE approach. The quality of evidence may be rated based on:

- Limitations in study design (risk of bias).
- Inconsistency of results (unexplained heterogeneity).
- Indirectness of evidence (interventions, populations and outcomes important to the patients with the condition).
- Imprecision (uncertainty about the results).
- Publication bias (selective publication of studies).

These five factors are additive and a reduction in one or more factors will reduce the certainty of the evidence for that outcome. The GRADE approach also includes methods for assessing observational studies. GRADE summaries in this monograph only include RCTs.

Treatment recommendations can also be assessed using the GRADE approach, but due to the diverse nature of CM practice, treatment recommendations were not included with the summary of findings. Therefore, the reader should interpret the evidence with reference to the local practice environment. It should also be noted that the GRADE approach requires judgements about the strength and quality of evidence and some subjective assessment. However, the experience of the panel members suggests that the judgements are reliable and transparent representations of the certainty of evidence.

The GRADE levels of evidence are grouped into four categories:

1. High certainty: We are very confident that the true effect lies close to that of the estimate of the effect.
2. Moderate certainty: We are moderately confident in the effect estimate: The true effect is likely to be close to the estimate of the effect, but there is a possibility that it is substantially different.
3. Low certainty: Our confidence in the effect estimate is limited: The true effect may be substantially different from the estimate of the effect.
4. Very low certainty: We have very little confidence in the effect estimate: The true effect is likely to be substantially different from the estimate of the effect.

References

1. Higgins J, Green S. (eds.) (2011) *Cochrane Handbook for Systematic Reviews of Interventions* Version 5.1.0 (The Cochrane Collaboration). http://www.cochrane-handbook.org
2. 中华医学会内分泌学分会. (2011) 中国成人肥胖症防治专家共识. 中国内分泌代谢杂志. **27(9):** 711–717.
3. Zhou BF. (2002) Cooperative Meta-Analysis Group of the Working Group on Obesity in China. Predictive values of body mass index and waist circumference for risk factors of certain related diseases in Chinese adults — study on optimal cut-off points of body mass index and waist circumference in Chinese adults. *Biomed Environ Science.* **15(1):** 83–96.
4. Garvey WT, Mechanick JI, Brett EM, *et al*. (2016) Reviewers of the AACE/ACE Obesity Clinical Practice Guidelines. American Association of Clinical Endocrinologists and American College of Endocrinology comprehensive clinical practice guidelines for medical care of patients with obesity. *Endocr Pract* **22(Suppl 3):** 1–203.
5. World Health Organization. Regional Office for the Western Pacific. (2000) The Asia-Pacific perspective: Redefining obesity and its treatment. http://iris.wpro.who.int/handle/10665.1/5379
6. Yumuk V, Tsigos C, Fried M, *et al*. (2015) Obesity Management Task Force of the European Association for the Study of Obesity. European Guidelines for Obesity Management in Adults. *Obes Facts* **8(6):** 402–424.
7. 中华人民共和国卫生部疾病控制司. (2003) 中国成人超重和肥胖症预防控制指南 (试行).
8. 危北海, 贾葆鹏. (1998) 单纯性肥胖病的诊断及疗效评定标准. 中国中西医结合杂志. **(05):** 317–319.
9. 中华人民共和国卫生部. (1995) 中药新药临床研究指导原则. 人民卫生出版社.
10. Schünemann H, Brozek J, Guyatt G, et al. (eds.) (2013) GRADE handbook for grading quality of evidence and strength of recommendations (The GRADE Working Group). http://www.guidelinedevelopment.org/handbook/
11. Schünemann HJ, Higgins JPT, Vist GE, *et al*. (2019) Completing 'summary of findings' tables and grading the certainty of the evidence. In: *Cochrane Handbook for Systematic Reviews of Interventions* version 6.0 (updated July 2019), (eds.) Higgins JPT, Thomas J, Chandler J, *et al*. Cochrane. www.training.cochrane.org/handbook

5

Clinical Evidence for Chinese Herbal Medicine

OVERVIEW

Chinese herbal medicine (CHM) has been widely used and researched for its effects on overweight and obesity. This chapter evaluates 232 clinical studies of CHM for obesity and includes 171 formulae and 212 herbs. The meta-analyses of 195 randomised controlled trials (RCTs) indicate that CHM combined with lifestyle therapies and/or drug therapies offer promising benefits for reducing weight and improving related metabolic parameters. In addition, CHM appears to be safe and well-tolerated by people with obesity.

Introduction

Chinese herbal medicine (CHM) for obesity includes oral preparations, such as decoctions, granules, capsules, pills and tablets. Many different herb combinations and formulae have been used to treat obesity, and the most commonly evaluated in clinical trials are presented in this chapter.

Previous Systematic Reviews

Previously, three systematic reviews and meta-analyses have evaluated the efficacy of CHM, either alone or in combination with lifestyle therapies and/or drug therapies for obesity. The efficacy and safety of CHM treatment for obesity were analysed by Sui and colleagues.[1] A total of 49 randomised controlled trials (RCTs) with 1,268 participants were included in the review. Results showed that people with obesity treated with CHM had greater body weight reduction and body mass index (BMI) reduction than those treated with a placebo or lifestyle modifications. The review also reported that CHM had similar changes in blood lipids and glucose levels compared to drug therapies. In terms of the safety of CHM, the adverse effects appeared to be mild and tolerable. However, despite some positive outcomes, the authors noted that the conclusions were limited by small sample sizes and poor methodologies.

In 2015, Tsang and colleagues reviewed the efficacy of CHM for obesity and included 17 RCTs and 1,587 participants.[2] They found that CHM was superior to drug therapies or lifestyle therapies in terms of effective rate. However, the methodological quality of the included trials was low according to the Jadad scale. In another review published in 2016, Zhou and colleagues reported similar results.[3] Eleven RCTs with 1,073 participants were included in the review. The results showed that CHM significantly improved the effective rate when compared to drug therapies or no treatment. But results were limited by poor quality individual studies and high heterogeneity in pooled results. The authors also published the frequency of herbs in this review, and the top three herbs used in the clinical trials were *fu ling* 茯苓, *bai zhu* 白术 and *cang zhu* 苍术.

Identification of Clinical Studies

Electronic database searches identified more than 70,000 citations. After removing duplicates and excluding ineligible studies by reviewing the titles, abstracts and full text, a total of 232 clinical studies (16,676 participants) were finally included in the systematic review. Among all clinical studies on CHM for obesity, 195 were RCTs, 13 were controlled clinical trials (CCTs), and 24 were non-controlled studies (Fig. 5.1). Most studies (219 studies) were conducted in

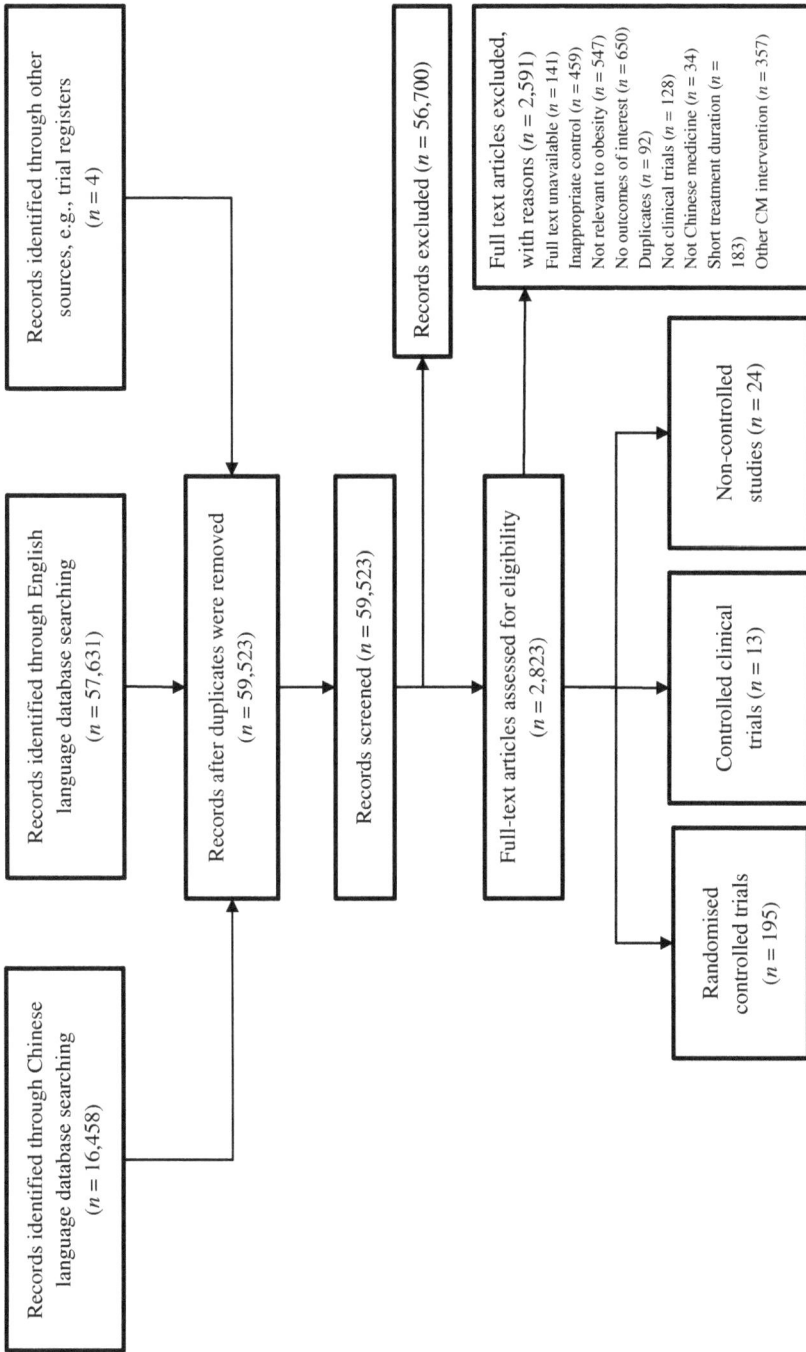

Fig. 5.1. Flow chart of the study selection process: Chinese herbal medicine

China, nine in Korea and one each in Australia, the United States (US), Japan and Iran. The effects of CHM generated from RCTs and CCTs were synthesised through meta-analyses. Non-controlled studies are summarised, but their results are not included in the evidence analysis.

The duration of obesity ranged from six months to 13 years and the ages of the participants ranged from 18 to 79 years. Fifty-nine studies assessed simple obesity and 173 studies assessed obesity with complications or comorbidities. Complications or comorbidities included diabetes or pre-diabetes (98 studies), polycystic ovarian syndrome (PCOS) (33), metabolic syndrome (17), hypertension (14), hyperlipidaemia (6), non-alcoholic fatty liver disease (3), hyperuricemia (1) and obstructive sleep apnoea/hypopnea syndrome (1). Chinese medicine syndrome differentiation was described in 135 studies. The most common syndromes were Spleen deficiency with dampness obstruction, dampness-heat in the Spleen and Stomach, phlegm-dampness, Kidney deficiency with phlegm-dampness, and *qi* deficiency with phlegm and stasis.

Chinese Herbal Medicine

CHM alone was assessed in 54 studies, and 178 studies combined CHM with drug therapies or non-drug therapies. Non-drug therapies included diet advice, physical exercise and health education. All CHM treatments were orally administrated. Oral preparation types included decoctions, capsules, granules, pills and tablets. A total of 171 distinct formulae and 212 different herbs were investigated in the clinical studies.

The most common formulae were *Wu ling san*五苓散 (10 studies), *Huang lian jie du tang* 黄连解毒汤 (7), *Shen ling bai zhu san* 参苓白术散 (6), *Ling gui zhu gan tang* 苓桂术甘汤 (5), *Pei lian ma huang fang* 佩连麻黄方 (4) and *Xiao zhi tang* 消脂汤 (4). The most frequently used herbs were *fu ling* 茯苓 (110 studies), *bai zhu* 白术 (98), *ban xia*半夏 (84), *chen pi* 陈皮 (78) and *ze xie* 泽泻 (77).

Randomised Controlled Trials of Chinese Herbal Medicine

A total of 195 RCTs (H1–195) assessing CHM for obesity were identified from the search. CHM alone was assessed in 38 studies, and 157 studies assessed a combination of CHM with drug therapies or non-drug therapies. Most studies (178 studies) were two-arm designs (i.e., CHM *vs.* control), 15 had three arms (i.e., CHM 1 *vs.* CHM 2 *vs.* control) and two had four arms (CHM 1 *vs.* CHM2 *vs.* control 1 *vs.* control 2). Comparators included drug therapies or/and non-drug therapies, such as a placebo, no treatment, diet, physical exercise, health education, etc.

In total, 15,172 participants were included in the RCTs. Among them, 7,780 were female, 5,992 were male, and the gender of the remaining 1,400 participants was not stated. The age range was from 18 to 79 years. Participants' duration of obesity ranged from six months to 13 years, and the treatment duration ranged from four weeks to 12 months. The studies mainly used the following diagnostic criteria to confirm obesity: the 2000 Obesity Report of the WHO Consultation (*Obesity: Preventing and managing the global epidemic*, World Health Organization, 2000), the *Chinese adults body mass index classification recommendation* by the Working Group on Obesity of China (WGOC) (2001年国际生命科学学会中国办事处中国肥胖问题工作组-中国成人体质指数分类推荐意见), the 2003 *Guidelines for prevention and control of overweight and obesity in Chinese adults* (2003 年中国成人超重和肥胖症预防控制指南 (试行)) or used the BMI.

Weight-related complications or comorbidities were common in obese people, and more than three-quarters of the RCTs assessed people with obesity and associated conditions, such as pre-diabetes or diabetes (90 studies), PCOS (26), metabolic syndrome (15), hypertension (12), hyperlipidaemia (3), non-alcoholic fatty liver disease (2) and obstructive sleep apnea/hypopnea syndrome (1).

Chinese medicine syndrome differentiation was described in 114 studies, and 109 studies specifically recruited participants with a pre-defined syndrome. The most common syndromes were Spleen deficiency with dampness obstruction, dampness-heat in the Spleen and Stomach and phlegm-dampness. Another five studies did not set strict inclusion criteria for syndromes, but they used individualised syndrome differentiation to allocate treatments to the participants.

In total, 149 distinct formulae (130 named and 19 unnamed) were assessed in the studies, and the most common were *Wu ling san* 五苓散, *Huang lian jie du tang* 黄连解毒汤 and *Pei lian ma huang tang* 佩连麻黄方 (Table 5.1). A total of 203 distinct herbs were used in the formulae, and the most common were *fu ling* 茯苓, *bai zhu* 白术, *ban xia* 半夏, *chen pi* 陈皮 and *huang lian* 黄连 (Table 5.2).

Risk of Bias

Although all 195 RCTs reported that they were randomised, only one-third (64 RCTs, 32.8%) provided sufficient details of sequence

Table 5.1.   Frequently Reported Formulae in Randomised Controlled Trials

Most Common Formulae	No. of Studies	Ingredients
Wu ling san 五苓散	8	*Ze xie* 泽泻, *zhu ling* 猪苓, *fu ling* 茯苓, *bai zhu* 白术, *gui zhi* 桂枝
Huang lian jie du tang 黄连解毒汤*	6	*Huang lian* 黄连, *huang qin* 黄芩, *huang bai* 黄柏, *zhi zi* 栀子
Pei lian ma huang fang 佩连麻黄方	4	*Pei lan* 佩兰, *huang lian* 黄连, *ma huang* 麻黄
Shen ling bai zhu san 参苓白术散*	4	*Lian zi* 莲子, *yi yi ren* 薏苡仁, *sha ren* 砂仁, *jie geng* 桔梗, *bai bian dou* 白扁豆, *fu ling* 茯苓, *ren shen* 人参, *gan cao* 甘草, *bai zhu* 白术, *shan yao* 山药
Ling gui zhu gan tang 苓桂术甘汤	4	*Fu ling* 茯苓, *gui zhi* 桂枝, *bai zhu* 白术, *gan cao* 甘草
Jue ming zi cha 决明子茶	3	*Jue ming zi* 决明子, *shan zha* 山楂, *ju hua* 菊花
Dao tan tang 导痰汤	3	*Ban xia* 半夏, *tian nan xing* 天南星, *zhi shi* 枳实, *chen pi* 陈皮, *fu ling* 茯苓
Shan zha xiao zhi jiao capsule 山楂消脂胶囊	3	*Shan zha* 山楂, *da huang* 大黄, *gan cao* 甘草

Table 5.1. (*Continued*)

Most Common Formulae	No. of Studies	Ingredients
Fang feng tong sheng san/wan 防风通圣散/丸	3	*Fang feng* 防风, *chuan xiong* 川芎, *dang gui* 当归, *shao yao* 芍药, *da huang* 大黄, *bo he* 薄荷, *ma huang* 麻黄, *lian qiao* 连翘, *mang xiao* 芒硝, *shi gao* 石膏, *huang qin* 黄芩, *jie geng* 桔梗, *hua shi* 滑石, *gan cao* 甘草, *jing jie* 荆芥, *bai zhu* 白术, *zhi zi* 栀子
Huang lian wen dan tang 黄连温胆汤*	3	*Huang lian* 黄连, *sheng jiang* 生姜, *ban xia* 半夏, *chen pi* 陈皮, *zhu ru* 竹茹, *zhi shi* 枳实, *gan cao* 甘草

Ingredients are referenced to the original studies where possible. If herb ingredients varied across studies, the herb ingredients were sourced from *Zhong Yi Fang Ji Da Ci Dian* 中医方剂大辞典.

* *Huang lian jie du tang* 黄连解毒汤, *Shen ling bai zhu san* 参苓白术散 and *Huang lian wen dan tang* 黄连温胆汤 were especially used for obesity complicated with pre-diabetes or diabetes.
Note: The use of some herbs, such as *ma huang* 麻黄, may be restricted in some countries. Readers are advised to comply with relevant regulations.

Table 5.2. Frequently Reported Herbs in Randomised Controlled Trials

Most Common Herbs	Scientific Name	Frequency of Use
Fu ling 茯苓	*Poria cocos* (Schw.) Wolf	90
Bai zhu 白术	*Atractylodes macrocephala* Koidz.	77
Ban xia 半夏	*Pinellia ternata* (Thunb.) Breit.	67
Chen pi 陈皮	*Citrus reticulata* Blanco	67
Huang lian 黄连	*Coptis chinensis* Franch.	64
Dan shen 丹参	*Salvia miltiorrhiza* Bge.	63
Shan zha 山楂	*Crataegus pinnatifida* Bge. var. *major* N.E. Br.	60
Ze xie 泽泻	*Alisma orientalis* (Sam.) Juzep.	59
Huang qi 黄芪	*Astragalus membranaceus* (Fisch.) Bge. var. *mongholicus* (Bge.) Hsiao	56
Cang zhu 苍术	*Atractylodes lancea* (Thunb.) DC.	55
Da huang 大黄	*Rheum palmatum* L.	43
Shan yao 山药	*Dioscorea opposita* Thunb.	38
Gan cao 甘草	*Glycyrrhiza uralensis* Fisch.	38

(*Continued*)

Table 5.2. (*Continued*)

Most Common Herbs	Scientific Name	Frequency of Use
Dang gui 当归	*Angelica sinensis* (Oliv.) Diels	28
He ye 荷叶	*Nelumbo nucifera* Gaertn.	28
Jue ming zi 决明子	*Cassia obtusifolia* L.	27
Yi yi ren 薏苡仁	*Coix lacryma-jobi* L. var. *mayuen* (Roman.) Stapf	25
Dang shen 党参	*Codonopsis pilosula* (Franch.) Nannf.	24
Ge gen 葛根	*Pueraria lobata* (Willd.) Ohwi	24
Huang qin 黄芩	*Scutellaria baicalensis* Georgi	24

Note: The use of some herbs may be restricted in some countries. Readers are advised to comply with relevant regulations.

generation methods and only 13 studies (6.7%) used appropriate methods to conceal allocation, such as envelopes or central allocation, and thus were judged to be at low risk of bias. The others were judged to be at an unclear risk of bias (Table 5.3).

Participants were blinded effectively in 20 studies (10.3%) that used a placebo as the control, but only 13 studies (6.7%) mentioned blinding of research personnel and were judged to be at low risk of bias. Information was not sufficient to judge whether the personnel were blinded in seven placebo-controlled studies (3.6%); therefore, they were at an unclear risk of bias for this domain. The other 175 studies (89.7%) were open-labelled and at high risk of bias in terms of the blinding of participants and personnel. Only one study (H2) stated that the outcome assessors were blind, and so this study was judged to be at low risk of bias. The others did not describe assessor blinding and were judged to be at an unclear risk of bias. In terms of the incomplete outcome data domain, all studies were judged to be at low risk of bias because they provided details on dropouts and used appropriate methods to impute data.

Five study protocols (H117, H174, H178, H179, H182) were available, and only two studies (1.0%) reported all pre-defined outcomes. Three studies did not report all the pre-defined outcomes and were judged to be at high risk of bias. The others (97.5%) did not

Table 5.3. Risk of Bias of Randomised Controlled Trials

Risk of Bias Domain	Low Risk *n* (%)	Unclear Risk *n* (%)	High Risk *n* (%)
Sequence generation	64 (32.8)	131 (67.2)	0
Allocation concealment	13 (6.7)	182 (93.3)	0
Blinding of participants	20 (10.3)	0	175 (89.7)
Blinding of personnel	13 (6.7)	7 (3.6)	175 (89.7)
Blinding of outcome assessors	1 (0.5)	194 (99.5)	0
Incomplete outcome data	195 (100)	0	0
Selective outcome reporting	2 (1.0)	190 (97.5)	3 (1.5)

provide sufficient information to permit judgement and thus were at an unclear risk of bias for selective outcome reporting (Table 5.3).

Results

Chinese Herbal Medicine Alone

In total, 45 studies (H1–2, H4, H8, H15, H26, H30, H35–36, H42, H51, H54, H64–65, H76, H80–81, H84, H86, H94–95, H105, H117, H130, H133, H145, H151, H158, H164, H173, H176, H178–180, H183–186, H188, H189, H191–195) assessed CHM therapy alone compared to a placebo, no treatment, lifestyle therapies or drug therapies. Nearly all the formulae were made by the researchers themselves according to their clinical experience. Among them, 13 studies evaluated simple obesity and the other 32 studies assessed obesity with complications or comorbidities, including diabetes (16 studies), PCOS (11), metabolic syndrome (4) and hyperlipidaemia (1). The treatment duration ranged from seven weeks to 24 weeks.

Chinese Herbal Medicine vs. Placebo

Compared to CHM, 10 studies (H2, H8, H35, H42, H86, H117, H133, H173, H176, H178) used a placebo as the control, including

Table 5.4. Chinese Herbal Medicine *vs.* Placebo

Outcomes	No. of Studies (Participants)	Effect Size MD [95% CI], I²%	Included Studies
Weight	5 (412)	−0.57 kg [−2.59, 1.45], 0	H8, H42, H86, H133 H178
BMI	8 (587)	0.34 kg/m² [−0.74, 0.07], 0	H2, H8, H35, H42, H86, H133, H176, H178
WC	4 (316)	1.75cm [−3.57, 0.07], 0	H8, H35, H86, H178
WHR	3 (202)	−0.01 [−0.05, 0.04], 80.3	H2, H35, H178
Body fat percentage	3 (240)	−1.20 [−2.46, 0.07], 0	H8, H86, H133

Abbreviations: BMI, body mass index; CI, confidence interval; MD, mean difference; WC, waist circumference; WHR, waist–hip ratio.

735 participants. All studies evaluated participants with simple obesity except for two (H35, H133) that evaluated obesity with metabolic syndrome. Treatment duration ranged from seven weeks to 12 weeks. Data from two studies (H117, H173) could not be analysed as relevant data was not provided. As for the other studies that were pooled into analysis, there was no difference in weight, BMI, waist circumference (WC), waist–hip ratio (WHR) and body fat percentage between the groups after treatment (Table 5.4).

Chinese Herbal Medicine vs. No Treatment

Three studies (H95, H192, H195) comprising 213 participants compared CHM to no treatment. All studies assessed the BMI, which was significantly reduced in the intervention group compared to the control (MD −2.37 kg/m² [95% CI −4.02, −0.71], I² = 69.8%). However, the WHR was not significantly different between the groups after treatment in two (H95, H195) of the studies (MD 0.09 [95% CI −0.24, 0.05], I² = 98.8%, 175 participants). Weight, WC and fat mass percentage were not reported in these three studies.

Chinese Herbal Medicine vs. Lifestyle Therapies

CHM was compared to diet therapy in two studies (H145, H184) comprising 133 participants. The BMI and WC were assessed, but neither showed a significant reduction between the groups after the treatment (MD −0.48 kg/m^2 [95% CI −1.15, 0.18], I^2 = 0% and MD −1.53 cm [95% CI −4.28, 1.23], I^2 = 55.4%, respectively). The weight and fat mass percentages were evaluated in one study (H184), but no significant difference was found.

Chinese Herbal Medicine vs. Drug Therapies

Thirty-two studies (H1, H4, H15, H26, H30, H36, H51, H54, H64–65, H76, H80–81, H84, H94, H105, H130, H151, H158, H164, H179, H180, H183, H185–186, H188–189, H191–195) comprising 2,826 participants used drug therapies as the control. Nearly all the studies compared CHM to metformin alone or alongside other therapies. One study (H26) used orlistat as a control, one simvastatin (H192), and one rosiglitazone (H164). Two studies used metformin alongside lifestyle therapies (H15) or ethinylestradiol cyproterone (H188), and two studies used simvastatin (H192) and rosiglitazone (H164), respectively. The results of these studies are presented in the weight-related complications and comorbidities section due to the participants having a diagnosis of obesity alongside a particular complication.

Chinese Herbal Medicine vs. Orlistat

Compared to orlistat (a lipase inhibitor), weight was reduced significantly in the CHM group (H26) after 12 weeks of treatment in 96 participants (MD −12.07 kg [95% CI −16.17, −7.97]). Other outcomes such as the BMI or WC were not reported.

Chinese Herbal Medicine vs. Metformin

Twenty-seven studies (H1, H4, H30, H36, H51, H54, H64–65, H76, H80–81, H84, H94, H105, H130, H151, H158, H179, H180, H183,

H185–186, H189, H191, H193–195) comprising 2,518 participants compared CHM to metformin. One study (H180) was not pooled in analysis due to different statistical methods. The weight, BMI and WC were reduced significantly in the CHM group compared to metformin. However, the WHR did not decrease. Indices of other obesity-related complications, such as blood glucose, insulin and cholesterol, were also evaluated and are presented in Table 5.5.

Table 5.5. Chinese Herbal Medicine *vs.* Metformin

Outcomes	No. of Studies (Participants)	Effect Size MD [95% CI], I^2%	Included Studies
Weight	5 (663)	−2.14 kg [−4.16, −0.01]*, 17.4	H51, H64, H65, H94, H158
BMI	23 (2,226)	−0.43 kg/m² [−0.67, −0.18]*, 38.9	H1, H4, H30, H36, H51, H54, H64–65, H76, H80, H81, H84, H105, H130, H158, H179, H183, H185, H189, H191, H193–195
WC	5 (893)	−1.74 cm [−4.31, −0.83]*, 81.5	H51, H64, H158, H179, H183
WHR	7 (389)	0.00 [−0.02, 0.02], 0	H1, H36, H54, H81, H189, H191, H195
Fasting blood glucose	22 (1,794)	−0.13 mmol/L [−0.33, 0.07], 83.0	H1, H4, H36, H54, H64–65, H76, H80–81, H84, H94, H105, H130, H151, H158, H183, H185–186, H191, H193-195
Postprandial blood glucose	13 (1,273)	−0.33 mmol/L [−0.69, 0.03], 46.4	H64–65, H80–81, H84, H94, H105, H130, H151, H158, H183, H186, H194
Hemoglobin A1c (HbA1c)	13 (1,269)	−0.17 [−0.40, 0.06], 66.5	H64–65, H80–81, H84, H105, H130, H151, H158, H183, H186, H194–195

Table 5.5.   (*Continued*)

Outcomes	No. of Studies (Participants)	Effect Size MD [95% CI], I²%	Included Studies
Fasting insulin	12 (705)	SMD 0.14 [−0.32, 0.37], 88.7	H1, H4, H36, H76, H81, H94, H183, H185, H191, H193–195
HOMA-IR	10 (571)	0.12 [−0.50, 0.74], 93.2	H4, H36, H81, H183, H185, H189, H191, H193–195
Total cholesterol	12 (1,239)	−0.189 mmol/L [−0.33, −0.05]*, 45.6	H36, H51, H64, H80, H81, H94, H179, H186, H189, H193–195
Total triglycerides	16 (1,510)	−0.23 mmol/L [−0.35, −0.11]*, 55.2	H1, H36, H51, H54, H64, H80, H81, H94, H151, H179, H183, H186, H189, H193–195
Low density lipoprotein cholesterol	13 (954)	−0.22 mmol/L [−0.33, −0.12]*, 62.7	H1, H36, H51, H54, H64, H80, H151, H185, H186, H189, H193-195
High density lipoprotein cholesterol	11 (814)	0.06 mmol/L [−0.02, 0.14], 76.8	H1, H36, H54, H64, H80, H151, H185–186, H189, H193, H195

Abbreviations: BMI, body mass index; CI, confidence interval; HOMA-IR, Homeostatic Model Assessment of Insulin Resistance; MD, mean difference; WC, waist circumference; WHR, waist–hip ratio.

* Statistically significant, see *Statistical Analysis* methods in Chapter 4.

Chinese Herbal Medicine plus Lifestyle Therapies

CHM administered alongside lifestyle therapies were evaluated in 71 studies (H6, H10–12, H16, H21, H23–24, H28, H32–33, H40, H44, H46–49, H53, H55, H58, H61, H63, H68–69, H71, H77, H83, H96–101, H103, H109, H112, H116, H118–121, H125–127, H131–132, H134–H136, H138, H140–141, H144–145, H155–156, H159, H163, H166–168, H171–172, H174–175, H177, H181–182, H184, H187, H190). Control groups included lifestyle therapies alone, placebo plus lifestyle therapies or drugs plus lifestyle therapies. Lifestyle therapies included diet and exercise programmes, behavioural therapies and health education. Thirty-three studies assessed simple obesity while the other 38 studies evaluated obesity with complications or comorbidities, including pre-diabetes or diabetes (21 studies), metabolic syndrome (8), PCOS (3), hypertension (3), non-alcoholic fatty liver disease (1), hyperlipidaemia (1) and obstructive sleep apnea/hypopnea syndrome (1). The treatment duration ranged from 4 to 36 weeks.

Chinese Herbal Medicine plus Lifestyle Therapies vs. Lifestyle Therapies

Compared to lifestyle therapies, 44 studies (H6, H10–12, H24, H33, H40, H44, H47-49, H53, H58, H61, H63, H68–69, H77, H83, H96, H98, H103, H112, H118–H121, H125, H127, H131–132, H134–H136, H138, H140, H144, H153, H163, H167–168, H177, H184, H187) comprising 2,903 participants assessed CHM combined with lifestyle therapies. More than half of the studies (25 studies) evaluated simple obesity, while the remaining studies (19) assessed obesity with complications or comorbidities, such as diabetes (11), metabolic syndrome (2), hypertension (2), PCOS (1), non-alcoholic fatty liver disease (1), hyperlipidaemia (1) and obstructive sleep apnea/hypopnea syndrome (1). The weight, BMI, WC, WHR, fat mass percentage, and effective rate showed a significant reduction after treatment in the CHM plus lifestyle therapies group compared to the control. Other related metabolic outcomes were also improved in the CHM plus lifestyle therapies groups (Table 5.6).

Chinese Herbal Medicine plus Lifestyle Therapies vs. Placebo plus Lifestyle Therapies

Ten studies (H28, H32, H71, H100, H141, H172, H174–175, H181–182) evaluated 509 participants comparing CHM plus lifestyle therapies to placebo plus lifestyle therapies. Two studies (H32, H181) were not pooled in the analysis due to data not being presented in a

Table 5.6.   Chinese Herbal Medicine plus Lifestyle Therapies *vs.* Lifestyle Therapies

Outcomes	No. of Studies (Participants)	Effect Size MD [95% CI], I²%	Included Studies
Weight	28 (1,936)	−3.68 kg [−4.52, −2.84]*, 42.7	H10, H12, H24, H33, H40, H44, H47–49, H53, H58, H61, H68–69, H77, H83, H96, H103, H120–121, H131, H135–136, H140, H144, H153, H167–168
BMI	40 (2,685)	−1.52 kg/m² [−1.90, −1.14]*, 81.9	H10–12, H24, H33, H40, H44, H47–49, H53, H58, H61, H63, H68–69, H77, H83, H96, H98, H103, H112, H118, H120–121, H125, H127, H131–132, H135, H138, H140, H144, H153, H163, H167–168, H177, H184, H187
WC	21 (1,384)	−3.08 cm [−3.47, −2.68]*, 0	H10, H12, H24, H44, H47–49, H53, H61, H69, H77, H83, H96, H135, H138, H144, H153, H163, H167–168, H184
WHR	18 (1,183)	−0.03[−0.04, −0.02]*, 78.4	H12, H33, H44, H47, H49, H58, H61, H77, H96, H118, H120, H121, H127, H135, H140, H144, H167, H187
Fat mass percentage	8 (694)	−2.07 [−3.46, −0.69]*, 76.6	H12, H47, H61, H68–69, H136, H167, H184
Effective rate‡	6 (380)	RR 1.33 [1.12,1.58]*, 61.3	H40, H58, H96, H119, H132, H136
Fasting blood glucose	22 (1,507)	−0.42 mmol/L [−0.60, −0.24]*, 89.7	H6, H10–12, H44, H48, H53, H58, H61, H69, H83, H98, H118, H125, H127, H134, H138, H144, H153, H163, H167, H168

(Continued)

Table 5.6. (Continued)

Outcomes	No. of Studies (Participants)	Effect Size MD [95% CI], I^2%	Included Studies
Postprandial blood glucose	11 (732)	−1.03 mmol/L [−1.51, −0.56]*, 85.6	H11–12, H48, H69, H98, H118, H125, H127, H134, H144, H153
Hemoglobin A1c (HbA1c)	7 (428)	−0.94 [−1.08, −0.79]*, 0	H44, H48, H118, H125, H127, H134–135
Fasting insulin	13 (1006)	SMD −0.28 [−0.49, −0.07]*, 62.7	H10, H12, H44, H58, H61, H68–69, H118, H125, H144, H153, H167–168
HOMA-IR	7 (448)	−0.46 [−0.80, −0.11]*, 34.4	H12, H58, H68–69, H144, H163, H168
Total cholesterol	29 (1,971)	SMD −0.68 [−0.99, −0.37]*, 90.2	H10–12, H24, H40, H44, H47–49, H53, H58, H69, H83, H96, H118–121, H132, H135–136, H138, H140, H144, H153, H167–168, H177, H187
Total triglycerides	35 (2,324)	SMD −0.89 [−1.18, −0.61]*, 90.2	H6, H10–12, H24, H40, H44, H47–49, H53, H58, H61, H69, H83, H96, H98, H103, H118–121, H125, H132, H135–136, H138, H140, H144, H153, H163, H167–168, H177, H187
Low density lipoprotein cholesterol	26 (1,724)	−0.14 mmol/L [−0.25, −0.03]*, 89.0	H10, H12, H24, H40, H47–49, H53, H58, H69, H83, H96, H103, H118–121, H132, H135, H140, H144, H153, H163, H167–168, H187

Table 5.6. (*Continued*)

Outcomes	No. of Studies (Participants)	Effect Size MD [95% CI], I²%	Included Studies
High density lipoprotein cholesterol	23 (1,561)	0.09 mmol/L [0.04, 0.14]*, 79.2	H6, H10–12, H24, H40, H47–49, H53, H69, H83, H96, H118–120, H135–136, H144, H153, H163, H167–168
Leptin	2 (119)	−1.82 ng/mL [−2.65, −0.98]*, 0	H61, H121

Abbreviations: BMI, body mass index; CI, confidence interval; HOMA-IR, Homeostatic Model Assessment of Insulin Resistance; kg, kilograms; MD, mean difference; RR, risk ratio; SMD, standard mean difference; WC, waist circumference; WHR, waist–hip ratio.
*Statistically significant, see *Statistical Analysis* methods in Chapter 4.
‡Effective rate was based on the 1997 China Obesity Efficacy Criteria.

Table 5.7. **Chinese Herbal Medicine plus Lifestyle Therapies *vs.* Placebo plus Lifestyle Therapies**

Outcomes	No. of Studies (Participants)	Effect Size MD [95% CI], I²%	Included Studies
Weight	3 (144)	2.50 kg [−1.11, 6.10], 0	H71, H172, H174
BMI	7 (407)	−0.84 kg/m² [−1.13, −0.54]*, 0	H28, H71, H100, H141, H172, H174, H175
WC	3 (166)	−2.78 cm [−5.19, −0.37]*, 0	H28, H172, H174
WHR	2 (124)	−0.01 [−0.02, 0.01], 0	H174, H175

Abbreviations: BMI, body mass index; CI, confidence interval; MD, mean difference; WC, waist circumference; WHR, waist–hip ratio.
*Statistically significant, see *Statistical Analysis* methods in Chapter 4.

usable format. The BMI and WC were reduced significantly at the end of the treatment between the intervention group and the control. However, the weight and WHR were not significantly different between the two groups (Table 5.7).

Chinese Herbal Medicine plus Lifestyle Therapies vs. Drugs plus Lifestyle Therapies

Eighteen studies (H16, H21, H23, H46, H55, H97, H99, H101, H109, H116, H126, H145, H156, H159, H166, H171, H187, H190) comprising 1,455 participants compared CHM plus lifestyle therapies to drug therapies plus lifestyle therapies. Drug therapies included orlistat, metformin alone or combined with lovastatin, and other antidiabetic drugs. Among them, two studies (H101, H187) assessed simple obesity and the other 16 studies evaluated obesity with complications or comorbidities such as diabetes (8 studies), metabolic syndrome (6) and PCOS (2). Results from studies that assessed drug therapies for defined comorbidities are presented in the weight-related complications and comorbidities section.

Chinese Herbal Medicine plus Lifestyle Therapies vs. Orlistat plus Lifestyle Therapies

The weight and BMI were reported in two studies (H101, H187), but no significant difference was found after the CHM plus lifestyle therapies were compared to the orlistat and lifestyle therapies. The WC and WHR were reported in one study each, but no significant reductions were observed.

Chinese Herbal Medicine plus Lifestyle Therapies vs. Metformin plus Lifestyle Therapies

Ten studies (H21, H23, H55, H97, H116, H126, H145, H156, H159, H190) compared CHM plus lifestyle therapies to metformin plus lifestyle therapies. There was no significant difference in terms of weight, BMI, WC and WHR after treatment between the groups. Other related metabolic outcomes were also evaluated and are presented in Table 5.8.

Chinese Herbal Medicine plus Drug Therapies

Thirty-four studies (H3, H7, H9, H22, H27, H37, H43, H50, H56–57, H62, H67, H75, H82, H85, H91–93, H104, H113, H115, H128,

Table 5.8. Chinese Herbal Medicine plus Lifestyle Therapies *vs.* Metformin plus Lifestyle Therapies

Outcomes	No. of Studies (Participants)	Effect Size MD [95% CI], I²%	Included Studies
Weight	1 (55)	−1.64 kg [−8.45, 5.17]	H21
BMI	9 (778)	−0.29 kg/m² [−0.67, 0.10], 51.7	H21, H23, H55, H97, H126, H145, H156, H159, H190
WC	3 (153)	−0.51 cm [−1.88, 0.86], 0	H21, H23, H97
WHR	4 (360)	−0.01 [−0.02, 0.01], 53.1	H21, H97, H156, H190
Fasting blood glucose	8 (730)	SMD −0.30 [−0.78, 0.17], 89.2	H21, H23, H55, H97, H116, H126, H145, H190
Postprandial blood glucose	7 (675)	SMD −0.49 [−0.84, −0.15]*, 77.8	H23, H55, H97, H116, H126, H145, H190
Hemoglobin A1c (HbA1c)	5 (557)	−0.56 [−0.90, −0.22]*, 70.5	H55, H97, H116, H145, H190
Fasting insulin	7 (692)	SMD −0.30 [−0.67, 0.08], 82.5	H21, H55, H97, H116, H126, H145, H190
HOMA-IR	3 (175)	−0.15 [−0.24, −0.06]*, 0	H21, H145, H159
Total cholesterol	7 (650)	SMD −0.20 [−0.98, 0.57], 95.2	H21, H23, H55, H97, H145, H159, H190
Total triglycerides	8 (730)	SMD −0.43 [−0.76, −0.09]*, 78.8	H21, H23, H55, H97, H126, H145, H159, H190
Low density lipoprotein cholesterol	8 (730)	SMD −0.41 [−0.77, −0.06]*, 80.8	H21, H23, H55, H97, H126, H145, H159, H190
High density lipoprotein cholesterol	7 (650)	SMD 0.58 [−0.25, 1.41], 95.6	H21, H23, H55, H97, H145, H159, H190

Abbreviations: BMI, body mass index; CI, confidence interval; HOMA-IR, Homeostatic Model Assessment of Insulin Resistance; kg, kilograms; MD, mean difference; SMD, standard mean difference; WC, waist circumference; WHR, waist–hip ratio.
*Statistically significant, see *Statistical Analysis* methods in Chapter 4.

H137, H142, H152, H157, H161–162, H185, H186, H188, H191, H194–195) compared CHM plus drug therapies to drug therapies alone. All of the studies evaluated obesity with complications or comorbidities, including pre-diabetes or diabetes (17 studies), PCOS (12), hypertension (3), metabolic syndrome (1) and non-alcoholic fatty liver disease (1). Drug therapies varied and included anti-diabetic drugs, anti-hypertension drugs as well as lipid regulating medications, depending on particular obesity comorbidities. Metformin alone was used in 20 studies, which was the most common drug among these studies. Results from studies that assessed drugs therapies for defined comorbidities are presented in the weight-related complications and comorbidities section.

Chinese Herbal Medicine plus Metformin vs. Metformin

Twenty studies (H43, H50, H56–57, H62, H67, H75, H82, H93, H104, H115, H128, H137, H142, H161, H185–186, H191, H194–195) comprising 1,559 participants compared CHM plus metformin with metformin alone. Participants had diabetes or PCOS in these studies. The BMI and WC were reduced significantly in the integrative medicine group compared to the control. Significant improvement was also found in terms of glucometabolic parameters, including blood glucose, insulin, etc. However, the weight and WHR did not reduce significantly between the groups at the end of treatment (Table 5.9).

Chinese Herbal Medicine plus Drug Therapies and Lifestyle Therapies

A total of 52 studies (H5, H13–14, H17–H20, H25, H29, H31, H34, H38, H39, H41, H45, H52, H59–60, H66, H70, H72–74, H78–79, H87–90, H102, H106–108, H110–111, H114, H122–124, H129, H139, H143, H147–150, H154–155, H160, H165, H169–170) comprising 3,672 participants compared CHM plus drug and lifestyle therapies to drug and lifestyle therapies. Drug therapies depended on different weight-related complications and comorbidities, such as

Table 5.9.   Chinese Herbal Medicine plus Metformin *vs.* Metformin

Outcomes	No. of Studies (Participants)	Effect Size MD [95% CI], I²%	Included Studies
Weight	3 (240)	−0.58 kg [−3.48, 2.31], 79.4	H82, H115, H142
BMI	17 (1,385)	−0.70 kg/m² [−1.19, −0.22]*, 89.6	H43, H50, H56–57, H62, H67, H82, H104, H115, H128, H137, H142, H161, H185, H191, H194–195
WC	3 (359)	−2.86 cm [−3.62, −2.10]*, 0	H56, H67, H104
WHR	5 (369)	−0.03 [−0.09, 0.02], 91.0	H62, H115, H142, H191, H195
Body fat mass	1 (60)	−0.76 [−1.36, −0.16]*	H142
Fasting blood glucose	17 (1,096)	−0.51 mmol/L [−0.74, −0.29]*, 95.2	H43, H50, H56–57, H62, H67, H75, H82, H93, H128, H142, H161, H185–186, H191, H194–195
Postprandial blood glucose	10 (698)	−1.22 mmol/L [−1.68, −0.76]*, 85.4	H50, H56–57, H62, H67, H82, H93, H128, H186, H194
Hemoglobin A1c (HbA1c)	11 (919)	−0.68 [−1.01, −0.36]*, 91.5	H50, H56–57, H62, H67, H93, H104, H128, H186, H194–195
Fasting insulin	10 (599)	SMD −0.97 [−1.44, −0.50]*, 86	H43, H57, H75, H93, H142, H161, H185, H191, H194, H195
HOMA-IR	8 (495)	−0.52 [−0.83, −0.21]*, 91.1	H43, H57, H142, H161, H185, H191, H194–195
Total cholesterol	12 (820)	−0.50 mmol/L [−0.71, −0.29]*, 80.7	H43, H50, H56–57, H62, H93, H128, H142, H161, H186, H194–195

(*Continued*)

Table 5.9.   (Continued)

Outcomes	No. of Studies (Participants)	Effect Size MD [95% CI], I²%	Included Studies
Total triglycerides	12 (820)	−0.62 mmol/L [−0.92, −0.32]*, 97.1	H43, H50, H56–57, H62, H93, H128, H142, H161, H186, H194–195
Low density lipoprotein cholesterol	7 (445)	−0.49 mmol/L [−0.82, −0.15]*, 89.7	H50, H57, H142, H161, H185–186, H195
High density lipoprotein cholesterol	9 (585)	0.11 mmol/L [−0.01, 0.23], 87.2	H50, H57, H128, H142, H161, H185–186, H194–195
Leptin	2 (180)	SMD −0.48 [−0.77, −0.18]*, 0	H115, H194

Abbreviations: BMI, body mass index; CI, confidence interval; HOMA-IR, Homeostatic Model Assessment of Insulin Resistance; kg, kilograms; MD, mean difference; SMD, standard mean difference; WC, waist circumference; WHR, waist–hip ratio.
*Statistically significant, see *Statistical Analysis* methods in Chapter 4.

anti-diabetic drugs, anti-hypertension drugs, lipid regulating drugs and hormones for PCOS. Only one study (H160) evaluated simple obesity, while the other 51 studies included people with related comorbidities, including pre-diabetes and diabetes (36 studies), PCOS (6), hypertension (6), metabolic syndrome (2) and hyperlipidaemia (1). The treatment duration ranged from 4 to 24 weeks. Metformin was the most common drug therapy, and lifestyle therapies included diet advice, exercise programs, education, etc.

Chinese Herbal Medicine plus Metformin and Lifestyle Therapies vs. Metformin and Lifestyle Therapies

Compared to metformin and lifestyle therapies, the weight, BMI, WC and WHR were reduced significantly in the CHM plus metformin and lifestyle therapies group at the end of the treatment. Glucometabolic parameters and serum lipid parameters were also significantly improved compared to the controls (Table 5.10).

Table 5.10. Chinese Herbal Medicine plus Metformin and Lifestyle Therapies *vs.* Metformin and Lifestyle Therapies

Outcomes	No. of Studies (Participants)	Effect Size MD [95% CI], I^2%	Included Studies
Weight	4 (236)	MD −2.31 kg [−3.67, −0.96]*, 0	H25, H31, H72, H170
BMI	33 (2,295)	−1.02 kg/m² [−1.35, −0.70]*, 86.2	H5, H13–14, H18–19, H25, H31, H34, H38, H45, H52, H59–60, H66, H70, H72–74, H78, H87–88, H102, H106, H108, H110, H122, H129, H139, H154–155, H165, H169–170
WC	8 (450)	−2.66 cm [−3.97, −1.53]*, 65.6	H25, H45, H72, H74, H129, H155, H160, H170
WHR	3 (232)	−0.07 [−0.12, −0.02]*, 89.4	H14, H74, H78
Fasting blood glucose	30 (2,151)	−0.53 mmol/L [−0.70, −0.35]*, 85.4	H5, H13–14, H18–19, H25, H31, H34, H38, H45, H52, H59–60, H70, H72–74, H87, H102, H106, H108, H110, H114, H122, H148, H154–155, H165, H169–170
Postprandial blood glucose	25 (1,853)	−1.63 mmol/L [−2.07, −1.19]*, 92.4	H13–14, H18–19, H25, H34, H38, H45, H52, H59–60, H70, H72, H74, H87–88, H102, H108, H114, H122, H148, H155, H165, H169–170
Hemoglobin A1c (HbA1c)	23 (1,718)	−0.63 [−0.78, −0.47]*, 84.4	H13, H18, H25, H31, H34, H45, H52, H59–60, H72, H74, H87–88,

(*Continued*)

Table 5.10. (*Continued*)

Outcomes	No. of Studies (Participants)	Effect Size MD [95% CI], I²%	Included Studies
			H102, H106, H108, H114, H148, H154–155, H165, H169–170
Fasting insulin	23 (1,630)	SMD −0.83 [−1.12, −0.53]*, 87.5	H5, H18, H25, H31, H34, H38, H45, H52, H59–60, H70, H72, H73, H78, H87–88, H102, H108, H139, H154, H155, H169–170
HOMA-IR	19 (1,243)	−0.77 [−1.06, −0.48]*, 89.4	H18, H25, H31, H34, H45, H52, H59–60, H70, H72–73, H78, H102, H108, H129, H139, H154–155, H170
Total cholesterol	23 (1,515)	−0.47 mmol/L [−0.60, −0.34]*, 72.6	H5, H13, H18, H25, H31, H34, H38, H45, H59, H66, H72, H74, H78, H102, H106, H108, H122, H129, H139, H155, H160, H169–170
Total triglycerides	23 (1,515)	−0.32 mmol/L [−0.41, −0.23]*, 68.8	H5, H13, H18, H25, H31, H34, H38, H45, H59, H66, H72, H74, H78, H102, H106, H108, H122, H129, H139, H155, H160, H169–170
Low density lipoprotein cholesterol	14 (929)	−0.15 mmol/L [−0.23, −0.07]*, 56.1	H13, H18, H25, H31, H45, H59, H66, H72, H102, H106, H108, H129, H169–170

Table 5.10. (*Continued*)

Outcomes	No. of Studies (Participants)	Effect Size MD [95% CI], I²%	Included Studies
High density lipoprotein cholesterol	13 (871)	0.13 mmol/L [0.03, 0.22]*, 86.7	H13, H18, H25, H31, H45, H59, H66, H102, H106, H108, H129, H169–170
Leptin	2 (152)	SMD −0.95 [−1.29, −0.62]*, 0	H18, H78

Abbreviations: BMI, body mass index; CI, confidence interval; HOMA-IR, Homeostatic Model Assessment of Insulin Resistance; kg, kilograms; MD, mean difference; SMD, standard mean difference; WC, waist circumference; WHR, waist–hip ratio.
*Statistically significant, see *Statistical Analysis* methods in Chapter 4.

Weight-related Complications and Comorbidities

Diabetes Mellitus

Diabetes and pre-diabetes appeared to be the most common comorbidity of obesity, including 90 studies (H1, H3, H5, H9–11, H13–14, H17–18, H21, H25, H28–29, H31, H34, H38, H41, H44–45, H48, H50, H52, H54–57, H59–60, H62, H64–67, H72, H74, H78–81, H84–85, H87–88, H91–94, H97–100, H102, H104–105, H108, H110, H114, H116, H118, H122, H124–128, H130, H134, H141–145, H148–149, H151–152, H154–155, H158–159, H163, H165–166, H169–170, H179–180, H186, H194) comprising 7,675 participants. Pre-diabetes refers to impaired glucose tolerance (IGT) or impaired fasting glucose (IFG).

Chinese Herbal Medicine Alone

Fifteen studies (H1, H54, H64, H80–81, H84, H94, H105, H130, H151, H158, H179–180, H186, H194) assessed CHM alone in the intervention group, using metformin as the control. The weight and BMI was reduced significantly in the CHM group compared to the control after treatment, but the WC and WHR were not. In terms of glucometabolic parameters, the postprandial blood glucose, fasting insulin and HOMA-IR, but not fasting blood glucose or HbA1c, were reduced significantly in the CHM group. Lipid metabolic parameters improved after the treatment between the groups except for HDL (Table 5.11).

Table 5.11. Chinese Herbal Medicine *vs.* Metformin

Outcomes	No. of Studies (Participants)	Effect Size MD [95% CI], I^2%	Included Studies
Weight	6 (1,059)	−2.48 kg [−4.77, −0.19]*, 23.1	H64, H65, H94, H158, H179–180
BMI	12 (1,510)	−0.57 kg/m² [−0.93, −0.21]*, 48.2	H1, H54, H64–65, H80–81, H84, H105, H130, H158, H179, H194
WC	3 (753)	−0.67 cm [−2.11, 0.77], 16.2	H64, H158, H179
WHR	3 (173)	−0.01 [−0.05, 0.02], 0	H1, H54, H81
Fasting blood glucose	14 (1,326)	−0.32 [−0.66, 0.02], 72.4	H1, H54, H64–65, H80–81, H84, H94, H105, H130, H151, H158, H186, H194
Postprandial blood glucose	12 (1,213)	−0.45 [−0.79, −0.12]*, 27.5	H64–65, H80–81, H84, H94, H105, H130, H151, H158–186, H194
Hemoglobin A1c (HbA1c)	11 (1,151)	−0.27 [−0.61, 0.07], 68.4	H64–65, H80–81, H84, H105, H130, H151, H158, H186, H194
Fasting insulin	3 (237)	SMD −0.53 [−0.96, −0.09]*, 64.1	H1, H81, H94
HOMA-IR	2 (120)	−0.98 [−1.62, −0.35]*, 45.4	H81, H194
Total cholesterol	7 (798)	−0.22 mmol/L [−0.43, −0.02]*, 47.2	H64, H80–81, H94, H179, H186, H194
Total triglycerides	10 (890)	−0.32 mmol/L [−0.48, −0.17]*, 52.7	H1, H54, H64, H80–81, H94, H151, H179, H186, H194

Table 5.11. (*Continued*)

Outcomes	No. of Studies (Participants)	Effect Size MD [95% CI], I^2%	Included Studies
Low density lipoprotein cholesterol	6 (543)	−0.29 mmol/L [−0.43, −0.14]*, 70.6	H1, H54, H64, H80, H151, H186
High density lipoprotein cholesterol	7 (603)	0.09 mmol/L [−0.02, 0.20], 87.3	H1, H54, H64, H80, H151, H186, H194

Abbreviations: BMI, body mass index; CI, confidence interval; HOMA-IR, Homeostatic Model Assessment of Insulin Resistance; kg, kilograms; MD, mean difference; SMD, standard mean difference; WC, waist circumference; WHR, waist–hip ratio.
*Statistically significant, see *Statistical Analysis* methods in Chapter 4.

Chinese Herbal Medicine plus Lifestyle Therapies

In total, 23 studies (H10, H11, H21, H28, H44, H48, H55, H97–100, H116, H118, H125–127, H134, H141, H144, H145, H159, H163, H166) evaluated CHM plus lifestyle therapies in the intervention group. Comparators were lifestyle therapies, a placebo plus lifestyle therapies or anti-diabetic drugs plus lifestyle therapies. In total, 681 obese people with pre-diabetes or diabetes received CHM combined with lifestyle therapies in the intervention group, using lifestyle therapies as a control in 11 studies (H10, H11, H44, H48, H98, H118, H125, H127, H134, H144, H163). The BMI, WC and glucometabolic parameters, such as fasting blood glucose, postprandial blood glucose and HbA1c, were significantly improved in the CHM group compared to the control:

- BMI: MD −1.33 kg/m² [95% CI −1.74, −0.92], I^2 = 38.9%, 10 studies, 643 participants.
- WC: MD −2.23 cm [95% CI −4.29, −0.17], I^2 = 0, 5 studies, 278 participants.
- Fasting blood glucose: MD −0.65 mmol/L [95% CI −0.90, −0.40], I^2 = 88.8%, 10 studies, 624 participants.
- Postprandial blood glucose: MD −1.26 mmol/L [95% CI −1.81, −0.72], I^2 = 88.5%, 8 studies, 523 participants.

- HbA1c: MD −0.94 [−1.08, −0.79], I^2 = 0, 6 studies, 355 participants.
- There was no significant difference in terms of weight, WHR, fasting insulin and HOMA-IR.

Compared to the placebo plus lifestyle therapies, there was a similar improvement in the BMI, fasting blood glucose, postprandial blood glucose and HbA1c in three studies (H28, H100, H141) comprising 206 participants:

- BMI: MD −0.93 kg/m^2 [95% CI −1.37, −0.50], I^2 = 23.9%.
- Fasting blood glucose: MD −0.66 mmol/L [95% CI −0.97, −0.34], I^2 = 43.9%.
- Postprandial blood glucose: MD −0.84 mmol/L [95% CI −1.17, −0.51], I^2 = 31.0%.
- HbA1c: MD −0.37 [95% CI −0.60, −0.14], I^2 = 49.1%.
- WC also was reduced significantly but only in one study (H28) with 60 participants (MD −4.24 mmol/L [95% CI −7.71, −0.77]).

Nine studies (H21, H55, H97, H99, H116, H126, H145, H159, H166) comprising 691 participants assessed CHM plus anti-diabetic drugs plus lifestyle therapies. In these studies, seven of them (H21, H55, H97, H116, H126, H145, H159) used metformin and the other two (H99, H166) used acarbose and repaglinide, respectively. The WHR, postprandial blood glucose and HOMA-IR improved after the treatment between the two groups:

- WHR: MD −0.02 [95% CI −0.03, −0.01], I^2 = 0, 2 studies, 115 participants.
- Postprandial blood glucose: MD −0.57 mmol/L [95% CI −1.12, −0.01], I^2 = 80.6%, 6 studies, 516 participants.
- HOMA-IR: MD −0.15 [95% CI −0.24, −0.06], I^2 = 0, 3 studies, 175 participants.
- There was no significant difference in terms of the BMI, weight, WC and other related parameters, including fasting blood glucose, fasting insulin or HbA1c.

Chinese Herbal Medicine plus Anti-Diabetic Drug Therapies

Seventeen studies (H3, H9, H50, H56, H57, H62, H67, H85, H91–93, H104, H128, H142, H152, H186, H194) comprising 1,764 participants compared CHM plus anti-diabetic drugs to anti-diabetic drugs. Anti-diabetic drugs included metformin, liraglutide, insulin, acarbose, repaglinide and gliclazide, used alone or in combination. The weight, BMI, WC, WHR, body fat mass as well as glucometabolic parameters all improved significantly in the integrative medicine group compared to the control (Table 5.12).

Table 5.12. Chinese Herbal Medicine plus Anti-diabetic Drugs *vs.* Anti-diabetic Drugs

Outcomes	No. of Studies (Participants)	Effect Size MD [95% CI], I^2%	Included Studies
Weight	2 (146)	−2.34 kg [−4.58, −0.09]*, 38.7	H142, H152
BMI	15 (1,634)	−1.30 kg/m² [−1.71, −0.88]*, 87.9	H3, H9, H50, H56–57, H62, H67, H85, H91–92, H104, H128, H142, H152, H194
WC	4 (448)	−1.96 cm [−3.63, −0.29]*, 56.2	H56, H67, H85, H104
WHR	3 (389)	−0.06 [−0.10, −0.02]*, 82.1	H62, H92, H142
Body fat mass	1 (60)	−0.76 [−1.36, −0.16]*	H142
Fasting blood glucose	16 (1,541)	−0.73 mmol/L [−0.98, −0.49]*, 93.6	H3, H9, H50, H56–57, H62, H67, H85, H91–93, H128, H142, H152, H186, H194
Postprandial blood glucose	15 (1,481)	−1.18 mmol/L [−1.52, −0.84]*, 85.0	H3, H9, H50, H56–57, H62, H67, H85, H91–93, H128, H152, H186, H194
Hemoglobin A1c (HbA1c)	15 (1,550)	−0.60 [−0.80, −0.41]*, 83.3	H3, H50, H56–57, H62, H67, H85, H91–93, H104, H128, H152, H186, H194

(*Continued*)

Table 5.12. (*Continued*)

Outcomes	No. of Studies (Participants)	Effect Size MD [95% CI], I²%	Included Studies
Fasting insulin	4 (261)	SMD −1.41 [−2.53, −0.30]*, 93.6	H57, H93, H142, H194
HOMA-IR	4 (287)	−1.16 [−2.14, −0.18]*, 99.1	H57, H142, H152, H194

Abbreviations: CI, confidence interval; MD, mean difference; SMD, standard mean difference; BMI, body mass index; HOMA-IR, Homeostatic Model Assessment of Insulin Resistance; kg, kilograms; WC, waist circumference; WHR, waist–hip ratio.
*Statistically significant, see *Statistical Analysis* methods in Chapter 4.

Chinese Herbal Medicine plus Anti-Diabetic Drugs and Lifestyle Therapies

A total of 36 studies (H5, H13–14, H17–18, H25, H29, H31, H34, H38, H41, H45, H52, H59–60, H66, H72, H74, H78–79, H87–88, H102, H108, H110, H114, H122, H124, H143, H148–149, H154–155, H165, H169–170) comprising 2,661 participants compared CHM plus anti-diabetic drugs and lifestyle therapies to anti-diabetic drugs and lifestyle therapies. Anti-diabetic drugs included metformin, insulin, acarbose, glimepiride, repaglinide and sitagliptin, used alone or in combination. The treatment duration varied from 45 days to 24 weeks. The weight, BMI, WC, WHR and related glucometabolic outcomes were reduced significantly in the integrative medicine group compared to the control (Table 5.13).

Polycystic Ovarian Syndrome

In total, 26 RCTs (H4, H15, H19, H22, H30, H36, H39, H43, H70, H73, H75–76, H112, H115, H129, H137, H139, H156, H161–162, H185, H188–189, H191, H193, H195) evaluated obesity complicated with PCOS, including 16 two-arm studies, 7 three-arm studies and 1 four-arm study. The treatment duration ranged from two to six months.

CHM alone was evaluated in 11 studies (H4, H15, H30, H36, H76, H185, H188–189, H191, H193, H195) compared to no

Table 5.13.   Chinese Herbal Medicine plus Drug and Lifestyle Therapies *vs.* Drug and Lifestyle Therapies

Outcomes	No. of Studies (Participants)	Effect Size MD [95% CI], I²%	Included Studies
Weight	8 (493)	−3.35 kg [−5.05, −1.66]*, 50.7	H17, H25, H29, H31, H72, H143, H149, H170
BMI	34 (2,454)	−1.09 kg/m² [−1.43, −0.76]*, 88.0	H5, H13–14, H17–18, H25, H29, H31, H34, H38, H41, H45, H52, H59–60, H66, H72, H74, H78–79, H87–88, H102, H108, H110, H122, H124, H143, H149, H154–155, H165, H169–170
WC	9 (553)	−2.08 cm [−2.95, −1.21]*, 28.5	H17, H25, H29, H45, H72, H74, H149, H155, H170
WHR	6 (361)	−0.07 [−0.11, −0.02]*, 91.1	H14, H17, H29, H74, H78–79
Fasting blood glucose	32 (2,133)	−0.69 mmol/L [−0.90, −0.48]*, 90.7	H5, H13–14, H17–18, H25, H29, H31, H34, H38, H41, H45, H52, H59–60, H72, H74, H87, H102, H108, H110, H114, H122, H124, H143, H148–149, H154–155, H165, H169–170
Postprandial blood glucose	29 (2,009)	−1.49 mmol/L [−1.82, −1.17]*, 90.7	H13–14, H17–18, H25, H29, H34, H38, H41, H45, H52, H59–60, H72, H74, H79, H87–88, H102, H108, H114, H122, H124, H143, H148, H155, H165, H169–170

(*Continued*)

Table 5.13. (*Continued*)

Outcomes	No. of Studies (Participants)	Effect Size MD [95% CI], I²%	Included Studies
Hemoglobin A1c (HbA1c)	27 (1,907)	−0.71 [−0.88, −0.53]*, 91.5	H13, H17–18, H25, H29, H31, H34, H41, H45, H52, H59–60, H72, H74, H87–88, H102, H108, H114, H143, H148–149, H154–155, H165, H169–170
Fasting insulin	24 (1675)	SMD −0.98 [−1.29, −0.67]*, 89.2	H5, H17–18, H25, H29, H31, H34, H38, H45, H52, H59–60, H72, H78, H87–88, H102, H108, H143, H149, H154–155, H169–170
HOMA-IR	17 (1186)	−0.76 [−0.99, −0.52]*, 91.7	H18, H25, H29, H31, H34, H45, H52, H59–60, H72, H78, H102, H108, H124, H154–155, H170

Abbreviations: BMI, body mass index; CI, confidence interval; HOMA-IR, Homeostatic Model Assessment of Insulin Resistance; kg, kilograms; MD, mean difference; SMD, standard mean difference; WC, waist circumference; WHR, waist–hip ratio.
*Statistically significant, see *Statistical Analysis* methods in Chapter 4.

treatment, or metformin alone, or metformin alongside lifestyle therapies or ethinylestradiol cyproterone (anti-androgen and pro-gestin medication). Compared to no treatment in one study (H195), the WHR, fasting insulin and HOMA-IR, but not the BMI or fasting blood glucose, were reduced significantly in the CHM group (WHR: MD −0.17 [95% CI −0.20, −0.14]; fasting insulin: MD −11.45 [95% CI −18.70, −4.2]; HOMA-IR: MD −2.57 [95% CI −4.39, −0.75], 55 participants). Compared to metformin alone (H4, H30, H36, H76, H185, H189, H191, H193, H195), metformin alongside lifestyle therapies (H15) or ethinylestradiol cyproterone (H188), the BMI, WHR, as well as metabolic parameters were not significantly improved in the CHM group compared to the control after the treatment.

Two studies (H112, H156) assessed CHM plus lifestyle therapies in the intervention group compared to lifestyle therapies. The BMI was significantly reduced in the intervention group after the treatment but only in one study (MD -2.49 kg/m^2 [95% CI -3.96, -1.02], H112). However, when compared to metformin combined with lifestyle therapies, neither the BMI nor WHR showed a significant difference between the groups at the end of the treatment.

Participants received CHM plus metformin alone, ethinylestradiol cyproterone alone or two drugs in combination in 11 studies (H22, H43, H75, H115, H137, H161–162, H185, H188, H191, H195). Compared to metformin alone, fasting insulin and HOMA-IR were reduced significantly in the CHM plus metformin group (SMD -0.71 [95% CI -1.06, -0.36], $I^2 = 57.9\%$, 6 studies, 338 participants, and MD -0.49 [95% CI -0.67, -0.31], $I^2 = 0$, 5 studies, 294 participants, respectively). However, the weight, BMI, WHR and other related parameters were not significantly improved in the CHM plus metformin group. Two studies (H22, H188) used metformin combined with ethinylestradiol and cyproterone acetate as the control. The BMI, HOMA-IR, luteinising hormone and follicle-stimulating hormone ratio (LH/FSH) and androgen levels were reported in one of the studies, and all outcomes were improved significantly after CHM plus metformin treatment compared to the control (BMI: MD -0.59 kg/m^2 [95% CI -0.79, -0.39]; HOMA-IR: MD -0.42 [95% CI -0.74, -0.1]; LH/FSH: MD -0.38 [95% CI -0.52, -0.24]; androgen: MD -0.09 ng/mL [95% CI -0.18, -0.01], H188). In another study (H22), the BMI and WHR were reduced significantly in the CHM plus the metformin and ethinylestradiol cyproterone group, but HOMA-IR and androgen levels were not (MD -3.37 kg/m^2 [95% CI -4.22, -2.52] and MD -0.04 [95% CI -0.06, -0.02], respectively). Compared to ethinylestradiol and cyproterone acetate alone, the WHR, fasting insulin and androgen levels were significantly improved after CHM plus ethinylestradiol and cyproterone acetate treatment in one study (H162) (WHR: MD -0.07 [95% CI -0.09, -0.05]; fasting insulin: MD −2.80 mIU/L [95% CI −5.49, −0.11]; androgen: MD −7.73 ng/dL [95% CI −13.92, −1.54]). However, there was no difference in terms of the BMI or the LH/FSH ratio.

Six studies (H19, H39, H70, H73, H129, H139) compared CHM plus drug and lifestyle therapies to drug and lifestyle therapies. The BMI and HOMA-IR were reduced significantly in the CHM plus metformin and lifestyle therapies group compared to metformin and lifestyle therapies in women with PCOS (MD −1.64 kg/m^2 [95% CI −2.17, −1.12], I^2 = 0, 5 studies, 261 participants and MD −0.47 [95% CI −0.81, −0.13], I^2 = 0, 4 studies, 204 participants, respectively). The WC was also significantly reduced in the intervention group compared to the control in one study (H129) of 54 participants (MD −3.31 cm [95% CI −6.29, −0.33]). Another study (H39) compared CHM combined with ethinylestradiol and cyproterone acetate and lifestyle therapies to ethinylestradiol and cyproterone acetate plus lifestyle therapies. The BMI and hormone levels, including LH/FSH ratio and androgen levels, were not significantly different between the groups at the end of the treatment.

Metabolic Syndrome

Fifteen RCTs (H6, H16, H20, H23, H35, H46, H106, H109, H113, H133, H135, H164, H171, H183, H190) assessed people with obesity and metabolic syndrome. Four studies (H35, H133, H164, H183) assessed CHM alone in the intervention group, compared to placebo or anti-diabetic drugs (metformin or rosiglitazone). There was no significant difference in terms of BMI, fasting blood glucose and total triglycerides when compared to the placebo group or to the anti-diabetic drugs group. When comparing CHM plus routine metabolic treatments to routine metabolic treatments alone in two studies (H6, H135) with 113 participants, no significant difference was found in terms of metabolic or lipid outcomes.

CHM plus routine metabolic treatments were compared to anti-metabolic disorder drugs and routine metabolic treatments in six studies (H16, H23, H46, H109, H171, H190) comprising 466 participants.

Among them, two studies (H23, H190) evaluated metformin alone, one (H16) used metformin combined with lovastatin and three (H46, H109, H171) assessed thiazolidinediones (TZDs) type drugs. The BMI, WC, blood glucose, insulin and blood pressure were reduced significantly at the end of the treatment between the groups:

- BMI: MD −0.82 kg/m^2 [95% CI −1.47, −0.17], I^2 = 64.9%, 6 studies, 424 participants.
- WC: MD −2.90 cm [95% CI −4.66, −1.14], I^2 = 0, 4 studies, 227 participants.
- Postprandial blood glucose: SMD −0.64 [95% CI −0.91, −0.37], I^2 = 21.3%, 4 studies, 300 participants.
- Fasting insulin: SMD −0.20 [95% CI −0.40, −0.00, I^2 = 0, 5 studies, 386 participants.
- Systolic blood pressure: MD −5.92 mmHg [95% CI −9.00, −2.83], I^2 = 47.9%, 5 studies, 317 participants.
- Diasolic blood pressure: MD −3.09 mmHg [95% CI −4.96, −1.21], I^2 = 36.4%, 5 studies, 317 participants.
- There was no significant difference in terms of weight, WHR or serum lipid levels.

Three studies (H20, H106, H113) compared CHM plus anti-metabolic drugs and routine therapies to anti-metabolic drugs and routine therapies alone. One study (H106) reported BMI, blood glucose and serum lipid parameters and compared CHM plus metformin and metabolic routine therapies to metformin and metabolic routine therapies. No significant difference was found between the two groups. Another study (H20) compared CHM plus anti-metabolic drugs, including metformin, perindopril and fenofibrate, plus routine therapies to the drugs and routine therapies. Lipids and blood pressure were significantly reduced in the intervention group compared to the control (LDL: MD −0.45 mmol/L [95% CI −0.75, −0.15]; HDL: MD 0.37 mmol/L [95% CI 0.24, 0.50]; systolic blood pressure: MD −9.83 mmHg [95% CI −11.67, −7.99]; diastolic blood pressure: MD −8.13 mmHg [95% CI −9.25, −7.01]). However, there was no significant difference in terms of weight, BMI, WC or glucometabolic parameters. Compared to irbesartan hydrochlorothiazide and atorvastatin plus routine treatment in one study (H113), the WC and blood pressure were reduced significantly in the integrative medicine group. However, lipids did not differ between the groups (WC: MD −3.53 cm [95% CI −6.34, −0.72]; systolic blood pressure: MD −7.33 mmHg [95% CI −10.80, −3.86]; diastolic blood pressure: MD −7.73 mmHg [95% CI −9.47, −5.99]).

Hypertension

People with obesity and hypertension were assessed in 12 studies (H7, H27, H89–90, H107, H111, H147, H150, H157, H159, H168, H177). Compared to hypertension routine therapies, the BMI did not significantly reduce in the CHM plus routine therapies group in two studies (H168, H177) comprising 168 participants. Blood pressure was reported in one of the studies (H168), where only the systolic blood pressure was significantly reduced in the intervention group (MD −7.38 mmHg [95% CI −14.20, −0.56]).

Compared to anti-hypertensive drug therapies, in which angiotensin receptor blockers were used as a control in the two groups (H7, H157), the BMI and blood pressure were significantly reduced in the CHM plus anti-hypertensive drug therapies groups compared to the control, as were serum lipid levels:

- BMI: MD −2.26 kg/m^2 [95% CI −2.84, −1.67], I^2 = 45.7%.
- Systolic blood pressure: MD −7.15 mmHg [95% CI −9.31, −4.99], I^2 = 0.
- Diastolic blood pressure: MD −4.73 mmHg [95% CI −6.38, −3.09], I^2 = 0.
- Total cholesterol: MD −0.48 mmol/L [95% CI −0.92, −0.05], I^2 = 84.0%.
- Total triglycerides: MD −0.51 mmol/L [95% CI −0.76, −0.26], I^2 = 50.1%.

Compared to nitrendipine plus fenofibrate, the BMI, blood pressure and serum lipid levels were significantly improved in the CHM plus nitrendipine group in one study (H27) assessing 60 participants:

- BMI: MD −1.01kg/m² [95% CI −1.49, −0.53].
- Systolic blood pressure: MD −2.00 mmHg [95% CI −5.31, −1.31].
- Diastolic blood pressure: MD −4.00 mmHg [95% CI −6.43, −1.57].
- Total cholesterol: MD −0.81 mmol/L [95% CI −1.26, −0.36].
- Total triglycerides: MD −0.97 mmol/L [95% CI −1.39, −0.55].

Six studies (H89–90, H107, H111, H147, H150) compared CHM plus anti-hypertension drugs and hypertension routine therapies to anti-hypertension drugs and hypertension routine therapies alone. There was a significant improvement in the intervention group in terms of the BMI, WC, blood pressure and serum lipid level, but no difference in terms of weight and WHR:

- BMI: MD −1.40 kg/m² [95% CI −2.19, −0.61], I² = 8.8%, 6 studies, 430 participants.
- WC: MD −1.87 cm [95% CI −2.68, −1.07], I² = 0, 2 studies, 140 participants.
- Systolic blood pressure: MD −7.30 mmHg [95% CI −9.64, −4.96], I² = 54.9%, 6 studies, 430 participants.
- Diastolic blood pressure: MD −5.47 mmHg [95% CI −8.97, −1.98], I² = 91.1%, 6 studies, 430 participants.

Another study (H159) compared CHM plus hypertension routine therapies to metformin and hypertension routine therapies. The BMI, systolic blood pressure and serum lipid levels were significantly improved in the CHM plus hypertension routine therapies group after eight weeks of the treatment, but the diastolic blood pressure was not significantly reduced:

- BMI: MD −0.91 kg/m² [95% CI −1.71, −0.11].
- Systolic blood pressure: MD −3.10 mmHg [95% CI −5.77, −0.43].
- Diastolic blood pressure: MD −0.94 mmHg [95% CI −2.78, 0.90].
- Total cholesterol: MD −0.58 mmol/L [95% CI −1.15, −0.01].
- Total triglycerides: MD −0.52 mmol/L [95% CI −0.86, −0.18].

Hyperlipidaemia

Three studies (H103, H123, H192) evaluated people with obesity and hyperlipidaemia. One study (H192) compared CHM to no treatment or simvastatin. Compared to no treatment, the BMI and serum lipid level were significantly reduced in the CHM group (BMI: MD −2.36 kg/m² [95% CI −4.02, −0.71]; total cholesterol: MD −3.37 mmol/L [95% CI −3.72, −3.02]; total triglycerides: MD −2.66 mmol/L [95% CI −3.42, −1.90]). However, when compared to simvastatin, only the BMI was significantly reduced after CHM treatment (MD −3.10 kg/m² [95% CI −4.79, −1.41]).

Another study (H103) using lifestyle therapies as the control showed a significant reduction in weight, BMI and lipid levels (weight: MD −5.00 kg [95% CI −7.97, −2.03]; BMI: MD −3.42 kg/m² [95% CI −3.94, −2.90]; total triglycerides: MD −1.32 mmol/L [95% CI −1.61, −1.03]). One study (H123) compared CHM plus simvastatin and lifestyle therapies to simvastatin and lifestyle therapies. The BMI and cholesterol were reduced but not the total triglycerides in the intervention group compared to the control in 80 participants (BMI: MD −2.09 kg/m² [95% CI −2.64, −1.54]; total cholesterol: MD −0.31 mmol/L [95% CI −0.60, −0.02]; total triglycerides: MD −0.07 mmol/L [95% CI −0.28, 0.14]).

Randomised Controlled Trial Evidence for Individual Formulae

A total of 149 distinct formulae (130 named and 19 unnamed) were reported in 195 RCTs. Evidence for the most common individual formulae (Table 5.1) used in three or more studies is separately analysed. Largely, these formulae overlap with those recommended in Chapter 2, that is, the commonly recommended herbal formulae in clinical practice guidelines. Some formulae such as *Xiao cheng qi tang*, *Bao he wan*, *Fang ji huang qi tang*, *Zhen wu tang* and *Xiao yao san* were not assessed in multiple RCTs. This is not surprising as these formulae are used for specific syndromes and are established traditional treatments. Furthermore, although many of the treatments assessed in the clinical trials did not specifically mention these formulae by name, the herbal ingredients were similar.

Wu ling san

Wu ling san 五苓散 was evaluated in eight studies (H14, H20, H24, H30, H41, H83, H92, H123). Standard *Wu ling san* contains the herbs *ze xie*, *zhu ling*, *fu ling*, *bai zhu* and *gui zhi*. One study (H30) compared a modified version of *Wu ling san* with metformin for women with obesity and PCOS. The BMI was reported, but there was no significant difference found between the groups after three months of the treatment. Two studies (H24, H83) administered *Wu ling san* plus diet and exercise therapies compared to diet and exercise. The BMI was significantly reduced in the *Wu ling san* group compared to the control (MD -2.10 kg/m^2 [95% CI -3.97, -0.23], I^2 = 51.1%). However, the weight and WC were not significantly different between groups.

One study (H92) compared modified *Wu ling san* plus repaglinide to repaglinide alone for obese people with diabetes. Both the BMI and WHR were significantly improved in the intervention group after the treatment (MD -1.35 kg/m^2 [95% CI -1.74, -0.96] and MD -0.06 [95% CI -0.09, -0.03], respectively). A similar result was reported when modified *Wu ling san* plus anti-diabetic drugs plus diabetes routine therapies were compared to anti-diabetic drugs plus diabetes routine therapies (BMI: MD -3.88 kg/m^2 [95% CI -4.63, -3.14], I^2 = 0, H14, H41, and WHR: MD -0.09 [95% CI -0.12, -0.06], H14). The BMI was also significantly reduced in the modified *Wu ling san* plus simvastatin and lifestyle therapies group for obese people with hyperlipidaemia compared to simvastatin and lifestyle therapies as the control (MD −2.09 kg/m² [95% CI −2.64, −1.54]) (H123). In another study (H20), there was no significant difference in terms of weight, BMI or WC for obese participants with metabolic syndrome when *Wu ling san* plus drug and lifestyle therapies were compared to drug and lifestyle therapies.

Huang lian jie du tang

Huang lian jie du tang 黄连解毒汤 was assessed in six studies (H59, H84, H105, H130, H145, H151). The formula contains *huang lian, huang qin, huang bai* and *zhi zi*. All of the studies were conducted in obese people with pre-diabetes or diabetes, using metformin alone or metformin alongside diabetes routine therapies as the control. The BMI was reported in five of the studies, but no significant difference was found between the *Huang lian jie du tang* group and the integrative medicine group. Weight, WC, WHR and fat mass percentage were not reported in these studies.

Pei lian ma huang fang

Pei lian ma huang fang 佩连麻黄方, containing *pei lan, huang lian* and *ma huang* was assessed in four studies (H58, H72, H140, H187). The weight, BMI and WHR were significantly reduced in the *Pei lian ma huang fang* plus lifestyle therapies group, compared to lifestyle therapies alone (weight: MD −4.71 kg [95% CI −8.04, −1.38], I² = 0 (H58, H140); BMI: MD −1.62 kg/m² [95% CI −2.23, −1.01], I² = 0 (H58, H140, H187); WHR: MD −0.04 [95% CI −0.05, −0.03], I² = 0 (H58, H140, H187)). However, none of the outcomes were significantly improved in the *Pei lian ma huang fang* plus lifestyle therapies group when compared to orlistat plus lifestyle therapies (H187). Another study (H72) compared *Pei lian ma huang fang* plus metformin and lifestyle therapies to metformin plus lifestyle therapies. Significant differences were found between the groups in weight, BMI and WC (weight: MD −2.80 kg [95% CI −5.27, −0.33]; BMI: MD −1.04 kg/m² [95% CI −1.57, −0.51]; WC: MD −1.22 cm [95% CI −2.36, −0.06]).

Shen ling bai zhu san

Shen ling bai zhu san 参苓白术散 was assessed in four studies (H3, H82, H127, H142), including obese people with pre-diabetes or diabetes. Key herbal ingredients included *lian zi, yi yi ren, sha ren, jie geng, bai bian dou, fu ling, ren shen, gan cao, bai zhu* and *shan yao*. The BMI and WHR were reduced significantly in the *Shen ling bai zhu san* plus diabetes routine therapies group, compared to diabetes routine therapies (MD -1.40 kg/m^2 [95% CI -2.21, -0.59] and MD -0.20 [95% CI -0.31, -0.09], respectively) (H127). However, when *Shen ling bai zhu san* plus anti-diabetic drugs were compared to anti-diabetic drugs alone, there was no significant difference in weight, BMI or WHR between the groups. The body fat mass percentage was reduced significantly in the integrative group but was only reported in one study (H142) (MD -0.76% [95% CI -1.36, -0.16]).

Ling gui zhu gan tang

Four studies (H40, H67, H111, H131) assessed *Ling gui zhu gan tang* 苓桂术甘汤 (*fu ling, gui zhi, bai zhu, gan cao*) in the intervention group. Among them, two studies (H40, H131) compared *Ling gui zhu gan tang* plus diet and exercise therapies to diet and exercise therapies alone. The weight but not BMI was significantly reduced in the integrative group (MD -3.77 kg [95% CI -5.88, -1.65], $I^2 = 0$). Both the BMI and WC were significantly reduced when *Ling gui zhu gan tang* plus metformin was compared to metformin alone in one study (H67) (MD -1.11 kg/m^2 [95% CI -1.39, -0.83] and MD -3.10 cm [95% CI -6.07, -0.13], respectively). There was also a significant difference in the BMI between *Ling gui zhu gan tang* plus anti-hypertension drugs and lifestyle therapies compared to the control in obese people with hypertension (MD -3.38 kg/m^2 [95% CI -4.22, -2.55]) (H111).

Jue ming zi cha

Jue ming zi cha 决明子茶, including *jue ming zi, shan zha* and *ju hua*, was evaluated in three studies (H49, H77, H135). *Jue ming zi cha* plus exercise therapy significantly reduced the weight, BMI, WC and WHR, compared to exercise therapy alone (weight: MD −4.85 kg [95% CI −9.47, −0.24], I^2 = 85.7%; BMI: MD −2.19 kg/m^2 [95% CI −3.64, −0.74], I^2 = 94.4%; WC: MD −3.46 cm [95% CI −3.99, −2.94], I^2 = 0; WHR: MD −0.03 [95% CI −0.05, −0.02], I^2 = 87.8%).

Dao tan tang

Three studies (H115, H125, H193) assessed *Dao tan tang* 导痰汤, including *ban xia, tian nan xing, zhi shi, chen pi* and *fu ling.* Two studies used metformin as the control. Among these two studies, there was a significant difference in weight and BMI but not the WHR in the *Dao tan tang* plus metformin group when compared to metformin (weight: MD −2.73 kg [95% CI −4.79, −0.67]); BMI: MD −1.25 kg/m^2 [95% CI −1.87, −0.63]) (H115). However, there was no significant difference in the BMI when *Dao tan tang* was compared to metformin (H193). Another study (H125) compared *Dao tan tang* plus lifestyle therapies to lifestyle therapies. At the end of the treatment, the BMI was reduced significantly in the intervention group (MD: −1.35 kg/m^2 [95% CI −2.11, −0.59]).

Shan zha xiao zhi jiao capsule

Shan zha xiao zhi jiao capsules 山楂消脂胶囊, containing *shan zha, da huang* and *gan cao* were assessed in three studies (H12, H68, H69) in participants with simple obesity and a BMI over 28 kg/m^2. *Shan zha xiao zhi jiao* capsules plus lifestyle therapies were not better than lifestyle therapies alone in terms of weight, BMI, WC, WHR or body fat mass in these studies.

Fang feng tong sheng san/wan

Three studies (H121, H122, H177) assessed *Fang feng tong sheng san/wan* 防风通圣散/丸. Formula ingredients included *fang feng, chuan xiong, dang gui, shao yao, da huang, bo he, ma huang, lian qiao, mang xiao, shi gao, huang qin, jie geng, hua shi, gan cao, jing jie, bai zhu* and *zhi zi.* Two studies (H121, H177) compared *Fang feng tong sheng san/wan* plus lifestyle therapies to lifestyle therapies alone. The BMI was not significantly reduced between the intervention and control groups. The weight and WHR reduced significantly in the integrative medicine groups but was only reported in one study (H121) (MD −4.53 kg [95% CI −8.51, −0.55] and MD −0.06 [95% CI −0.08, −0.04], respectively). There was a significant difference in the BMI after the treatment in another study (H122) that compared *Fang feng tong sheng san/wan* plus metformin and lifestyle therapies to metformin and lifestyle therapies (MD −0.86 kg/m^2 [95% CI −1.63, −0.09]).

Huang lian wen dan tang

Huang lian wen dan tang 黄连温胆汤 was assessed in three studies (H45, H97, H98) in obese participants with pre-diabetes or diabetes. Herbal ingredients included *huang lian, sheng jiang, ban xia, chen pi, zhu ru, zhi shi* and *gan cao.* Two studies (H45, H97) used metformin plus diabetes routine therapies as the control. Among them, the BMI and WHR, but not the WC, were significantly reduced in the *Huang lian wen dan tang* plus diabetes routine therapies group in one study (MD −0.81 kg/m^2 [95% CI −1.38, −0.24] and MD −0.02 [95% CI −0.03, −0.01], respectively). The BMI and WC were also improved in the *Huang lian wen dan tang* plus metformin and diabetes routine therapies group (MD −1.51 kg/m^2 [95% CI −2.19, −0.83] and MD −3.90 cm [95% CI −7.38, −0.42], respectively). Another study (H98) compared *Huang lian wen dan tang* plus lifestyle therapies to lifestyle therapies, and the BMI was significantly reduced in the intervention group compared to the control (MD −1.50 kg/m^2 [95% CI −2.48, −0.52]).

Assessment using GRADE

An assessment of the strength and quality (certainty) of the evidence from RCTs was made using GRADE. Interventions, comparators and outcomes were selected based on a consensus process, described in

Chapter 4. Outcomes included weight, BMI and WC. Three GRADE tables were produced:

- Table 5.14: CHM *vs.* placebo.
- Table 5.15: CHM plus lifestyle therapies *vs.* placebo plus lifestyle therapies.
- Table 5.16: CHM plus lifestyle therapies *vs.* lifestyle therapies.

Table 5.14.   GRADE: Chinese Herbal Medicine *vs.* Placebo

Outcome	Absolute Effect		Relative Effect (95% CI) No. of Participants & Studies	Certainty of the Evidence GRADE
	With CHM	Without CHM		
Weight Treatment duration: range 45 days to 12 weeks	**75.34** Average difference: 0.57 kg lower (95% CI: 2.59 lower to 1.45 higher)	**75.91**	**MD −0.57** (−2.59, 1.45) Based on data from 412 patients in 5 studies	⊕⊕⊡⊡ LOW[1,2]
Body mass index (BMI) Treatment duration: range 45 days to 12 weeks	**27.35** Average difference: 0.34 kg/m² higher (95% CI: 0.74 lower to 0.07 higher)	**27.01**	**MD 0.34** (−0.74, 0.07) Based on data from 587 patients in 8 studies	⊕⊕⊡⊡ LOW[1,2]
Waist circumference Treatment duration: range 45 days to 12 weeks	**90.37** Average difference: 1.75 cm higher (95% CI: 3.57 lower to 0.07 higher)	**88.62**	**MD 1.75** (−3.57, 0.07) Based on data from 316 patients in 4 studies	⊕⊕⊡⊡ LOW[1,2]

Abbreviations: BMI, body mass index; CI, confidence interval; CHM, Chinese herbal medicine; cm, centimetres; kg, kilograms; MD, mean difference. The risk in the intervention group (and its 95% confidence interval) is based on the assumed risk in the comparison group and the relative effect of the intervention (and its 95% CI).

1. Inadequacy of allocation concealment.
2. Difference in population and interventions.

References

Weight: H8, H42, H86, H133, H178
Body mass index: H2, H8, H35, H42, H86, H133, H176, H178
Waist circumference: H8, H35, H86, H178

Table 5.15. GRADE: Chinese Herbal Medicine plus Lifestyle Therapies *vs.* Placebo plus Lifestyle Therapies

Outcome	Absolute Effect		Relative Effect (95% CI) No. of Participants & Studies	Certainty of the Evidence GRADE
	With CHM	Without CHM		
Weight Treatment duration: range 8 to 12 weeks	**76.14** Average difference: 2.50 kg higher (95% CI: 1.11 lower to 6.10 higher)	**73.64**	**MD 2.50** (−1.11, 6.10) Based on data from 144 patients in 3 studies	⊕⊕▢▢ LOW[1,2]
Body mass index (BMI) Treatment duration: range 8 to 12 weeks	**26.07** Average difference: 0.84 kg/m² lower (95% CI: 0.13 lower to 0.54 lower)	**26.91**	**MD −0.84** (−0.13, −0.54) Based on data from 407 patients in 7 studies	⊕⊕⊕▢ MODERATE[3]
Waist circumference Treatment duration: range 8 to 12 weeks	**84.81** Average difference: 2.78 cm lower (95% CI: 5.19 lower to 0.37 lower)	**87.59**	**MD −2.78** (−5.19, −0.37) Based on data from 166 patients in 3 studies	⊕⊕▢▢ LOW[2,3]

Abbreviations: BMI, body mass index; CI, confidence interval; CHM, Chinese herbal medicine; cm, centimetres; kg, kilograms; MD, mean difference. The risk in the intervention group (and its 95% confidence interval) is based on the assumed risk in the comparison group and the relative effect of the intervention (and its 95% CI).

1. Difference in population and intervention.
2. Small sample size.
3. Inadequacy of allocation concealment.

References

Weight: H71, H172, H174
Body mass index: H28, H71, H100, H141, H172, H174, H175
Waist circumference: H28, H172, H174

Frequently Reported Herbs in Meta-analyses Showing Favourable Effect

The most frequently used herbs in meta-analyses showing favourable effects were calculated according to outcome category and comparator type. Table 5.17 includes the list of herbs.

Table 5.16. GRADE: Chinese Herbal Medicine plus Lifestyle Therapies *vs.* Lifestyle Therapies

Outcome	Absolute Effect		Relative Effect (95% CI) No. of Participants & Studies	Certainty of the Evidence GRADE
	With CHM	Without CHM		
Weight Treatment duration: range 4 to 36 weeks	**71.28** Average difference: 3.68 kg lower (95% CI: 4.52 lower to 2.84 lower)	**74.96**	**MD −3.68** (−4.52, −2.84) Based on data from 1,936 patients in 28 studies	⊕⊕⊕⊡ MODERATE[1]
Body mass index (BMI) Treatment duration: range 4 weeks to 12 months	**25.33** Average difference: 1.52 kg/m² lower (95% CI: 1.90 lower to 1.14 lower)	**26.85**	MD −1.52 (−1.90, −1.14) Based on data from 2,685 patients in 40 studies	⊕⊡⊡⊡ VERY LOW[1-3]
Waist circumference Treatment duration: range 4 to 36 weeks	**84.34** Average difference: 3.08 cm lower (95% CI: 3.47 lower to 2.68 lower)	**87.42**	**MD −3.08** (−3.47, −2.68) Based on data from 1,384 patients in 21 studies	⊕⊕⊕⊡ MODERATE[1]

Abbreviations: BMI, body mass index; CI, confidence interval; CHM, Chinese herbal medicine; cm, centimetres; kg, kilograms; MD, mean difference. The risk in the intervention group (and its 95% confidence interval) is based on the assumed risk in the comparison group and the relative effect of the intervention (and its 95% CI).

1. Unclear sequence generation and allocation concealment. Lack of blinding of participants and personnel.
2. Considerable statistical heterogeneity.
3. Difference in measured time.

References

Weight: H10, H12, H24, H33, H40, H44, H47–49, H53, H58, H61, H68, H69, H77, H83, H96, H103, H120, H121, H131, H135, H136, H140, H144, H155, H167, H168
Body mass index: H10–12, H24, H33, H40, H44, H47–49, H53, H58, H61, H63, H68, H69, H77, H83, H96, H98, H103, H112, H118, H120, H121, H125, H127, H131, H132, H135, H138, H140, H144, H155, H163, H167, H168, H177, H184, H187
Waist circumference: H10, H12, H24, H44, H47–49, H53, H61, H69, H77, H83, H96, H135, H138, H144, H155, H163, H167, H168, H184

Table 5.17. Frequently Reported Herbs in Meta-Analyses Showing Favourable Effect

Herbs	Scientific Name	Frequency of Use
Outcomes — Weight and BMI: 7 meta-analyses (121 studies)[a]		
Fu ling 茯苓	*Poria cocos* (Schw.) Wolf	58
Bai zhu 白术	*Atractylodes macrocephala* Koidz.	50
Chen pi 陈皮	*Citrus reticulata* Blanco	42
Huang lian 黄连	*Coptis chinensis* Franch.	42
Shan zha 山楂	*Crataegus pinnatifida* Bge. var. *major* N.E. Br.	40
Ban xia 半夏	*Pinellia ternata* (Thunb.) Breit.	39
Dan shen 丹参	*Salvia miltiorrhiza* Bge.	36
Ze xie 泽泻	*Alisma orientalis* (Sam.) Juzep.	34
Huang qi 黄芪	*Astragalus membranaceus* (Fisch.) Bge. var. *mongholicus* (Bge.) Hsiao	34
Cang zhu 苍术	*Atractylodes lancea* (Thunb.) DC.	33
Outcomes — WC and WHR: 5 meta-analyses (50 studies)[b]		
Huang lian 黄连	*Coptis chinensis* Franch.	19
Shan zha 山楂	*Crataegus pinnatifida* Bge. var. *major* N.E. Br.	18
Fu ling 茯苓	*Poria cocos* (Schw.) Wolf	18
Bai zhu 白术	*Atractylodes macrocephala* Koidz.	17
Ze xie 泽泻	*Alisma orientalis* (Sam.) Juzep.	14
Da huang 大黄	*Rheum palmatum* L.	13
Chen pi 陈皮	*Citrus reticulata* Blanco	13
Ban xia 半夏	*Pinellia ternata* (Thunb.) Breit.	12
Dan shen 丹参	*Salvia miltiorrhiza* Bge.	11
He ye 荷叶	*Nelumbo nucifera* Gaertn.	11
Huang qi 黄芪	*Astragalus membranaceus* (Fisch.) Bge. var. *mongholicus* (Bge.) Hsiao	11

Note: The use of some herbs may be restricted in some countries. Readers are advised to comply with relevant regulations.

Abbreviations: BMI, body mass index; WC, waist circumference; WHR, waist–hip ratio.

Meta-analysis pools:

a. CHM *vs.* no treatment, CHM *vs.* orlistat, CHM *vs.* metformin, CHM plus lifestyle therapies *vs.* placebo plus lifestyle therapies, CHM plus lifestyle therapies *vs.* lifestyle

(Continued)

Table 5.17. (*Continued*)

therapies, CHM plus metformin *vs.* metformin, CHM plus metformin and lifestyle therapies *vs.* metformin and lifestyle therapies.

b. CHM *vs.* metformin, CHM plus lifestyle therapies *vs.* placebo plus lifestyle therapies, CHM plus lifestyle therapies *vs.* lifestyle therapies, CHM plus metformin *vs.* metformin, CHM plus metformin and lifestyle therapies *vs.* metformin and lifestyle therapies.

Safety of Chinese Herbal Medicine in Randomised Controlled Trials

Adverse events were mentioned in 98 studies. Among them, 39 studies reported that no adverse events occurred, and 50 studies provided specific details about the adverse events (Table 5.18). In total, 194 adverse events were reported after CHM treatment. In 10 studies that administered CHM alone, the total number of adverse events was 41, and the most common event was headache (9 cases). In 20 studies assessing CHM plus lifestyle therapies, 98 adverse events were reported. Diarrhoea was the most common adverse event (40 cases), followed by an upset stomach — such as stomachache or nausea (11) — musculoskeletal symptoms (11), etc.

In patients receiving CHM plus drug therapies with or without lifestyle therapies in 20 studies, 55 adverse events were reported. Drug therapies included metformin, repaglinide, telmisartan, liraglutide, fenofibrate, acarbose, gliclazide and perindopril. The most common adverse events in the integrative medicine groups were nausea with or without vomiting (15 cases), diarrhoea (14) and gastrointestinal symptoms (without specific details) (11). In the control groups, 301 adverse events were reported. After a placebo with or without lifestyle therapies, 43 adverse events were reported, and the most common were gastrointestinal symptoms (10 cases, without specific details). Other events included upper respiratory tract infections, diarrhoea, increased appetite, constipation, palpitations, etc. Participants receiving lifestyle therapies in 11 studies reported 9 adverse events, including dizziness (3 cases), insomnia (2), gastrointestinal symptoms (without specific details) (2), nausea and vomiting (1) and palpitation (1).

Table 5.18.   Adverse Events

Interventions		
CHM	**CHM plus Lifestyle Therapies**	**CHM plus Drug Therapies**
N = 10	*N* = 20	*N* = 20
Total AEs = 41	Total AEs = 98	Total AEs = 55
• Headache (9) • Diarrhoea (7) • Nausea (6) • Increased appetite (4) • Increased flatulence (3) • Common cold (2) • Stomach ache (2) • Other (8)	• Diarrhoea (40) • Upset stomach symptoms (11), including stomachache or stomach discomfort (6), nausea with or without vomiting (5) • Musculoskeletal symptoms (11) • Gastrointestinal symptoms (no details) (7) • Upper respiratory tract infections (6) • Headache and dizziness (4) • Oral symptoms (4) • Skin rash (2) • Other (13)	• Nausea with or without vomiting (15) • Diarrhoea (14) • Gastrointestinal symptoms (no details) (11) • Upset stomach (3) • Liver dysfunction (2) • Irritability (2) • Other (8)
Placebo	**Lifestyle Therapies**	**Drug Therapies**
N = 7	*N* = 11	*N* = 32
Total AEs = 43	Total AEs = 9	Total AEs = 249
• Gastrointestinal symptoms (no details) (10) • Upper respiratory tract infections (4) • Diarrhoea (3) • Increased appetite (3) • Constipation (2) • Palpitations (2)	• Dizziness (3) • Insomnia (2) • Gastrointestinal symptoms (no details) (2) • Other (2)	• Upset stomach symptoms (99), including nausea with or without vomiting (62), loss of appetite (22), stomachache or stomach discomfort (10), belching (5) • Gastrointestinal symptoms (no details) (56)

(*Continued*)

Table 5.18. (*Continued*)

Placebo	Lifestyle Therapies	Drug Therapies
• Nausea and vomiting (2) • Neurologic symptoms (2) • Loss of appetite (2) • Stomachache (2) • Other (11)		• Diarrhoea (35) • Facial flush (8) • Headache (7) • Increased flatulence (5) • Skin rash (5) • Liver dysfunction (5) • Oedema of lower extremity (4) • Fatigue (4) • Urinary tract infection (3) • Fatty stools (3) • Irritability (3) • Palpitations (2) • Neurological symptoms (2) • Other (8)

Other events include individual cases where the symptom or sign only occurred on one occasion. Abbreviations: AE, adverse event; CHM, Chinese herbal medicine.

Drug therapies with or without lifestyle therapies were administered in 32 studies, including metformin, repaglinide, telmisartan, liraglutide, fenofibrate, acarbose, gliclazide, perindopril, orlistat, rosiglitazone, pioglitazone, glimepiride and polyene phosphatidylcholine. Adverse events were various, and the most common were upset stomach symptoms (99 cases), such as nausea, loss of appetite, stomachache and belching.

Controlled Clinical Trials of Chinese Herbal Medicine

Controlled clinical trials (CCTs) used a non-random process for allocating participants to interventions. Thirteen CCTs (H196–H208) investigated the effect of CHM in 997 participants. Twelve studies assessed a combination of CHM with drug therapies or non-drug therapies and one study assessed CHM alone. Eight studies were two-arm designs and five studies had three arms, usually including a CHM group, an integrative medicine group and a control group. Drug therapies with or without lifestyle therapies were used as the control in all studies.

The participants were aged from 27 to 67 years, the duration of obesity was 1.5 to 15 years, and the treatment duration ranged from four weeks to six months. Two studies assessed simple obesity and 11 studies assessed obesity with complications or comorbidities. Complications included pre-diabetes or diabetes (7 studies) and one study each for PCOS, metabolic syndrome, hyperlipidaemia and hyperuricemia. Eight studies reported CM syndromes, including Spleen deficiency with dampness obstruction (5 studies), dampness-heat in the Spleen and Stomach (1), phlegm-dampness (1) and *qi* deficiency with phlegm obstruction (1).

Twelve distinct formulae were assessed in the studies. Among them, *Xiao zhi tang* 消脂汤 was evaluated in two studies (H204, H207), which mainly consisted of *huang qi, bai zhu, ze xie, pei lan* and *dan shen*. The other 11 formulae were evaluated in one study each. All formulae were orally administrated. A total of 44 distinct herbs were used in the formulae, and the most common were *huang qi, he ye, ze xie, bai zhu* and *fu ling* (similar to the RCTs).

Controlled Clinical Trials Results

Chinese Herbal Medicine Alone

Three studies (H201, H205, H206) assessed CHM alone in the intervention group, compared to atorvastatin, rosiglitazone and liraglutide, respectively. Included participants were diagnosed with obesity and hyperlipidaemia or diabetes. The CHM group was superior to the atorvastatin group in terms of the BMI, WC and total triglycerides after one month of the treatment, but other serum lipid parameters were not significantly different in people with obesity and hyperlidemia (H201):

- BMI: MD −4.80 kg/m^2 [95% CI −5.26, −4.34].
- WC: MD −4.90 cm [95% CI −6.98, −2.82].
- Total triglycerides: MD −0.40 mmol/L [95% CI −0.70, −0.11].

As for people with diabetes, CHM therapy was superior to lira-glutide in terms of the BMI, but was inferior to liraglutide in reducing blood glucose and HbA1c (H206):

- BMI: MD −1.50 kg/m² [95% CI −1.62, −1.38].
- Fasting blood glucose: MD 0.30 mmol/L [95% CI 0.20, 0.40].
- Postprandial blood glucose: MD 0.30 mmol/L [95% CI 0.15, 0.45].
- HbA1c: MD 0.51 [95% CI 0.34, 0.68]).

BMI and glucometabolic outcomes did not differ in the integrative medicine group of CHM and rosiglitazone (H205).

Chinese Herbal Medicine plus Routine Treatments

Three studies (H204, H207, H208) compared CHM plus routine treatments to exenatide (glucagon-like peptide-1 receptor agonist) plus routine treatments over three months. All three studies assessed obesity with complications or comorbidities, including diabetes, metabolic syndrome and hyperuricemia. For obese people who suffered from metabolic syndrome, no outcomes except HDL were significantly improved in the CHM plus routine group compared to the control (HDL: MD 0.07 mmol/L [95% CI 0.02, 0.12]) (H204). The BMI and WC, but not weight, were reduced significantly in the intervention group for obese people with hyperuricemia (MD −1.90 kg/m² [95% CI −2.32, −1.48] and MD −1.96 cm [95% CI −3.57, −0.35], respectively) (H207). The integrative medicine treatments were not superior to exenatide plus routine treatments in terms of weight, BMI or glucometabolic parameters for participants with diabetes (H208).

Chinese Herbal Medicine plus Drug Therapies

Five studies (H196, H197, H200, H205, H206) assessed CHM plus drug therapies compared to drug therapy control. Four studies (H196, H197, H205, H206) evaluated obesity with pre-diabetes or diabetes and one (H200) assessed obesity with PCOS. Compared to anti-diabetic drugs, the BMI and related glucometabolic parameters except fasting blood glucose were significantly reduced in the CHM plus anti-diabetic drug group compared to the control:

- BMI: MD −3.77 kg/m² [95% CI −5.70, −1.83], I² = 85.5%, 3 studies, 200 participants.
- Postprandial blood glucose: MD −0.90 mmol/L [95% CI −1.08, −0.72], I² = 13.5%, 4 studies, 293 participants.
- Fasting insulin: MD −2.98 mIU/L [95% CI −4.55, −1.42], I² = 0, 2 studies, 120 participants.
- HOMA-IR: MD −0.98 [95% CI −1.34, −0.62], I² = 86.7%, 2 studies, 153 participants.
- HbA1c: MD −0.38 [95% CI −0.51, −0.26], I² = 0, 2 studies, 140 participants.

One study (H200) evaluated obesity with PCOS and compared CHM plus ethinylestradiol and cyproterone acetate to ethinylestradiol and cyproterone acetate. After six months of the treatment, the BMI, fasting blood glucose and fasting insulin were reduced significantly in the intervention group, but the WHR and serum hormone levels, including LH/FSH and androgen, were not.

- BMI: MD −2.38 kg/m² [95% CI −3.70, −1.06].
- Fasting blood glucose: MD −0.32 mmol/L [95% CI −0.56, −0.08].
- Fasting insulin: MD −4.97 mIU/L [95% CI −7.39, −2.55].

Chinese Herbal Medicine plus Drug and Lifestyle Therapies

Seven studies (H198, H199, H202–204, H207, H208) compared CHM plus drug and lifestyle therapies to drug and lifestyle therapies. Two studies assessed simple obesity and five studies evaluated obesity with complications or comorbidities, including pre-diabetes or diabetes (3 studies), metabolic syndrome (1 study) and hyperuricemia (1 study).

Compared to orlistat and lifestyle therapies, no outcomes except the BMI reduced significantly in the CHM add-on group (MD −2.81 kg/m² [95% CI −4.89, −0.73]) (H198). In another study (H203) that compared CHM plus metformin and lifestyle therapies to metformin plus lifestyle therapies for simple obesity, the BMI and body fat mass did not differ between the two groups after the treatment.

Three studies (H199, H202, H208) comprising 193 people with diabetes compared CHM plus anti-diabetic drugs and diabetes routine treatments to anti-diabetic drugs and diabetes routine treatments alone. There was a significant difference in terms of the BMI, WHR, blood glucose and HbA1c, but not weight, insulin or HOMA-IR:

- BMI: MD −1.57 kg/m^2 [95% CI −2.96, −0.19], I^2 = 79.9%, 3 studies, 160 participants.
- WHR: MD −0.05 [95% CI −0.09, −0.01], 1 study, 100 participants.
- Fasting blood glucose: MD −0.28 mmol/L [95% CI −0.50, −0.05], I^2 = 67.4%, 3 studies, 160 participants.
- Postprandial blood glucose: MD −0.80 mmol/L [95% CI −1.55, −0.05], I^2 = 72.4%, 2 studies, 93 participants.
- HbA1c: MD −0.31 [95% CI −0.49, −0.12], I^2 = 33.0%, 3 studies, 160 participants.

For obese people with metabolic syndrome, the CHM plus exenatide and routine treatment group (H204) was superior to the exenatide plus routine treatment group in the WHR but not in weight, BMI and WC. In terms of metabolic parameters, blood glucose, HOMA-IR and total cholesterol were significantly reduced in the intervention group compared to the control, but insulin and total triglycerides were not.

- WHR: MD −0.03 [95% CI −0.05, −0.02].
- Fasting blood glucose: MD −0.76 mmol/L [95% CI −0.97, −0.55].
- Postprandial blood glucose: MD −1.25 mmol/L [95% CI −1.61, −0.90].
- HOMA-IR: MD −1.16 mIU/L [95% CI −1.25, −1.07].
- Total cholesterol: MD −0.34 mmol/L [95% CI −0.56, −0.12].

CHM plus exenatide and routine treatment were also given to obese people with hyperuricemia in one study (H207), but it was not superior to the control group in terms of weight, BMI or WC.

Safety of Chinese Herbal Medicine in Controlled Clinical Trials

Eight studies reported adverse events. Among them, one study (H202) reported that no adverse events occurred. One study (H204) reported that slight nausea and diarrhoea occurred in both the CHM group and integrative medicine group. Six studies (H197, H198, H201, H206–208) reported specific details about the event types and numbers. One study (H201) compared *Qu tan tiao zhi tang* 祛痰调脂汤 to atorvastatin. No adverse events occurred in the CHM group, while two adverse events — transient fever and stomach distension — occurred in the control group. In five integrative medicine studies (H197, H198, H206–208), there were 111 adverse events. A total of 34 adverse events occurred in the integrative medicine group, including nausea with or without vomiting (15 cases), gastrointestinal symptoms (without specific details) (6), diarrhoea (3), constipation (3), hypoglycaemia (3), loss of appetite (2), dizziness (1) and fatigue (1). In the drug therapy control groups, 77 adverse events were reported, including nausea with or without vomiting (31 cases), gastrointestinal symptoms (without specific details) (11), diarrhoea (10), dizziness (8), loss of appetite (6), fatigue (5), constipation (3), abdominal distention (2) and hypoglycaemia (1).

Non-controlled Studies of Chinese Herbal Medicine

Twenty-four non-controlled studies (H209–232) evaluated the effect of CHM in 507 participants. Fifteen studies assessed CHM alone and nine studies assessed a combination of CHM with drug therapies or lifestyle therapies.

The participants' age ranged from 19 to 77 years, duration of obesity was from 3 to 10 years, and the treatment duration ranged from 6 weeks to 6 months. Eleven studies assessed simple obesity and 13 studies assessed obesity with complications or comorbidities. Complications included PCOS (6 studies), hyperlipidaemia (2), hypertension (2), pre-diabetes or diabetes (1), metabolic syndrome (1) and non-alcoholic fatty liver disease (1). Thirteen studies reported CM syndromes and the most common syndromes were Spleen deficiency with dampness obstruction, dampness-heat in the Spleen and Stomach and phlegm-dampness.

Twenty-three distinct formulae were assessed in the studies. Among them, only *Qi gong wan* 启宫丸 was evaluated in more than one study (H221, H226), which consists of *chuan xiong, bai zhu, ban xia, xiang fu, fu ling, shen qu, chen pi* and *gan cao*. All formulae were administrated orally. A total of 97 distinct herbs were used in the formulae, and the most common were *ban xia, bai zhu, fu ling, ze xie* and *shan zha* (Table 5.19).

Table 5.19. Frequently Reported Herbs in Non-controlled Studies

Most Common Herbs	Scientific Name	Frequency of Use
Ban xia 半夏	*Pinellia ternata* (Thunb.) Breit.	15
Bai zhu 白术	*Atractylodes macrocephala* Koidz.	15
Fu ling 茯苓	*Poria cocos* (Schw.) Wolf	13
Ze xie 泽泻	*Alisma orientalis* (Sam.) Juzep.	12
Shan zha 山楂	*Crataegus pinnatifida* Bge. var. *major* N.E. Br.	10
Gan cao 甘草	*Glycyrrhiza uralensis* Fisch.	9
Chen pi 陈皮	*Citrus reticulata* Blanco	8
Chuan xiong 川芎	*Ligusticum chuanxiong* Hort.	6
Sheng jiang 生姜	*Zingiber officinale* Rosc.	6
Cang zhu 苍术	*Atractylodes lancea* (Thunb.) DC.	6
Huang qin 黄芩	*Scutellaria baicalensis* Georgi	6

Note: The use of some herbs may be restricted in some countries. Readers are advised to comply with relevant regulations.

Safety of Chinese Herbal Medicine in Non-controlled Studies

Among 24 studies, only three mentioned adverse events. Two of the studies (H230, H231) reported no adverse events. One study (H214) reported slight diarrhoea, an upset stomach and belching after taking the CHM decoction, but the number of cases was not specified.

Summary of Chinese Herbal Medicine Clinical Evidence

In total, 232 clinical studies were included that evaluated the efficacy and safety of CHM for overweight and obesity. Most of the studies were RCTs (195 studies), 13 were CCTs, and 24 were non-controlled studies. The majority of the studies (74.6%) assessed obesity with complications or comorbidities, such as PCOS and diabetes, and only 59 studies (25.4%) assessed simple obesity. This is not surprising since being overweight and obese is often associated with various metabolic disorders. Chinese medicine syndrome differentiation was reported in more than half of the studies (58.2%), and the most common syndromes were Spleen deficiency with dampness obstruction, dampness-heat in the Spleen and Stomach, and phlegm-dampness, which is in accordance with the clinical guidelines (see Chapter 2).

A total of 171 distinct formulae and 212 different herbs were investigated in the clinical studies. The most common formula was *Wu ling san*, and the most frequently used herbs were *fu ling, bai zhu, ban xia* and *chen pi*. In addition, several formulae were developed by researchers according to their clinical experience rather than traditional prescribing practices.

Previous systematic reviews and meta-analyses indicate that CHM can reduce weight, BMI and total effective rate significantly more than a placebo, lifestyle modifications or drug therapies.[1-3] In addition, CHM appears to be safe for the treatment of obesity. However, conclusions are limited due to the poor methodological quality of the included studies.

In this chapter, 195 RCTs and 15,172 participants were included in the analysis. The participants' age ranged from 18 to 79 years, and the treatment duration ranged from four weeks to 12 months (mode: 12 weeks). There were more female participants (7,780) than males (5,992). The gender of 1,400 participants was not described.

An analysis of 195 RCTs showed that CHM alongside lifestyle therapies was superior to lifestyle therapies in reducing weight, BMI, WC and WHR. There were also significant reductions in the BMI and WC when compared to a placebo alongside lifestyle therapies. However, in terms of CHM alone, the results were divergent. When CHM was compared to no treatment or metformin, the BMI was reduced significantly in the CHM groups after the reatment. However, there was no significant difference in weight, BMI and WC when CHM was compared to a placebo or diet therapy. This may be because CHM has a more holistic effect to induce weight loss rather than just targeting fat or lipid metabolism. In addition, the pathogenesis of overweight and obesity is closely related to an unhealthy diet and insufficient exercise. Therefore, holistic treatment with CHM combined with lifestyle interventions is more favourable for weight reduction.

As for weight-related complications or comorbidities, pre-diabetes and diabetes, PCOS and metabolic syndrome appeared to be the most common in the included studies. Metformin, rather than the traditional drugs for obesity, such as orlistat, appeared to be the most common drug therapy for obesity, and related complications. For people with obesity and pre-diabetes or diabetes, CHM alongside lifestyle therapies was superior to lifestyle therapies alone, with or without a placebo, in reducing the BMI, WC and glucometabolic parameters, such as fasting blood glucose, postprandial blood glucose and HbA1c. There were similar reductions in weight, BMI, WC, WHR and glucometabolic outcomes when CHM plus anti-diabetic drugs were compared to anti-diabetic drugs, with or without lifestyle therapies. As for obesity with PCOS or with metabolic syndrome, the BMI and related metabolic outcomes — such as HOMA-IR, LH/FSH and androgen level for PCOS, and the serum glucose level, lipid level and blood pressure for metabolic syndrome — were also significantly reduced in the CHM groups or the integrative medicine groups. However, there were only a small number of studies included in these results.

Safety

CHM appears to be safe for the treatment for overweight and obesity. Gastrointestinal symptoms were the most frequent adverse events according to the analysis of the RCT studies, such as nausea, vomiting, diarrhoea, stomachache, etc. These symptoms were generally mild, tolerated and self-resolving. From another point of view, events like increased flatulence or loose stools may be one of the effects of CHM to increase gastrointestinal peristalsis and help lose weight. Other adverse events included headaches and skin rash, etc., but they were few in number.

Limitations

Despite the positive results, the studies were not free from bias. Most studies (89.7%) were open-label and at high risk of bias in terms of blinding of the participants and personnel. As for sequence generation, allocation concealment, blinding of outcome assessors and selective outcome reporting, it was hard to make judgements due to insufficient information. Therefore, these four domains were mainly judged to be an unclear risk of bias. Besides the bias, heterogeneity was high in many meta-analysis results. Furthermore, many studies only evaluated CHM over a short period. Any follow-up for longer than three months was seldom reported.

Best Available Evidence

CHM combined with diet and exercise resulted in a greater weight reduction than diet and exercise alone. Results showed a 3.68 kg reduction (about 5%) (moderate certainty evidence). This validates existing recommendations that exercise combined with dietary change can reduce weight by about 1–1.5 kg,[4] indicating that CHM has an added benefit in the short-term reduction of weight and meeting the threshold for a clinically important effect.[5] Furthermore, CHM plus lifestyle therapies reduced the WC by 3.08 cm more than lifestyle therapies alone (moderate certainty evidence). Overall, the results support the use of CHM combined with exercise and dietary change and are associated with reduced weight and improved cardiovascular disease risk factors.

References

1. Sui Y, Zhao HL, Wong VCW, *et al.* (2012) A systematic review on use of Chinese medicine and acupuncture for treatment of obesity. *Obesity Reviews* **13(5):** 409–30.
2. 曾鸿孟, 唐乾利, 唐红珍, *et al.* (2015) 中药治疗单纯性肥胖有效性的 Meta 分析. *世界复合医学*. **1(02):** 134–139.
3. 周静波, 孙心怡, 张舒, 叶丽芳. (2016) 中药复方治疗单纯性肥胖的 Meta 分析. *东南国防医药*. **18(01):** 62–64.
4. Shaw K, Gennat H, O'Rourke P, *et al.* (2006) Exercise for overweight or obesity. *Cochrane Database Syst Rev* **18(4):** CD003817.
5. Jensen MD, Ryan DH, Apovian CM, *et al.* (2014) 2013 AHA/ACC/TOS Guideline for the management of overweight and obesity in adults: A report of the American College of Cardiology/American Heart Association Task Force on Practice Guidelines and The Obesity Society. *Circulation* **129(25 suppl 2):** S102–S138.

References for Included Chinese Herbal Medicine Clinical Studies

Study No.	Reference
H1	安其, 李朝敏, 程斌. (2003) 安一胶囊治疗胰岛素抵抗综合征的临床观察. 成都中医药大学学报. **26(1):** 10–12.
H2	毕桂芝. (2006) "络通" 对超重和肥胖者血管内皮功能障碍的防治作用研究. 北京中医药大学.

(Continued)

Study No.	Reference
H3	曹福建, 张翠玲. (2016) 中西医结合治疗肥胖型 2 型糖尿病临床研究. *中医学报*. **31(11):** 1688–1690.
H4	曹红霞, 徐浪, 邱英明, 贺支文. (2015) 芪精丹兰汤对痰湿肥胖型多囊卵巢综合征患者内分泌紊乱的影响. *中国社区医师*. **31(11):** 73–75.
H5	曾英, 龙晓静, 江涛. (2007) 血府逐瘀汤合二陈汤治疗肥胖 2 型糖尿病疗效观察. 辽宁中医杂志. **34(8):** 1089–1090.
H6	陈晶. (2006) 调理三焦法治疗代谢综合征的临床研究. 广州中医药大学.
H7	陈利群. (2007) 半夏白术天麻汤合泽泻汤加味对痰湿壅盛型高血压病体重指数, 降压效果的影响. *中国中医急症*. **16(6):** 650–651.
H8	陈亮, 竹剑平. (2008) 芦荟治疗单纯性肥胖症 50 例临床疗效观察. *浙江临床医学*. **10(2):** 219–220.
H9	陈宁, 黄培颖, 吴华. (2013) 保和丸联合阿卡波糖对糖耐量异常的肥胖者血清铁蛋白水平的影响. 光明中医. **28(12):** 2597–2599.
H10	陈蔷, 吴佳丽. (2007) 金芪降糖片对肥胖型空腹血糖升高者的干预治疗. 现代中西医结合杂志. **16(17):** 2370–2371.
H11	陈少仕. (2011) 保和丸加减治疗肥胖型糖耐量减低 60 例临床观察. *中国热带医学*. **11(8):** 1000–1001.
H12	陈诗慧, 梁绮君, 胡晨鸣, *et al.* (2017) 山楂消脂胶囊对非酒精性脂肪性肝病合并肥胖症患者的疗效观察. *时珍国医国药*. **28(12):** 2946–2948.
H13	陈文实, 王汉伟, 刘继松. (2013) 益气活血汤联合二甲双胍治疗 2 型糖尿病疗效观察. *中华全科医学*. **11(4):** 564, 585.
H14	陈晓辉, 石鹤峰. (2012) 五苓散加味联合盐酸二甲双胍片治疗肥胖型 2 型糖尿病 40 例. *中医研究*. **25(4):** 26–27.
H15	陈燕, 刘何玥, 杨冰馨, 唐岚. (2015) 补肾活血化痰中药治疗肥胖型多囊卵巢综合征 30 例临床观察. 实用中西医结合临床. **15(10):** 36–38.
H16	陈元. (2011) 自拟三降散治疗代谢综合征 50 例. 光明中医. **26(11):** 2230–2231.
H17	陈子欢. (2014) 参芎荷叶汤治疗肥胖 2 型糖尿病气虚痰瘀证的临床研究. 南京中医药大学.
H18	程妍. (2012) 祛胰抵方对肥胖型 T2DM 胰岛素抵抗患者血清瘦素及抵抗素的影响. 黑龙江中医药大学.
H19	刁亚红, 鄢慧妤, 黄泳, 亓鲁光. (2017) 中西医结合治疗多囊卵巢综合征合并胰岛素抵抗肥胖患者临床疗效观察. 中国中医基础医学杂志. **23(8)**.

(Continued)

(*Continued*)

Study No.	Reference
H20	范玉网. (2012) 五苓散治疗代谢综合征的理论和临床研究. 广州中医药大学.
H21	冯博. (2014) 健脾调肝化浊法治疗单纯性肥胖症合并糖调节受损的实验研究及临床疗效评价. 山东中医药大学.
H22	冯彩凤. (2009) 中西药联合治疗痰湿型多囊卵巢综合征 50 例. *中医学报*. **24(6):** 60–61.
H23	冯大勇. (2007) 消脂汤治疗代谢综合征肥胖及相关指标的临床研究. 成都中医药大学.
H24	冯少玲, 何采辉, 李文纯, 刘思雅. (2015) 脾虚痰湿型单纯性肥胖症应用五苓散治疗的 bmi 及血脂变化观察. *中国医药科学*. **5(9):** 67–69.
H25	付贵珍. (2017) 葛根芩连汤治疗肥胖 2 型糖尿病 (湿热内蕴型) 的临床观察. 河南中医药大学.
H26	高舜天. (2018) 化痰祛瘀减肥汤用于痰瘀型肥胖症患者治疗中的临床效果观察. *中医临床研究*. **10(9):** 56–57.
H27	高志扬. (2007) 平肝祛痰化瘀治疗高血压伴肥胖 30 例临床研究. *中西医结合心脑血管病杂志*. **5(8):** 679–680.
H28	宫畅. (2017) 解毒通络调肝方加减治疗肥胖 2 型糖尿病伴非酒精性脂肪肝患者的临床观察. 长春中医药大学.
H29	顾庆奎. (2009) 中西医结合优化方案对超重/肥胖 2 型糖尿病临床疗效的观察. 广州中医药大学.
H30	顾映玉. (2015) 桂葛五苓散治疗肥胖型多囊卵巢综合征 60 例的临床观察. *内蒙古中医药*. **34(11):** 24–25.
H31	郭晓洁. (2010) 益气解毒汤对肥胖型 2 型糖尿病患者胰岛素抵抗的干预性临床研究. 山东中医药大学.
H32	Kang JH, Jeong IS, Kim MY. (2018) Antiangiogenic herbal composition Ob-X reduces abdominal visceral fat in humans: A randomized, double-blind, placebo-controlled study. *Evid Based Complementary Altern Med* **28(2018):** 4381205.
H33	韩静, 王亚平, 张炜, *et al.* (2017) 中药健脾祛湿法结合运动干预肥胖症临床疗效观察. *时珍国医国药*. **28(8):** 1924–1926.
H34	韩笑, 朴春丽, 仝小林. (2010) 连梅汤治疗肥胖 2 型糖尿病 40 例. *中医研究*. **23(6):** 26–27.
H35	何春燕, 王文健, 李玢, *et al.* (2007) 益气散聚方治疗代谢综合征肥胖高危人群的临床研究. *中西医结合学报*. **5(3):** 263–267.

(Continued)

Study No.	Reference
H36	洪寅雯, 孙薛亮, 周玉珍. (2016) 健脾祛痰通络方治疗肥胖型多囊卵巢综合征 23 例. *江西中医药.* **47(10):** 48–50.
H37	侯光华, 汪慧兰, 周红星, *et al.* (2013) 二甲双胍片联合健脾调脂化瘀方治疗肥胖症并非酒精性脂肪性肝炎的临床疗效观察. *中国中西医结合消化杂志.* **21(1):** 11–14
H38	胡梅芳. (2008) 七味白术散合补阳还五汤治疗肥胖 2 型糖尿病及改善胰岛素抵抗的研究. *现代中西医结合杂志.* **17(22):** 3415–3416.
H39	胡燕, 薛晓玲, 周海悦. (2018) 奥利司他联合益肾化痰方治疗肥胖型多囊卵巢综合征不孕患者临床研究. *河北医药.* **40(18):** 2743–2747.
H40	黄蔚, 潘丰满, 黄江荣. (2017) 加味苓桂术甘汤治疗脾虚湿阻型单纯性肥胖症临床研究. *长江大学学报 (自科版).* **14(4):** 4–6.
H41	黄翌, 李妍妍. (2014) 五苓散联合瑞格列奈治疗肥胖型 2 型糖尿病临床分析. *白求恩医学杂志.* **12(1):** 89–90.
H42	Park SH, Huh TL, Kim SY, *et al.* (2014) Antiobesity effect of Gynostemma pentaphyllum extract (actiponin): A randomized, double-blind, placebo-controlled trial. *Obesity (Silver Spring).* **22(1):** 63–71.
H43	黄长盛, 冯婷, 管雁丞. (2016) 补肾化痰行气方联合二甲双胍治疗肥胖型多囊卵巢综合征伴胰岛素抵抗的临床研究. *深圳中西医结合杂志.* **26(10):** 46–48.
H44	黄中一. (2005) 健脾滋阴利湿活血法治疗肥胖型 II 型糖尿病的研究. 南京中医药大学.
H45	姬广慧. (2017) 黄连温胆汤治疗腹型 2 型糖尿病伴胰岛素抵抗的临床观察. 山东中医药大学.
H46	季菲. (2017) 王文友老师学术思想与临床经验总结及从少阳论治代谢综合征的理论与临床研究. 北京中医药大学.
H47	金琴. (2017) 健脾化湿方治疗脾虚湿阻型肥胖症的临床研究. 浙江中医药大学.
H48	康稚宜. (2010) 苦酸通调法治疗早期肥胖的 2 型糖尿病的临床观察. 长春中医药大学.
H49	赖学鸿. (2011) 决明子茶和运动双重干预对老年女性的减肥效果. *中国老年学杂志.* **31(13):** 2402–2404.
H50	郎宁, 文俊, 余洁. (2015) 自拟益气固本方联合二甲双胍缓释片对初诊超重肥胖 2 型糖尿病代谢指标的影响. *医学综述.* **21(19):** 3611–3613.

(Continued)

(Continued)

Study No.	Reference
H51	郎宁, 余洁, 文俊. (2015) 自拟益气固本方治疗单纯性肥胖的效果及其对患者血清炎症因子的影响. *广东医学.* **36(1):** 136–138.
H52	雷枭, 张博达, 任继刚, 李宗林. (2017) 健脾化浊散联合二甲双胍治疗肥胖2型糖尿病的临床研究. *重庆医科大学学报.* **42(10):** 1336–1340.
H53	李奥杰. (2014) 补气消痰饮治疗脾肾两虚型超重和单纯性肥胖的临床观察. 北京中医药大学.
H54	李朝敏, 文俊. (2003) 安一胶囊治疗2型糖尿病合并高脂血症及肥胖的临床观察. *中药药理与临床.* **19(4):** 45–46.
H55	李红霞, 关得安, 史红霞. (2007) 化痰逐瘀法治疗肥胖型2型糖尿病临床研究. *长治医学院学报.* **21(1):** 59–61.
H56	李惠林, 刘玲, 赵恒侠, *et al.* (2013) 三仁汤治疗湿热蕴脾型肥胖2型糖尿病疗效观察. *新中医.* **45(6):** 108–110.
H57	李吉武, 孟立锋. (2013) 温阳益气活血方治疗初发肥胖2型糖尿病临床观察. *新中医.* **45(3):** 105–107.
H58	李健. (2015) 佩连麻黄方治疗单纯性肥胖的疗效观察及对 INS, GLP-1, IAPP 的影响. 黑龙江中医药大学.
H59	李丽. (2013) 黄连解毒汤对初发肥胖2型糖尿病患者的临床干预研究. 山东中医药大学.
H60	李娜, 贺红梅, 王齐有, 美娜, 虞梅. (2017) 消渴健脾胶囊治疗肥胖痰湿型2型糖尿病40例临床观察. *湖南中医杂志.* **33(5):** 4–6.
H61	李松伟, 宰军华, 王又红, *et al.* (2007) 减肥调脂胶囊对单纯性肥胖症 (胃热湿阻证) 的临床研究. *新中医.* **39(02):** 28–29.
H62	李小忠. (2018) 二甲双胍+逍遥散加减治疗肥胖型2型糖尿病的临床效果. *临床合理用药杂志.* **11(5):** 7–8, 15.
H63	李艳斐. (2014) 健脾化痰方治疗阻塞性睡眠呼吸暂停低通气综合征的疗效研究. 中国中医科学院.
H64	连凤梅, 仝小林, 白煜, *et al.* (2008) 中药降糖复方与二甲双胍对照治疗2型糖尿病的临床研究. *中国临床药理学杂志.* **24(6):** 501–504.
H65	连凤梅, 仝小林, 白煜, *et al.* (2009) 清热降浊方治疗超重2型糖尿病疗效分析. *中国中医药信息杂志.* **16(2):** 17–18.
H66	连真, 屠亦文, 孙鼎. (2014) 肥胖1号方治疗脾虚痰湿型肥胖症合并胰岛素抵抗疗效观察. *河北中医.* **36(12):** 1783–1785.
H67	梁厚策, 王松林. (2016) 苓桂术甘汤+干预生活方式联合二甲双胍治疗痰湿壅盛糖尿病肥胖随机平行对照研究. *实用中医内科杂志.* **30(11):** 40–42.

Study No.	Reference
H68	梁绮君, 胡晨鸣, 黄容, *et al.* (2017) 山楂消脂胶囊对肥胖症患者炎性状态及脂多糖水平的影响. 国际内分泌代谢杂志. **37(4):** 236–238.
H69	梁绮君, 胡晨鸣, 黄容, *et al.* (2016) 山楂消脂胶囊对肥胖症患者内脏脂肪的影响. 广东医学. **37(17):** 2669–2671.
H70	林寒梅, 逯克娜, 赵柯杭, *et al.* (2017) 化痰通脉饮联合二甲双胍治疗肥胖型多囊卵巢综合征的临床研究. 辽宁中医杂志. **44(7):** 1416–1418.
H71	林志燕, 田怀平, 李方, *et al.* (2017) 舒肝祛脂胶囊治疗成人单纯性肥胖的临床疗效及安全性评价. 中国药学 · 英文版. **26(12):** 890–894.
H72	刘美娜. (2018) 佩连麻黄方治疗肥胖 T2DM 胃热湿阻证的疗效观察及对 TNF-α 的影响. 黑龙江中医药大学.
H73	刘美琪. (2017) 补肾化痰方联合二甲双胍治疗肥胖型多囊卵巢综合征的临床研究. 南京中医药大学.
H74	刘梦瑶, 张家林, 裴瑞霞. (2014) 中西医结合治疗肥胖型 2 型糖尿病 30 例临床观察. 四川中医. **32(8):** 93–95.
H75	刘声乐. (2009) 补肾祛痰法结合二甲双胍治疗痰湿型多囊卵巢综合征伴胰岛素抵抗的临床研究. 南京中医药大学.
H76	刘舒婷, 陈木柯, 李冰. (2015) 补肾化痰祛瘀方治疗肥胖型多囊卵巢综合征 35 例临床观察. 中国民族民间医药杂志. **24(22):** 60–61.
H77	刘天晓, 刘佳, 张冠华. (2012) 有氧运动伴决明子茶饮对肥胖女大学生身体形态及血脂代谢的影响. 山东体育科技. **34(3):** 34–38.
H78	陆聆韵. (2018) 苍柴调中方对肥胖合并胰岛素抵抗患者干预效果的临床研究. 中国中医药科技. **25(2):** 162–164, 167.
H79	陆聆韵, 沈小珩. (2016) 苍柴调中汤联合西格列汀治疗胰岛素抵抗合并肥胖患者的疗效及其糖代谢的影响研究. 环球中医药. **9(9):** 1111–1113.
H80	马迪. (2006) 降脂减肥汤治疗 2 型糖尿病并肥胖的临床研究. 云南中医学院.
H81	马国庆, 寇吉友, 贾英丽, *et al.* (2010) 芪术饮对新诊断肥胖 2 型糖尿病患者胰岛 β 细胞功能的影响. 中医药信息. **27(3):** 45–46.
H82	马秀. (2015) 参苓白术散加减治疗脾虚湿盛证糖尿病前期肥胖疗效观察. 中医药临床杂志. **27(11):** 1583–1585.
H83	麦熙. (2008) 五苓散治疗脾虚痰湿型单纯性肥胖症的临床观察. 广州中医药大学
H84	牛韬, 石敏. (2011) 黄连解毒合剂治疗肥胖 2 型糖尿病 32 例疗效观察. 山东医药. **51(37):** 103–104.

(*Continued*)

(*Continued*)

Study No.	Reference
H85	潘海洋. (2015) 康脾燥湿汤联合西医治疗超重和肥胖老年 2 型糖尿病患者的疗效. *中国老年学杂志*. **35(4):** 1074–1075.
H86	潘玲, 李德良, 雷茂茹, *et al*. (2005) 藕节, 绿茶及三七微丸制剂干预成年性肥胖. *中国临床康复*. **9(15):** 231–233.
H87	潘善余. (2011) 健脾化湿祛痰法治疗肥胖 2 型糖尿病 50 例观察. *浙江中医杂志*. **46(12):** 891.
H88	潘善余. (2018) 健脾化湿清热导滞法治疗肥胖型糖耐量受损 42 例观察. *浙江中医杂志*. **53(3):** 198.
H89	全毅红, 雷学剑. (2011) 加味六君子汤对肥胖相关性高血压病患者血清瘦素的影响. *南京中医药大学学报*. **27(2):** 181–183.
H90	全毅红, 庹玲玲, 杨雅琴. (2013) 加味六君子汤对肥胖相关高血压患者血清瘦素及血管活性物质含量的影响研究. *中国全科医学*. **16(31):** 3746–3748.
H91	尚祥岭. (2017) 健脾降糖汤治疗肥胖型 2 型糖尿病痰瘀气虚证临床研究. *中医学报* **32(5):** 743–746.
H92	申香莲. (2016) 五苓散加减联合瑞格列奈治疗肥胖型 2 型糖尿病疗效观察. *现代中西医结合杂志*. **25(13):** 1425–1427.
H93	盛立红. (2012) 消渴脂平胶囊治疗肥胖 2 型糖尿病合并血脂异常 (气阴两虚挟痰瘀证) 的临床观察. 长春中医药大学.
H94	石珺, 胡衍园, 王清华. (2005) 复方苍术汤治疗老年肥胖或超重合并糖耐量异常 32 例临床观察. 中医杂志. **46(1):** 24–25.
H95	史志萍, 刘霄霞, 陆君, *et al*. (2015) 补肾健脾方对围绝经期及绝经期肥胖妇女体质量及性激素水平的影响. *河北中医*. **37(4):** 497–500.
H96	司银梅, 向楠. (2014) 温肾健脾化痰方治疗单纯性肥胖症疗效观察. *湖北中医杂志*. **36(2):** 11–12.
H97	苏小芳. (2014) 从胆郁论治中心肥胖型胰岛素抵抗患者的临床干预研究. 河南中医药大学; 河南中医学院.
H98	随子云. (2009) 黄连温胆汤对肥胖型糖耐量减低的干预. *四川中医*. **27(4):** 69–70.
H99	孙昊. (2011) 加味连梅汤治疗早期肥胖 2 型糖尿病的临床观察. 长春中医药大学.
H100	孙璐, 唐咸玉, 张鹏, *et al*. (2017) 益气化痰活血法改善超重/肥胖 2 型糖尿病患者糖脂代谢紊乱及肥胖抑制素的临床观察. *中国实验方剂学杂志*. **23(6):** 180–185.

Study No.	Reference
H101	唐红珍, 宋宁, 刘鹏. (2013) 壮医调气畅龙内服方对超重, 肥胖的疗效. *中国实验方剂学杂志*. **19(9):** 291–293.
H102	陶静怡, 李敏, 胡利江, 杨颖. (2018) 健脾祛湿方联合盐酸二甲双胍片治疗肥胖型 2 型糖尿病临床观察. *新中医*. **50(1):** 48–52.
H103	田麒, 顾淑英, 刘玉伏. (2013) 荷丹片对肥胖合并高脂血症人群的干预. *中西医结合心脑血管病杂志*. **11(11):** 1290–1291.
H104	仝小林, 连凤梅, 黎明, *et al.* (2009) 黄连组方对 2 型糖尿病患者血清瘦素, 脂联素的影响. *中国糖尿病杂志*. **17(3):** 171–173.
H105	涂春联, 李红胜. (2015) 黄连解毒汤治疗肥胖型 2 型糖尿病临床研究. *中医学报*. **30(5):** 644–646.
H106	涂志芳. (2012) 扶阳祛痰化瘀疗法治疗代谢综合征血糖异常的临床疗效观察. 福建中医药大学.
H107	汪春, 程志清. (2007) 平肝益肾涤痰饮治疗高血压肥胖 31 例临床观察. *中医杂志*. **48(2):** 135–137.
H108	王爱秋. (2016) 健脾化痰, 通腑泄浊法改善肥胖型 2 型糖尿病胰岛素抵抗临床观察. 山东中医药大学.
H109	王斌胜. (2009) 化浊行血兼以温阳法治疗代谢综合征的临床和实验研究. 山东中医药大学.
H110	王春红. (2013) 血府逐瘀汤合二陈汤治疗肥胖 2 型糖尿病疗效观察. *中外医疗*. **32(15):** 6–7.
H111	王吉元, 李树斌, 谢相智, *et al.* (2017) 加味苓桂术甘汤联合替米沙坦治疗老年肥胖型高血压疗效观察. *现代中西医结合杂志*. **26(17):** 1898–1900.
H112	王静. (2016) 中药配合健康指导对痰湿血瘀型 PCOS 患者体重的影响. 黑龙江中医药大学.
H113	王亮友. (2014) 滋潜化痰汤联合西医常规对腹型肥胖者血压, 血脂的影响. 黑龙江中医药大学.
H114	王婷婷, 张雪锋. (2014) 中药联合二甲双胍对超重人群糖代谢的影响. *浙江中医药大学学报*. **38(6):** 722–724.
H115	王小燕. (2018) 加减苍附导痰汤对肥胖型多囊卵巢综合征患者性激素水平及受孕率的影响. *吉林中医药*. **38(4):** 421–425.
H116	王雪莹. (2013) 苦酸通络调肝方治疗肥胖 2 型糖尿病 (肝胃郁热证) 的临床研究. 长春中医药大学.

(Continued)

(*Continued*)

Study No.	Reference
H117	Zhou Q, Chang B, Chen XY, *et al.* (2014) Chinese herbal medicine for obesity: A randomized, double-blinded, multicenter, prospective trial. *Am J Chin Med* **42(6):** 1345–1356.
H118	魏玲玲. (2011) 清热利湿中药对肥胖 2 型糖尿病患者胰岛素抵抗的影响. *国际中医中药杂志.* **33(9):** 777–779.
H119	魏岳斌, 郝建军, 黄海英, 李进友. (2008) 肥可消方治疗老年单纯性肥胖症的临床研究. *实用中西医结合临床.* **8(3):** 6–7.
H120	文秀英, 刘浩, 张彩艳, 潘青云. (2010) 决明子减肥的临床疗效评价及对脂代谢的影响. *中国医院药学杂志.* **30(24):** 2097–2100.
H121	吴文妙. (2016) 防风通圣丸治疗单纯性肥胖的临床疗效观察及对 LP 、APN 的影响. 黑龙江中医药大学.
H122	吴艳, 郑承红. (2011) 防风通圣散联合二甲双胍片治疗腹型肥胖 2 型糖尿病临床观察. *湖北中医杂志.* **33(2):** 23–24.
H123	武永华. (2018) 五苓散加味治疗单纯性肥胖合并脂代谢异常 40 例. *河南中医.* **38(1):** 42–44.
H124	肖一公, 张玉福, 徐霖, 孙斌. (2017) 加味小陷胸汤治疗肥胖型糖耐量减低临床观察. *山西中医.* **33(6):** 18–20.
H125	徐霖. (2013) 导痰汤加减治疗肥胖型糖耐量异常的临床观察. *黑龙江医药.* **26(3):** 493–495.
H126	徐宁. (2015) 应用化浊解毒法治疗超重合并糖耐量减低分析. *实用中西医结合临床.* **15(5):** 8–9, 14.
H127	徐小娟, 刘丹, 王静. (2015) 参苓白术散加减辅助治疗 2 型糖尿病伴肥胖症 80 例临床观察. *海南医学.* **26(24):** 3612–3614.
H128	徐艳文. (2015) 六味地黄丸联合二甲双胍治疗 2 型糖尿病伴肥胖的临床观察. *中国药房.* **26(15):** 2077–2079.
H129	许金榜, 王小云, 纪峰, *et al.* (2017) 痰脂消颗粒联合二甲双胍治疗肥胖型多囊卵巢综合征伴胰岛素抵抗的临床观察. *中华中医药学刊.* **35(06):** 1431–1434.
H130	旋宝泰. (2010) 黄连解毒汤治疗肥胖 2 型糖尿病 30 例疗效观察. *河北中医.* **32(10):** 1460–1461.
H131	鄢琪. (2014) 苓桂术甘汤加味治疗脾虚痰湿型肥胖症研究. 南京中医药大学.
H132	杨国伟. (2010) 健脾祛湿化痰法治疗肥胖症 24 例. *中国中医药现代远程教育.* **8(7):** 28–29.

Study No.	Reference
H133	杨叔禹. (2012) 代谢综合征中医病理特征及泽泻汤加味方的疗效观察和机制研究. 福建中医药大学.
H134	杨秀萍. (2017) 中西药联合治疗 2 型糖尿病合并超重或肥胖患者 19 例. *光明中医*. **32(17):** 2544–2546.
H135	杨杨, 刘佳, 赖学鸿. (2013) 决明子茶结合步行锻炼对中老年人减肥效果观察. *现代预防医学*. **40(13):** 2468–2470, 2474.
H136	杨一文. (2016) 祛痰清胃方治疗湿热阻滞型单纯性肥胖症临床观察. *上海中医药杂志*. **50(2):** 62–63.
H137	杨志琴, 闫冰. (2018) 桂枝茯苓丸合当归芍药汤联合二甲双胍片对肥胖型多囊卵巢综合征卵巢体积及卵泡数目的影响. *国际中医中药杂志*. **40(5):** 398–401.
H138	叶丽芳, 尚文斌, 赵娟, *et al.* (2016) 三黄汤治疗单纯性肥胖症临床观察. *南京中医药大学学报*. **32(03):** 242–244.
H139	叶丽芳, 邵鑫, 刘苏, *et al.* (2017) 三黄汤加减治疗痰湿热结型多囊卵巢综合征临床观察. *南京中医药大学学报*. **33(5):** 480–483.
H140	于洪宇. (2016) 佩连麻黄方治疗单纯性肥胖的疗效观察及对脂多糖（LPS）的影响. 黑龙江中医药大学.
H141	于淼. (2017) 解毒通络调肝方加减改善肥胖 2 型糖尿病患者糖脂代谢的临床研究. 长春中医药大学.
H142	于征. (2011) 健脾运湿法对单纯性肥胖糖调节受损脾虚不运证患者血清胰高血糖素样肽 -1、抵抗素、胰岛素水平的影响. 山东中医药大学.
H143	俞芳芳. (2012) 参术麦冬饮治疗肥胖 2 型糖尿病气阴两虚夹湿证的临床研究. 南京中医药大学.
H144	袁朵. (2012) 糖消汤联合生活方式干预痰湿体质超重, 肥胖 IGT 患者的临床观察. 湖北中医药大学.
H145	张春燕. (2011) 健脾化浊法治疗老年单纯性肥胖临床观察. *老年医学与保健*. **17(6):** 378–380.
H146	张芳. (2015) 加味黄连解毒汤对初发肥胖 2 型糖尿病患者的临床研究. 山东中医药大学.
H147	张佳琪. (2014) 自拟芪术汤治疗肥胖相关性高血压病的临床观察及对饮食诱导肥胖的实验机理研究. 山东中医药大学.
H148	张珂炜. (2017) 化痰祛瘀中药治疗肥胖 2 型糖尿病的疗效观察. *中医临床研究*. **9(16):** 70–72.

(Continued)

Study No.	Reference
H149	张昆. (2012) 茯苓颗粒对超重糖尿病患者体重的影响. *中西医结合研究.* **4(4):** 169–171.
H150	张玲玲. (2013) 通脉降压汤治疗肥胖型高血压病临床疗效观察. 山东中医药大学.
H151	张森乐. (2018) 黄连解毒汤加味对肥胖 2 型糖尿病患者血糖、血脂及胰岛 β 细胞功能的影响. *实用糖尿病杂志.* **14(1):** 54–55.
H152	张卫欢, 李秋云, 杨春伟, *et al.* (2018) 大柴胡汤加减联合利拉鲁肽对肥胖 2 型糖尿病患者胰岛素抵抗、β- 细胞功能和低度炎症反应的影响. *现代中西医结合杂志.* **27(1):** 23–26, 30.
H153	张晓冉. (2014) 三黄丹参饮治疗代谢综合征（痰湿瘀滞型）的有效性及安全性研究. 成都中医药大学.
H154	张秀琴, 王素莉. (2015) 血脂康对新发 2 型糖尿病合并超重患者胰岛素抵抗的影响. *中国实验方剂学杂志.* **21(21):** 185–188.
H155	赵晨男. (2017) 自拟平脂降糖增敏汤治疗肥胖 2 型糖尿病胰岛素抵抗的临床研究. 山东中医药大学.
H156	赵春梅, 罗喜平, 陈秀廉. (2013) 中药结合健康生活模式对多囊卵巢综合征肥胖患者体重的影响. *新中医.* **45(11):** 65–67.
H157	赵华云, 黄嘉文, 王文会, 罗翠芬. (2016) 半夏白术天麻汤干预治疗肥胖型高血压疗效观察. *辽宁中医药大学学报.* **18(12):** 14–17.
H158	赵锡艳. (2013) 降糖调脂方对 2 型糖尿病患者的糖脂肥同调疗效分析. 中国中医科学院.
H159	郑立虎. (2012) 疏肝运脾法对肥胖合并高血压的降压疗效及对胰岛素抵抗的影响. 山东中医药大学.
H160	周翠红. (2015) 益气祛湿化瘀丸联合盐酸二甲双胍治疗成人单纯性肥胖症疗效观察. *实用中医药杂志.* **31(12):** 1128–1129.
H161	周道成, 赵恒侠, 李惠林, *et al.* (2017) 荷芪散联合二甲双胍治疗肥胖型多囊卵巢综合征临床研究. *国际中医中药杂志.* **39(7):** 592–596.
H162	周海悦, 胡燕, 薛晓玲. (2018) 奥利司他治疗肥胖型多囊卵巢综合征不孕患者的疗效观察. *河北医药.* **40(17):** 2598–2602.
H163	周欢. (2016) 平陈汤对肥胖痰湿型 2 型糖尿病前期患者胰岛素抵抗指数干预的临床研究. 甘肃中医药大学.
H164	周晖. (2007) 化瘀降浊合剂干预代谢综合征的疗效评价及其对部分致动脉粥样硬化因子的影响. 北京中医药大学.

(Continued)

Study No.	Reference
H165	周辉林. (2014) 中药降糖 3 号合二甲双胍治疗 2 型糖尿病 32 例. *中国中医药现代远程教育*. **12(24):** 64–65.
H166	周晓燕, 韦湘林, 黄艳. (2011) 泻心承气汤治疗 2 型糖尿病湿热困脾证临床研究. *新中医*. **43(6):** 32–33.
H167	周雄根, 顾雯艳, 钱风华, 钱义明. (2011) 宣肺降脂方治疗单纯性肥胖疗效观察. *上海中医药杂志*. **45(4):** 43–44.
H168	周训杰, 姚磊, 符德玉, *et al.* (2017) 活血潜阳祛痰方干预肥胖高血压患者左室重构的临床观察. *上海中医药杂志*. **51(09):** 43–47.
H169	朱建伟, 留菁菁. (2013) 升阳利湿法对肥胖的糖耐量受损人群的干预性治疗效果. *中国慢性病预防与控制*. **21(2):** 226–228.
H170	朱益丽. (2017) 三黄苓术汤治疗肥胖T2DM湿热困脾证的疗效观察及对血清RBP4 的影响. *黑龙江中医药大学*.
H171	朱智琦. (2014) 益气活血降浊方对代谢综合征患者慢性亚临床炎症的临床研究. *河南中医学院*.
H172	Cho YG, Jung JH, Kang JH, *et al.* (2017) Effect of a herbal extract powder (YY-312) from Imperata cylindrica Beauvois, Citrus unshiu Markovich, and Evodia officinalis Dode on body fat mass in overweight adults: A 12-week, randomized, double-blind, placebo-controlled, parallel-group clinical trial. *BMC Complement Altern Med* **17(1):** 375.
H173	Yang Y, Wu H, Chang Y, *et al.* (2018) The effect of decoction Xiang-sha Six Jun-zi on weight reduction in subjects with simple obesity — A pilot study. *Obesity Facts* **11:** 297.
H174	Namazi N, Alizadeh M, Mirtaheri E, Farajnia S. (2017) The effect of dried Glycyrrhiza Glabra L. Extract on obesity management with regard to PPAR-gamma2 (Pro12Ala) gene polymorphism in obese subjects following an energy restricted diet. *Adv Pharm Bull* **7(2):** 221–228.
H175	Kim HJ, Park JM, Kim JA, Ko BP. (2008) Effect of herbal Ephedra sinica and Evodia rutaecarpa on body composition and resting metabolic rate: A randomized, double-blind clinical trial in Korean premenopausal women. *J Acupunct Meridian Stud* **1(2):** 128–138.
H176	Cho Y H, Ahn SC, Lee SY, *et al.* (2013) Effect of Korean red ginseng on insulin sensitivity in non-diabetic healthy overweight and obese adults. *Asia Pac J Clin Nutr* **22(3):** 365–371.

(Continued)

(Continued)

Study No.	Reference
H177	Azushima K, Tamura K, Haku S, *et al.* (2015) Effects of the oriental herbal medicine Bofu-tsusho-san in obesity hypertension: A multicenter, randomized, parallel-group controlled trial (ATH-D-14-01021.R2). *Atherosclerosis* **240(1):** 297–304.
H178	Lenon GB, Li KX, Chang YH, *et al.* (2012) Efficacy and safety of a Chinese herbal medicine formula (RCM-104) in the management of simple obesity: A randomized, placebo-controlled clinical trial. *Evid Based Complement Alternat Med* **2012:** 1–11.
H179	Yu X, Lian F, Tong X. (2016) The efficacy and safety of Chinese herbal formula JTTZ (jiangtangtiaozhi) for type 2 diabetes patients with obesity and hypertriglyceridemia: A multicenter randomized, positive controlled, open-label clinical trial. *J Altern Complement Med* **22(6):** A56–A57.
H180	Shi J, Hu Y, Wang Q. (2006) Fufang Cangzhu Tang for treatment of senile obesity or overweight complicated with impaired glucose tolerance — A clinical observation in 32 cases. *J Tradit Chin Med* **26(1):** 33–35.
H181	Greenway FL, Liu Z, Martin CK, *et al.* (2006) Safety and efficacy of NT, an herbal supplement, in treating human obesity. *Int J Obes (Lond)* **30(12):** 1737–1741.
H182	Song MY, Wang JH, Eom T, Kim H. (2015) Schisandra chinensis fruit modulates the gut microbiota composition in association with metabolic markers in obese women: A randomized, double-blind placebo-controlled study. *Nutr Res* **35(8):** 655–663.
H183	董晗硕. (2015) "通经调脏" 治疗代谢综合征 (肝胃郁热证) 的临床疗效观察. 长春中医药大学.
H184	贺飞, 吴卉丽, 蔡文, *et al.* (2017) 茶饮方联合中低热量饮食治疗脾肾阳虚型产后肥胖的临床疗效. 广西医学. **39(8):** 1146–1149.
H185	焦楠, 石亚萍, 郭志强, 王必勤. (2013) 燥湿化痰补肾方治疗肥胖型多囊卵巢综合征 26 例. 山东中医杂志. **32(02):** 86–88.
H186	刘作东, 郁萍. (2018) 津力达颗粒联合盐酸二甲双胍缓释片对初诊肥胖 2 型糖尿病糖脂代谢的临床效果观察. 中外女性健康研究. **(2):** 39–40.
H187	马建, 余海燕, 赵娜, 王云芳. (2014) 佩连麻黄方治疗单纯性肥胖的临床研究. 中医药信息 **31(1):** 46–49.
H188	马媛美. (2015) 中西医结合治疗肥胖伴胰岛素抵抗型多囊卵巢综合征的临床研究. 扬州大学.

Study No.	Reference
H189	庞颖. (2018) 基于斡旋中州法针药联合治疗肥胖型 PCOS-IR 的临床研究. 北京中医药大学.
H190	朴信映. (2004) 开郁清胃颗粒对代谢综合征胰岛素敏感性的影响. 北京中医药大学.
H191	宋艳华, 廖英, 夏亦冬, 潘芳. (2015) 益肾化痰方联合二甲双胍治疗肥胖型多囊卵巢综合征临床研究. *上海中医药杂志.* **49(05):** 66–69.
H192	谭锦萍, 张海艇, 倪建新, *et al.* (2013) 荷叶对痰湿型体质高脂血症伴肥胖影响随机平行对照研究. *实用中医内科杂志.* **27(8):** 12–13.
H193	王晨晔, 孙忻, 丁彩飞, 沈瑛红. (2016) 苍附导痰汤加减联合针刺对肥胖型多囊卵巢综合征患者糖脂代谢及排卵率的影响. *现代中西医结合杂志.* **25(36):** 4056–4058.
H194	张彤, 盖云, 冯雯, 徐诗静. (2016) 运脾活血方对脾虚湿阻型肥胖型 2 型糖尿病脂肪激素及胃肠激素的调节研究. *辽宁中医杂志.* **43(01):** 82–86.
H195	朱妍桦. (2014) 调周法联合苍附导痰汤改善肥胖型 PCOS 内分泌代谢异常的临床研究. 南京中医药大学
H196	马宁宁. (2017) 参苓白术散加减治疗肥胖型2型糖尿病脾虚湿困证的疗效观察. *中医药导报.* **23(12):** 74–76.
H197	沙开香. (2015) 自拟益气固本方联合二甲双胍缓释片对初诊超重肥胖 2 型糖尿病代谢指标的影响. *内蒙古中医药.* **34(11):** 74–75.
H198	孙丹萍. (2017) 清热降脂方联合奥利司他治疗单纯性肥胖临床研究. *陕西中医药大学学报.* **40(6):** 47–49.
H199	翁玮潞. (2017) 健脾化痰活血方对肥胖 2 型糖尿病胰岛素敏感性的影响. 辽宁中医药大学.
H200	叶慧君, 江延姣, 李爱萍, 俞渊. (2013) 桂枝茯苓胶囊联合达英 -35 治疗多囊卵巢综合征疗效观察. *浙江医学.* **17(06):** 63–65.
H201	叶金池. (2016) 祛痰调脂汤治疗腹型肥胖伴血脂异常 50 例临床观察. *中国民族民间医药.* **25(4):** 120–121.
H202	虞寒芬. (2014) 五苓散加味联合二甲双胍治疗肥胖型 2 型糖尿病 48 例疗效观察. *新中医.* **46(10):** 92–94.
H203	王文婷, 金涛. (2018) 荷叶降脂汤治疗痰湿阻滞型肥胖症疗效观察. *新中医.* **50(3):** 81–83.
H204	陈继杰. (2014) 消脂汤联合艾塞那肽治疗脾虚痰湿型代谢综合征的临床研究. 成都中医药大学.

(*Continued*)

(Continued)

Study No.	Reference
H205	姜国良, 申国明, 周萍. (2007) 三黄脂消饮改善糖耐量减低患者胰岛肽功能的临床研究. *齐齐哈尔医学院学报.* **28(21):** 2573–2574.
H206	刘雪梅, 李惠林, 赵恒侠, *et al.* (2016) 荷芪散联合利拉鲁肽治疗肥胖 2 型糖尿病 30 例. *江西中医药大学学报.* **28(1):** 50–53.
H207	罗净. (2014) 消脂汤联合艾塞那肽注射液治疗肥胖伴高尿酸血症的临床研究. 成都中医药大学.
H208	薛玉坤. (2013) 益气健脾化浊法对肥胖 2 型糖尿病的临床疗效观察. 成都中医药大学.
H209	侯丽辉, 杨新鸣, Risto Erkkola, 吴效科. (2006) 金芪降糖片治疗多囊卵巢综合征的临床研究. *中西医结合学报.* **4(6):** 579–584.
H210	陈慧, 高雅文, 陈羡人, *et al.* (2013) 参苓白术散加味治疗女性单纯性肥胖症 32 例. *浙江中医杂志.* **48(11):** 813.
H211	黄慧芹. (2010) 加味温胆汤治疗单纯性肥胖症 52 例临床观察. *中医临床研究.* **2(16):** 58–59.
H212	李成刚, 周丽, 李霜, 李晓. (2018) 加味补中益气汤治疗肥胖型多囊卵巢综合征临床疗效观察. *湖北医药学院学报.* **37(2):** 136–139.
H213	李小清, 朱小宝, 徐红. (2007) 二甲双胍结合中药治疗肥胖型多囊卵巢综合征疗效观察. *现代中西医结合杂志.* **16(13):** 1799.
H214	林敏. (2008) 化痰活血汤治疗肥胖型多囊卵巢综合征临床疗效观察. 北京中医药大学.
H215	刘新敏, 郑冬雪, 程冉. (2016) 清胃健脾法治疗超重并胰岛素抵抗型多囊卵巢综合征 52 例. *世界中医药.* **11(3):** 418–421, 426.
H216	彭小菊, 于振英, 汪川, 辛兆洋. (2014) 蒲参胶囊减肥降脂作用临床观察 — 70 例分析. *内蒙古中医药.* **33(35):** 56–57.
H217	唐红珍. (2007) 减肥方治疗单纯性肥胖症 60 例临床观察. *湖南中医杂志.* **23(4):** 17–18.
H218	熊翡. (2012) 丹溪治湿痰方加味治疗肥胖型多囊卵巢综合征 46 例. *浙江中医药大学学报.* **36(3):** 265–266.
H219	李春生. (1984) 《金匮》防己黄芪汤治疗单纯性肥胖病合并高脂血症 2 例. *传统老年医学研究论文集.* **5(2):** 136–138.
H220	黄蔚, 陈广, 黄江荣. (2018) 黄祥武以健脾祛湿, 活血化瘀法治疗单纯性肥胖症的经验. *辽宁中医杂志.* **45(6):** 1157–1159.
H221	李旭. (2008) 孙定隆运用启宫丸治疗代谢性疾病的临床经验. *辽宁中医药大学学报.* **10(5):** 72–73.

(Continued)

Study No.	Reference
H222	李智滨, 崔志梅. (2015) 王淑玲健脾化湿法治疗单纯性肥胖经验. *中医临床研究*. **7(18):** 8–9.
H223	刘永平. (2014) 防风通圣丸的临床应用. *内蒙古中医药*. **33(9):** 75–76.
H224	王媛媛, 冯志海. (2017) 冯志海教授治疗湿热型肥胖验案 2 则. *中国中医药现代远程教育*. **15(4):** 129–131.
H225	徐彦飞, 刘津, 李振华. (2011) 李振华教授治疗单纯性肥胖病经验. *中华中医药杂志*. **26(7):** 1542–1543.
H226	许振伟. (2000) 启宫丸加减治疗单纯性肥胖症举隅. *实用中医药杂志*. **16(11):** 40.
H227	周强, 张家成, 夏乐, 仝小林. (2010) 仝小林教授运用小陷胸汤治疗单纯性肥胖症验案解析. *中国美容医学*. **19(z4):** 173–174.
H228	段阳泉. (2009) 二陈汤加味治疗肥胖验案 2 则. *江苏中医药*. **41(2):** 41–42.
H229	陆西宛, 陆曙. (2011) 陆曙教授治疗代谢综合征验案 2 则. *现代中医药*. **31(6):** 1–2.
H230	Kwon S, Jung W, Byun AR, *et al*. (2015) Administration of Hwang-Ryun-Haedok-tang, a herbal complex, for patients with abdominal obesity: A case series. *Explore (NY)*. **11(5):** 401–406.
H231	Han K, Bose S, Kim YM, *et al*. (2015) Rehmannia glutinosa reduced waist circumferences of Korean obese women possibly through modulation of gut microbiota. *Food Funct*. **6(8):** 2684–2692.
H232	Kim HJ, Gallagher D, Song MY. (2005) Comparison of body composition methods during weight loss in obese women using herbal formula. *Am J Chin Med*. **33(6):** 851–858.

6

Pharmacological Actions of Frequently Used Herbs

OVERVIEW

This chapter reviews the available experimental evidence to explore the possible biological activities and mechanisms of the 10 most frequently used herbs from randomised clinical trials in Chapter 5. The herbs showed anti-obesity actions and regulated gut microbiota, which are important mechanisms underlying their effects on weight loss and weight maintenance.

Introduction

The evidence from clinical studies included in Chapter 5 have shown the benefits of Chinese herbal medicines (CHMs) in reducing weight and waist circumference and improving metabolic outcomes. If such treatments play a role in the clinical management of obesity, it is important to examine how CHMs exert their clinical effects. This chapter reviews experimental evidence from *in vitro* experimental cells and *in vivo* animal models for some of the most frequently used herbs in clinical trials.

The pathological processes and mechanisms of obesity are complicated and have been described in Chapter 1. The basic pathogenesis of obesity involves either up-regulation of appetite or down-regulation of calorie utilisation governing cellular functions, physical activity, etc., to cause the accumulation of extra body fat into adipocytes with an increase in the number and size.

Various animal models have been well established and used to study obesity and type 2 diabetes mellitus (T2DM). In this chapter, spontaneous and targeted monogenic models include the *ob/ob* and *db/db* mice and *fa/fa* rats. The *ob/ob* mouse model has a mutated leptin receptor showing mild diabetes but severe obesity. The *db/db* mouse model has leptin deficiency; it is more moderately obese but still severely diabetic. Zucker (*fa/fa*) rats, similar to the *ob/ob* mouse, lead to hyperphagia and become profoundly obese. In addition, diet-induced obesity (DIO) rodents are typically given free access to calorie-dense foods highly enriched in fats, known as high-fat diets (HFDs), to induce obesity and T2DM.[1]

Methods

The key herbs reviewed were *fu ling* 茯苓, *bai zhu* 白术, *ban xia* 半夏, *chen pi* 陈皮, *huang lian* 黄连, *dan shen* 丹参, *huang qi* 黄芪, *da huang* 大黄, *he ye* 荷叶 and *ge gen* 葛根. To identify experimental studies on their pharmacological actions of relevance to obesity, the activities of each herb and/or main compounds were examined to identify their therapeutic effects on the prevention of obesity, including regulatory effects on adipocyte differentiation and lipid metabolism, lipase inhibitory effects, increase in energy expenditure, appetite suppressant effects and related brain and gut hormones that modulate body weight and food intake. Regulatory effects on gut microbiota were also examined.

The constituent compounds were identified by searching herbal monographs, high-quality reviews of CHM, *materia medica* and the PubMed biomedical database. To identify pre-clinical studies, a literature search in PubMed, Google Scholar and PubMed Central was undertaken. Search terms included the scientific names of the plant as well as the Chinese pinyin and names of the main compounds found in the plants. These were combined with terms for obesity, 3T3-L1 adipocytes, body weight, body fat, lipid metabolism, lipase inhibition, thermogenesis, energy expenditure, browning of white adipose tissue, brown adipose tissue, brain and gut hormones related to appetite and body weight, gut microbiota and obese rodent models.

Experimental Studies on *fu ling*

Fu ling 茯苓 is derived from the dried sclerotium of the fungus *Poria cocos* (Schw.) Wolf (*Polyporaceae*). The major compounds in *P. cocos* are triterpenoids (lanostane and 3,4-secolanostane skeletons) and polysaccharides (beta-pachyman). Pharmacological activities include anti-inflammatory, anti-oxidative and anti-apoptotic effects, and anti-viral activities.[2] Other pharmacological effects in relation to obesity are discussed.

Anti-obesity Actions

Being one of the most commonly used herbs in clinical studies included in Chapter 5, most available studies on *P. cocos* are mainly related to T2DM, although it is strongly associated with obesity actions that may be relevant to the pathogenesis of obesity. These studies have been summarised below.

3T3-L1 adipocytes are commonly used to study fat metabolism. The crude polysaccharides from *P. cocos* exert the effects of lipogenesis suppression and bi-directional regulation of adipogenesis with stimulating differentiation of 3T3-L1 preadipocyte at lower concentration and inhibiting differentiation at a high concentration.[3] Anti-obesity activity of *P. cocos* was mainly attributed to its function in lipid metabolism. *P. cocos* was reported to regulate lipid metabolism in HFD-fed rats by improving HFD-induced hyperlipidaemia, such as the elevation of plasma triglyceride (TG) and total and low-density lipoprotein cholesterol (LDL-C) concentrations, and the associated abnormalities of the lipid metabolites in the plasma fatty acids and sterols.[4] In addition to crude extracts of *P. cocos*, dehydro-trametenolic acid, one triterpene constituent of *P. cocos*, was demonstrated to reduce hyperglycaemia in obese *db/db* mice through activating the peroxide proliferator-activated receptor γ (PPARγ), a regulator of lipid metabolism predominately expressed in adipose tissue that stimulates adipose differentiation to ameliorate dyslipidemia and improve adiposity.[5]

Regulation of Gut Microbiota

In recent decades, substantial evidence has indicated that numerous species of gut microbiota play a vital role in the development and onset of obesity in animals and humans. Of particular interest is a reduction in *Bacteroidetes* and the ratio of *Bacteroidetes* to *Firmicutes*, where various species of *Lactobacillus*, *Bifidobacterium* and *Akkermansia muciniphila* are strongly associated with obesity.[6]

Oral administration with water insoluble polysaccharide from *fu ling* in obese *ob/ob* mice greatly modulated the composition of gut microbiota by increasing the abundance of *Bacteroidetes* and decreasing the abundance of *Megamonas* and *Proteus* that play important roles in pro-inflammatory responses and obesity. The polysaccharide was also demonstrated to enhance butyrate production, which is involved in the maintenance of gut homeostasis. Even more, faecal transplantation with the microbiota of *fu ling* polysaccharide-treated mice to *ob/ob* mice could ameliorate hyperglycaemia and lipid metabolism through improving glucose and lipid homeostasis.[7] In addition, carboxymethylated pachyman (CMP), a polysaccharide isolated from the *P. cocos*, was reported to reverse chemotherapeutic agent 5-fluorouracil-induced intestinal microflora disorders in the CT26 colon tumour-bearing mice by increasing the proportion of *Bacteroidetes*, *Lactobacilli* and butyric acid-producing and acetic acid-producing bacteria, and restoring the intestinal flora diversity.[8]

Experimental Studies on *bai zhu*

Bai zhu 白术 is from the rhizome of *Atractylodes macrocephala* Koidz. Sesquiterpenoids, polyacetylenes and polysaccharides are the major bioactive constituents that contribute much of the pharmacological activities, including anti-inflammatory, anti-oxidative, anti-osteoporotic, anti-bacterial, anti-tumour, anti-ageing, anti-obesity and neuroprotective activities, gonadal hormone regulation and energy-enhancing metabolism.[9]

Anti-obesity Actions

A. macrocephala demonstrated an anti-adipogenic effect by inhibiting 3T3-L1 adipocyte differentiation in a dose-dependent manner with a concomitant decrease in lipid accumulation through the inhibition of the PI3/Akt pathway. In addition to this *in vitro* study, administration of *A. macrocephala* to DIO rats significantly reduced the body weight gain along with decreased plasma TG levels via affecting adipogenesis and energy expenditure.[10] More interestingly, the fermented *A. macrocephala* (FRAM) showed more potent anti-adipogenic activity in differentiated 3T3-L1 adipocytes and greater anti-obesity activity in HFD plus liposaccharide-treated rats by effectively reducing body weights and abdominal and total fat pads with an attenuation of serum total cholesterol (TC) and TG levels and an increase in the serum high-density lipoprotein (HDL) content.[11]

Stimulating energy expenditure in muscle and brown fat offers a strategy to reduce body weight for treating obesity by the induction of non-shivering thermogenesis. The root of *A. macrocephala* was found to improve lipid and glucose metabolism by enhancing the activities of peroxisome proliferator-activated receptor gamma coactivator 1 alpha (PGC1α) and adenosine monophosphate-activated protein kinase (AMPK) in C_2C_{12} skeletal muscle cells.[12] A further study indicated that atractylenolide III was the responsible compound for the activities.[13] More recently, the administration of aqueous *A. macrocephala* extracts in DIO mice not only decreased body weight and serum TC levels with increases in the expression of PGC1α and AMPK but also increased the brown adipocyte count and the expression of uncoupling protein 1 (UCP1), a marker of non-shivering thermogenesis in mitochondria-rich brown adipose tissue. These data suggested that *A. macrocephala* could prevent diet-induced obesity by increasing the metabolic rate in skeletal muscle and brown adipose tissue.[14]

Regulation of Gut Microbiota

The root of *A. macrocephala* has been known to adjust disordered intestinal flora due to its abundant polysaccharides and atractylenolides. It was found that the consumption rate of reducing sugar was increased *in vitro* when *A. macrocephala* was incubated with human/rat intestinal bacterial mixture from faeces. In the *C. angustifolia* extract (CAE)-induced disordered model of intestinal flora, *A. macrocephala* could significantly improve disordered intestinal flora evaluated by the ERIC-PCR fingerprinting method.[15] Furthermore, FRAM showed a great beneficial impact on the distribution profile of intestinal bacteria by reversing the HFD plus LPS-induced reduction in the relative abundance of *Bifidobacterium* spp., *Akkermansia* spp., *Bacteroidetes* and *Lactobacillus* spp., as well as the *Bacteroidetes/Firmicutes* ratio, which were reported to reverse HFD-induced obesity.[11]

Experimental Studies on *ban xia*

Ban xia 半夏 (*Pinellia ternata* (Thunb.) Breit.) contains many bioactive compounds, including alkaloids, lectins, fatty acids, cerebrosides, volatile oils, phenylpropanoids, sterols, flavonoids, furans and others. Pharmacological activities include anti-tumour, anti-emetic, anti-tussive, anti-microbial, anti-fungal, anti-viral, sedative, hypnotic and anti convulsant activities.[16]

The thermogenic effect of *P. ternata* has been believed to contribute to anti-obesity. Treatment with the water extract of *P. ternata* in Zucker (*fa/fa*) rats slightly reduced body weight, remarkably lowered the levels of TG and free fatty acids in the blood of the obese rats, and significantly increased the expression of both UCP1 in brown adipose tissue and PPARα and PGC1α in visceral white adipose tissue, indicating that the anti-obesity effect of *P. ternata* was through affecting thermogenesis and fatty acid oxidation by leading the white fat deposits to convert into thermogenically active brown adipose tissue.[17] Moreover, an extract of petroleum ether processed rhizomes of *P. ternata* was confirmed to have a moderate reduction of TNF-α-induced NF-κB activity and a strong PPARα and PPARα activity due to containing fatty acids as PPAR-agonists to combat obesity.[18] Due to the limited number of studies assessing *ban xia*'s effects on obesity-related cell or animal models, the full extent of its benefits is yet to be elucidated.

Experimental Studies on *chen pi*

Chen pi 陈皮 is derived from the dried peel of *Citrus reticulata* Blanco. Alkaloids, flavonoids and essential oils are the main bioactive compounds. *Chen pi* possesses wide beneficial effects on the cardiovascular system, digestive system, respiratory system, as well as liver protective effects, neuroprotective effects, anti-tumour, anti-oxidant, and anti-inflammatory properties.[19] Other pharmacological effects in relation to obesity are discussed.

Anti-obesity Actions

It was reported that an extract of *C. reticulata* reduced HFD-induced body weight gain in mice without affecting food intake, reduced abdominal fat mass, shifted the adipocyte size to a smaller and more condensed range and exhibited significantly lower plasma TC, plasma apoB-100 and the production of very low-density lipoprotein (VLDL)/LDL. These beneficial anti-obesity effects might be associated with the activation of AMPK in adipose tissue and be due to a high content of 5-demethylated polymethoxyflavones (5-OH PMFs), including 5-OH nobiletin and 5-OH tangeretin in *C. reticulata*.[20]

Indeed, citrus polymethoxyflavones (PMFs), such as nobiletin, tangeretin (TAN), hydroxylated polymethoxyflavones (HPMFs) and 3,5,6,7,8,3',4'-heptamethoxyflavone (HMF), have been of increasing interest due to their promising therapeutic effects for metabolic disorders. In 3T3-L1 adipocytes, nobiletin was observed to lower lipid accumulation in cultured cells and decrease the expression of the key transcription regulators of adipogenesis C/EBPβ and PPARγ.[21] *In vivo*, nobiletin improved adiposity and dyslipidemia, supported by decreasing body weight gain, white adipose tissue weight and plasma TG, and increasing fatty acid oxidation in DIO mice through regulating the expression of lipid metabolism-related and adipokine genes, such as PPARα and PPARγ, as well as their target genes sterol regulatory element-binding protein-1c (SREBP-1c), fatty acid synthase, stearoyl-CoA desaturase-1 (SCD-1), carnitine palmitoyltransferase-1 (CPT-1 — the rate-limiting enzyme in mitochondrial β-oxidation for reducing body fat), uncoupling protein 2 (UCP2 — a mitochondrial proton transporter to influence body temperature, energy expenditure and fat mass) and adiponectin.[22]

Tangeretin also demonstrates an effect on human hepatoma HepG2 cell lipoprotein and lipid metabolism *in vitro.*[23] Substantial hypolipidemic responses in diet-induced hypercholesterolemia hamsters *in vivo* were shown by a reduced serum total and VLDL and LDL cholesterol and TG through activating PPAR to positively regulate fatty acid oxidation.[24] Additionally, HPMFs were shown to effectively suppress the accumulation of lipid droplets in adipocytes and decrease HFD-induced weight gain and relative fat weight in C57BL/6 mice with the decreased serum levels of aspartate aminotransferase, alanine aminotransferase, TG and TC through modulating PPARγ, SREBP-1c, fatty acid-binding protein 2 (aP2), fatty acid synthase and acetyl-coenzyme A carboxylase (ACC).[25]

More recently, HMF was reported to prevent rats from developing HFD-induced obesity and hyperlipidaemia. Treatment with HMF not only significantly reduced body weight gain and adipose tissue weight but also markedly decreased serum TC, TG and LDL-C levels, as well as the decreased weight, TG levels and lipid droplets in the liver through downregulating genes related to adipogenesis transcription and inflammatory responses, and upregulating genes related to fatty acid oxidation and energy expenditure.[26]

A pronounced effect on obesity of immature *C. reticulata* extract, which contains synephrine, was proven to exert adipose thermogenesis through promoting browning of white adipose tissue to maintain energy homeostasis in C57BL/6 mice fed a HFD. It demonstrated a decrease in body weight gain, epididymal fat weight, serum TG and TC, as well as an improvement in cold tolerance during acute cold challenge.[27]

Experimental Studies on *huang lian*

Huang lian 黄连 is derived from the dried rhizome of *Coptis chinensis* Franch. Chemical constituents include alkaloids, lignans, phenylpropanoids, flavonoids, phenolic acids, saccharides and steroids. Among them, protoberberine type alkaloids, such as berberine, palmatine, coptisine, epiberberine, jatrorrhizine and columamine, are the main bioactive components. *Huang lian* and its main alkaloids exhibit many biological activities, including anti-inflammatory, anti-pathogenic microorganisms, anti-cancer, anti-hyperglycaemic, anti-diabetic, neuroprotective and cardioprotective effects.[28]

Anti-obesity Actions

Huang lian and its alkaloids, in particular berberine, have been extensively studied from many aspects of pathogenesis of obesity, including regulation of adipocyte differentiation, lipid metabolism, lipase inhibition, energy expenditure and brain and gut hormones (such as glucagon-like peptide-1 [GLP-1] and neuropeptide Y to modulate body weight and appetite/food intake).

It has been revealed that in 3T3-L1 cells, the methanol extract of *huang lian*, together with its five isolated alkaloids (berberine, coptisine, palmatine, epiberberine and magnoflorine), were found to significantly inhibit adipocyte differentiation and cellular TG accumulation through downregulating protein levels of PPARγ and C/EBP,[29] which was consistent with the reported mechanism for the anti-adipogenic activity of berberine via suppressing PPARγ pathway[30] and decreasing CREB transcriptional activity.[31] It has been well known that adipose TG lipase and hormone-sensitive lipase (HSL) control the hydrolysis of TG to increase lipolysis to counteract obesity. Berberine was also reported to increase the expression of p-HSL and adipose TG lipase in differentiated 3T3-L1 adipocytes through the AMPK pathway.[32]

The anti-obesity potential of *huang lian* has also been demonstrated in *in vivo* studies. Treatment with *huang lian* and berberine in DIO mice resulted in significant reduction of body and visceral adipose weight through the activation of fasting-induced adipose factor and related gene expressions of mitochondrial energy metabolism such as AMPK, PGC1α, UCP2 and CPT-1α in visceral adipose tissue.[33] In addition to berberine, other alkaloids derived from *huang lian*, including coptisine, palmatine, epiberberine and jatrorrhizine, also prevented body weight gain, reduced the serum levels of TC, TG and LDL-C, and increased HDL-C in diet-induced hyperlipidaemic hamsters[34] and in a DIO mouse model.[35]

Down-regulation of adiponectin and its two main receptors (AdipoR1 and AdipoR2) is involved in the development of obesity. Berberine was reported to upregulate the expression of AdipoR1 and AdipoR2, consequently elevating the production of adiponectin and induced lipolysis. It is also reported to directly upregulate lipolysis-related genes, such as those encoding lipoprotein lipase (LPL), PPARα, CPT-1 and medium-chain acyl-CoA dehydrogenase.[36]

Several studies of berberine on increasing energy expenditure through stimulating energy-dissipation via brown adipose tissue activation and white-to-brown adipose tissue conversion were reported. The treatment with berberine significantly protected the obese *db/db* mice from weight gain, inhibited fat accumulation, increased energy expenditure and adaptive thermogenesis, improved cold tolerance, enhanced brown adipose tissue activity by promoting thermogenic programme in brown adipose tissue. Berberine also induced the development of brown-like adipocytes in inguinal adipose depots by inducing the activation of a network of genes (such as UCP1, PGC-1α, estrogen-related receptor-α and nuclear respiratory factor 1), fatty acid oxidation and other classical brown adipose tissue marker genes, controlling energy expenditure and thermogenic programme in white and brown adipose tissue and primary adipocytes via a mechanism involving AMPK and PGC-1α signalling.[37] Collectively, berberine dramatically enhanced thermogenic stimuli by switching the existing white adipocytes to beige adipocytes in subcutaneous fat (white-to-brown adipose tissue conversion) and by forming new beige adipocytes from adipogenic progenitor cells.[38]

AMPK, an energy sensor, is the master regular of energy metabolism by activating ATP-generating catabolic processes (such as glycolysis, lipolysis and fatty acid oxidation) and by inhibiting ATP-consuming anabolic processes (such as gluconeogenesis, fatty acid synthesis and cholesterol synthesis). A large body of evidence indicated that berberine could modulate central and peripheral AMPK activity to combat obesity.[39] It has been demonstrated that berberine exerted anti-obesity effects in obese *db/db* mice and HFD-fed Wistar rats through the activation of AMPK in both myotubes and adipocytes *in vitro* and in peripheral tissues (such as liver, muscle and adipose tissues) to directly increase energy expenditure.[40] The peripheral AMPK activation was confirmed and AMPK activation in the central nervous system was further explored as well in obese *db/db* and *ob/ob* mice to indirectly increase whole-body energy homeostasis.[41]

Modulation of Microbiota-gut-brain Axis

As berberine was reported to be able to cross the blood-brain barrier to modulate AMPK activity in the central nervous system,[42] it might regulate food intake and body weight in the hypothalamus through neuropeptide expressions.[43]

The administration of berberine-reduced *Firmicutes* abundance moderately increased *Bacteroidetes* abundance, resulting in a higher *Bacteroidetes*-to-*Firmicutes* (B/F) ratio in DIO rats. It also could increase the proportion of short-chain fatty acid-producing bacteria such as *Bacteroides* and *Bilophila*. These changes of gut microbiota could stimulate gut hormone production to promote an elevated level of GLP-1 expression in gut L cells and GLP-1 receptor (GLP-1R) expression in the hypothalamus, leading to an increase in serum GLP-1 level and a decrease in neuropeptide Y (NPY, appetite/food intake-stimulator). GLP-1 is a target of a number of drugs for T2DM — it can stimulate the satiety centre of the hypothalamus to reduce appetite and also bind to receptors on islet β-cells, and increase insulin secretion. Meanwhile, ultra-structural changes were revealed that berberine intervention could reverse HFD feeding that had caused structural distortion and cytoplasm swelling of the cellular body of the hypothalamus. All of the above changes resulted in decreased weight gain, endogenous glucose production and lipolysis of HFD-fed rats.[44]

Regulation of Gut Microbiota

Berberine has been an over-the-counter drug in China for microbial diarrhoea treatment for many years. Its regulation of gut microbiota has been extensively studied and proven to counteract obesity through suppressing calorie intake, HFD-induced weight gain, adipogenesis and *de novo* lipogenesis.

Although the bioavailability of berberine is very low, with 5–10% of the absorption rate in the intestinal tract, it could be able to modulate the structure and diversity of gut microbiota to restore the balance of disrupted gut microflora associated with the obese condition. It may enrich beneficial microbes and inhibit harmful microbes, as evidenced by significantly reducing the activity of disaccharidase and α-glucosidase in the intestinal tract, resulting in a reduction in the absorption of glucose and postprandial hyperglycaemia.[45,46] Furthermore, it may significantly increase the abundance of microbial species negatively associated with obesity; namely, *Sporobacter termitidis*, *Alcaligenes faecalis* and *Akkermansia muciniphila*, and decrease the abundance of the microbial species positively associated with obesity; namely, *Escherichia coli*, *Desulfovibrio C21-c20*, and *Parabacteroides distasonis* in high-fat and high-cholesterol induced hyperlipidaemic B6 mice.[47]

Several studies on rats and mice have shown that the administration of *huang lian* demonstrated similar reverting effects as metformin on the HFD-induced structural changes of gut microbiota through enriching short-chain fatty acid-producing bacteria and normalising microbial diversity, resulting in decreased degradation of dietary polysaccharides, lower additional calorie intake in the gut and *de novo* lipogenesis.[33,48,49]

It is believed that adiposity was associated with the downregulated intestinal B/F ratio that might increase the capacity to harvest energy from the diet.[6] Other studies demonstrated that berberine could modulate gut microbiota by restoring the relative level of *Bifidobacteria* and the B/F abundance ratio.[44,50]

Experimental Studies on *dan shen*

Dan shen 丹參 is derived from the dried root of *Salvia miltiorrhiza* Bunge (SM). Based on their structural characteristics, the principal bioactive constituents can be classified into two groups. A lipid-soluble lipophilic group (known as tanshinones) includes tanshinone I, tanshinone IIA, tanshinone IIB, cryptotanshinone and dihydrotanshinone. A water-soluble polyphenolic group (known as salvianolic acids/depsides) includes salvianolic acid B (Sal B), salvianolic acid A (Sal A) and danshensu.[51] Pharmacological activities include anti-inflammatory, anti-oxidant, anti-neuropathic pain, anti-diabetes, anti-cancer, anti-fibrotic, anti-hepatocyte and neuroprotective activities.[51]

Anti-obesity Actions

Tanshinone IIA, a lipophilic diterpene, was reported to prevent 3T3-L1 preadipocyte differentiation and adipogenesis through suppressing PPARγ and C/EBPα activities and the PPARγ-related gene expression, such as αP2, CD36, LPL and UCP-2. It also inhibits lipogenesis and glucose uptake through increasing phosphorylation of AMPKα and its downstream effector of ACC in 3T3-L1 cells.[52] This tanshinone IIA-mediated strong anti-adipogenic effect was further confirmed through downregulation of the expression and/or phosphorylation levels of C/EBPα, PPARγ, fatty acid synthase, perilipin A and phosphorylation levels of the signal transducer and activator of transcription-3/5 (STAT-3/5) in 3T3-L1 preadipocytes and zebrafish.[53] Sal B, a water-soluble ingredient, was reported to reduce glycerol release, enhance adipocytes glycolysis capacity and mitochondrial respiration through PGC-1α.[54]

In vivo, tanshinone IIA showed anti-obesity effects on DIO mice with a significant reduction of body weight, fat to body weight ratio, the size of the adipocytes in white adipose tissue and TG, HDL, as well as LDL levels in obese mice through the regulation of AMPK/ACC signalling pathways and inhibition of PPARγ activity.[52] More recently, a similar anti-obesity effect as tanshinone IIA was observed in HFD-fed obese mice with Sal B treatment involving the regulation of adipogenic differentiation through PPARγ, c/EBP α and SREBP-1 in adipose tissues,[55] and the regulation of the expression of mRNA, circular ribonucleic acid (circRNA) and long non-coding RNA lncRNA) in epididymal white adipose tissue induced by a high-fat diet in obese mice.[56]

In addition, tanshinone IIA was demonstrated to promote white adipose tissue browning supported by significantly upregulating ectopic expression of PGC-1α in white adipose tissue of tanshinone-treated mice, resulting in weight loss.[52] Sal B was reported, similar to metformin, to enhance adipogenesis in interscapular brown adipose tissue, thereby promoting energy utilisation through non-shivering thermogenesis, evidenced by increased protein expression levels of C/EBPα, PPARγ, PPARα and SREBP-1.[55]

Regulation of Gut Microbiota

It has been shown that the aerial parts of *S. miltiorrhiza* Bge., rich in salvianolic acids similar to the rhizome, could repair the intestinal barrier damage of streptozocin (STZ)-induced diabetic mice. The STZ-caused lower level of vasoactive intestinal peptide, a stimulator for the secretion of pancreatic and intestinal juice, was significantly increased by *S. miltiorrhiza*, while the STZ-induced higher level of advanced glycation end products, a useful non-invasive marker for tissue damage, was significantly decreased. More importantly, treatment with *S. miltiorrhiza* could normalise the STZ-caused lower level of microbial community alpha diversity of gut microbiota and modulate the gut microbiota imbalance of diabetic mice induced by STZ by significantly improving the *Firmicutes/Bacteroidetes* ratio and the relative abundance of *Deferribacteres* in diabetic mice.[57]

Experimental Studies on *huang qi*

Huang qi 黄芪 is from the dried root of *Astragalus membranaceus* (Fisch.) Bunge var. *mongholicus*. More than 200 compounds have been identified, including saponins, flavonoids, polysaccharides and amino acids. Among them, the triterpenoid saponin astragaloside IV is a principal active component. Pharmacological activities include anti-inflammatory, anti-oxidative, anti-fibrotic, anti-asthma, anti-cancer, anti-diabetic, anti-hyperglycaemic, anti-ageing, anti-tumour, anti viral, immunostimulant, cardioprotective and hepatoprotective effects.[58]

Anti-obesity Actions

Huang qi and its saponins, in particular, astragaloside IV, has attracted great attention in the last decade for its strong pharmacological effects on obesity, diabetes and hyperlipidaemia.[59]

Hypolipidaemic effects were observed in *huang qi* and its compounds. Although *huang qi* treatment showed no effect on body weight and intra-abdominal white adipose tissue mass when normalised to body weights in the DIO rats, it did result in a decrease in adipocyte size, improved lipid metabolic parameters and decreased infiltration of macrophages. This consequently alleviated the inflammatory state of white adipose tissue, which is associated with HFD-induced obesity. In addition, the mammalian target of rapamycin complex 1 (mTORC1) activation by *huang qi* treatment led to an enhanced expression of PPARγ in differentiated 3T3-L1 cells, indicating beneficial effects through the upregulation of the mTORC1-PPARγ signalling pathway.[60] *A. membranaceus* polysaccharides were reported to effectively reduce the metabolic stress-induced increase of body weight, leptin and hepatic TG levels in metabolically stressed transgenic mice.[61] Astragaloside IV also ameliorated adipose dysfunction and inhibited adipose lipolysis in HFD-fed mice by reducing cAMP accumulation via regulation of Akt phosphodiesterase 3B (PDE3B).[62]

More interestingly, the anti-obesity effect of astragaloside IV reversed leptin resistance and thermogenic disorder and modulated the leptin-mediated appetite-associated gene expression in the hypothalamus.

In DIO mice, it effectively reduced body weight gain and food intake, lessened adipocyte size and decreased adipose tissue weight with notably diminished serum TG and TC levels. Moreover, it also increased energy expenditure with the elevated carbon dioxide production and oxygen uptake and decreased the amplitude of the circadian respiratory exchange ratio of DIO mice. Further, mechanism studies showed that astragaloside IV modulated energy homeostasis through upregulating thermogenesis associated gene expressions in brown adipose tissue such as ADRβ3, PPARα, PPARγ, PGC-1α, PGC-1β, UCP1 and UCP2, and enhanced leptin sensitivity and appetite-associated genes, such as an elevated protein level of melanin-concentrating hormone receptor 4 (MC4R, appetite/food intake — inhibition) and a reduced protein level of NPY (appetite/ food intake — stimulation) in the hypothalamus of DIO mice. While astragaloside IV did not change body weight gain and appetite-associated genes in leptin receptor-deficient *db/db* mice, lower TG and TC were observed.[63]

Formononetin derived from *huang qi* was found to induce adipocyte thermogenesis *in vitro* and reduce body weight gain and increase energy expenditure in DIO mice with an increase of adipocyte UCP1 expression through a non-classical PPARγ agonist to regulate PPARγ activity.[64]

Regulation of Gut Microbiota

The effect of *huang qi* on the gut-microbiota composition was explored in T2DM mice. *Huang qi* could alter the relative abundance of several key bacterial species, such as the increased abundance of *Lactobacillus* and *Bifidobacterium*, a decreased abundance of *Clostridium cluster XI* and the normalisation of the microbial diversity and richness. These changes of gut microbiota resulted in a significantly reduced body weight of T2DM mice.[65]

Experimental Studies on *da huang*

Da huang 大黄 is derived from the dried root and rhizome of *Rheum palmatum* L., *Rheum tanguticum* Maxim. ex Balf or *Rheum officinale* Baill. Anthraquinones (mainly including emodin, rhein, chrysophanic acid and physcion), bianthrone, stilbenes, polysaccharides and tannins are the main bioactive compounds that exert anti-inflammatory, anti-bacterial, anti-fungal, anti-tumour, anti-oxidant, anti-fibrosis, hepatoprotective and nephroprotective activities.[66]

Anti-obesity Actions

The anti-obesity effects of *da huang* are largely attributed to its active compounds. The effects of rhein (4,5-dihydroxyanthraquinone-2-carboxylic acid) on the inhibition of 3T3-L1 preadipocyte differentiation and lipogenesis were observed through downregulating the expressions of adipogenesis-specific transcription factors PPARγ and C/EBPα, and their downstream target genes involved in adipocyte differentiation, such as CD36, aP2, acyl-CoA oxidase, UCP2, ACC and fatty acid synthase, in both 3T3-L1 preadipocytes and mice. In DIO mice, HFD-induced weight gain and adiposity were also reversed by rhein.[67] Rhein demonstrated not only to block HFD-induced obesity with decreases in fat mass, the size of white and brown adipocytes, and lower serum cholesterol and LDL in DIO mice but also to reduce the fat weight of *db/db* mouse through inhibiting PPARγ trans-activity and the expression of its target genes.[68] Further mechanism studies indicated that rhein suppressed the expression levels of liver X receptor target genes in both 3T3-L1 and HepG2 cells *in vitro* by directly binding to these receptors that play important roles in regulating cholesterol homeostasis and energy metabolism. Moreover, *in vivo*, rhein increased adaptive thermogenesis by activating the UCP1 expression in brown adipose tissue in wild-type mice and reprogrammed the expression of liver X receptor target genes related to adipogenesis and cholesterol metabolism in white adipose tissue, muscle and liver of mice, indicating that rhein protected against obesity and related metabolic disorders through liver X receptor antagonism and the regulation of thermogenesis.[69]

Emodin (1,3,8-trihydroxy-6-methylanthraquinone) is a potent and selective inhibitor of 11β-hydroxysteroid dehydrogenase type 1 (11β-HSD1) with the ability to ameliorate metabolic disorders in DIO mice. The effects of emodin on adipocyte function *in vitro* demonstrated that it inhibited the 11β-HSD1 activity in 3T3-L1 adipocytes and suppressed 11-dehydrocorticosterone-induced adipogenesis and lipolysis. In *ob/ob* mice, long-term emodin administration decreased 11β-HSD1 activity in mesenteric adipose tissues.[70] It was also suggested that the anti-obesity effect of emodin involved the regulation of the sterol regulatory element-binding proteins (SREBP) pathway to reduce body weight and the size of white and brown adipocytes and decrease blood lipids during administration to DIO mice.[71]

The anti-obesity effect of chrysophanic acid was examined in *in vitro* models (of 3T3-L1 adipocytes and primary cultured brown adipocytes) and *in vivo* models of DIO mice and zebrafish. Chrysophanic acid inhibited lipid accumulation in 3T3-L1 adipocytes, accompanied by the decreased expression of adipogenic and lipogenic genes, such as PPARγ and C/EBP. It also activated the thermogenesis of brown adipocytes with the increased expression of thermogenic factors, such as UCP1 and PGC1α. *In vivo*, administration of chrysophanic acid to DIO mice resulted in decreases in body weight, food intake, TC, TG, LDL-C and cholesterol. These data suggested that chrysophanic acid ameliorated obesity through the activation of AMPK to regulate the adipogenic and thermogenic pathways.[72]

Physcion was also observed to reduce body and white adipose tissue weights of DIO mice, enhance energy expenditure, suppress lipid accumulation in white adipose tissue by decreasing fatty acid synthesis and increase lipolysis and fatty acid oxidation.[73] As to the anti-lipase effects of *da huang,* it has been reported to exert *in vitro* lipase inhibitory activity against porcine pancreatic lipase (PPL, triacylglycerol lipase) to inhibit adsorption of dietary lipids and reduce body weight gain, indicating a rich source of anti-lipase compounds.[74]

Regulation of Gut Microbiota

It was shown that oral administration of rhein remarkably stimulated gut hormone production to promote an elevated level of GLP-1 (appetite/food intake — inhibition) expression in the L-cells of the gut terminal ileum, leading to an increase in the plasma active GLP-1 in *db/db* mice. Furthermore, rhein treatment maintained the diversity of gut microbiota communities of diabetic mice with a relative abundance of *Bacteroides* and *Akkermansia*, while antibiotics reduced the diversity of the community significantly.[75]

A purified anthraquinone-glycoside preparation from *da huang* was also demonstrated in diabetic rats induced by HFD combined with STZ to ameliorate gut dysbiosis with a greater abundance of probiotic *Lactobacillus* and short-chain fatty acid-producing bacteria that stimulated intestinal L cells to secrete more GLP-1, and also by reducing the abundance of the *Lachnospiraceae* NK4A136 group and LPS-producing *Desulfovibrio* to enhance intestinal integrity that would suppress chronic systemic inflammation responses.[76]

Experimental Studies on *he ye*

He ye 荷叶 (*Nelumbo nucifera* Gaertn), also known as lotus, contains diverse natural compounds, including alkaloids, flavonoids, glycosides, terpenoids, steroids, fatty acids, proteins, minerals and vitamins. Pharmacological activities target stress, cancer, microbial infection, diabetes, inflammation, oxidation, atherosclerosis and obesity.[77]

Anti-obesity Actions

He ye has been widely used in weight-loss foods to prevent obesity in China. Its beneficial effects have been extensively investigated *in vitro* and *in vivo*.

In vitro treatment with both nuciferine and pronuciferine derived from *he ye* significantly decreased the lipid droplets and the intracellular TG contents but increased the glucose uptake in the insulin-resistant 3T3-L1 adipocytes by activating the AMPK-signalling pathway.[78] Kaempferol, the main component, inhibited lipogenic transcription factors and lipid accumulation during adipocyte differentiation through binding to PPARα to stimulate fatty acid oxidation in adipocytes.[79]

It was reported that a *he ye* seed ethanol extract exerted anti-obesity and hypolipidaemic effects in human pre-adipocytes and HFD-fed rats. *In vitro*, it inhibited the differentiation of pre-adipocytes into adipocytes shown by the inhibition of lipid accumulation and the decreased expression of PPARγ and leptin in cultured human adipocytes. *In vivo*, administration of a *he ye* extract significantly reduced body weight gain and adipose tissue weight in rats with lower levels of serum TG and leptin.[80] These anti-obesity and hypolipidaemic effects were also observed in treatment with a *he ye* leaf extract to HFD-fed rats with taurine supplementation,[81] and treatment with a flavonoid-enriched extract, showing reduced obesity and body fat accumulation by stimulating lipolysis and hypolipidemic activity through the regulation of fatty acid synthase, ACC and AMPK.[82] In addition, the anti-obesity efficacy of *he ye* has been explored to attribute its actions to its active constituents with strong inhibitory effects on pancreatic lipase and adipocyte differentiation.[83]

Regulation of Gut Microbiota

Lotus seed resistant starch type 3 (LRS3) from *he ye* was demonstrated to modulate gut microbiota. Its intake could enhance the proliferation of *Lactobacillus* and increase the contents of starch-utilising and butyrate-producing bacteria, such as *Lactobacillus*, *Bifidobacterium*, *Lachnospiraceae*, *Ruminococcaceae* and *Clostridium*, and decrease *Rikenellaceae* and *Porphyromonadaceae* in mice. It also promoted the production of short-chain fatty acids, lactic acid and mineral absorption. These changes of gut microbiota resulted in reduced body weight gain and food intake and increased the satiety of mice assessed by the feed conversion ratio that was used to describe the relationship between the total weight increment and total feed intake of mice.[84] Indeed, lotus seed oligosaccharides and purified lotus seed oligosaccharides were also found to effectively promote the growth of *Bifidobacterium adolescentis* to potentially combat obesity.[85]

Experimental Studies on *ge gen*

Ge gen 葛根 (*Pueraria lobata* (Willd.) Ohwi) includes over 70 chemical constituents, such as isoflavones, isoflavone glycosides, coumarins, puerarols, oleanane-type triterpenes and triterpenoid glycosides. Among the isolated isoflavone constituents, puerarin, daidzin and daidzein are the three most abundant components. Pharmacological activities include anti-inflammatory, anti-oxidant, anti-cancer, anti-osteoporotic, anti-pyretic, anti-diabetic, cardioprotective, neuroprotective and phytoestrogenic activities.[86]

Anti-obesity Actions

Puerarin, a major isoflavone glycoside from *ge gen*, has drawn much attention due to its comprehensive pharmacological action for the treatment of metabolic disorder–related diseases.

Conflicting data were reported *in vitro* in terms of the regulation of puerarin-mediated adipocyte differentiation and adipogenesis, which might be related to the different duration and concentrations of puerarin supplementation. A study reported that puerarin suppressed adipogenesis, and intracellular TG levels decreased the expression levels of C/EBPα, PPARγ and adipocyte lipid-binding protein 4 (FABP4) through an Akt/GSK-3β/β-catenin signalling pathway.[87] While other studies indicated that puerarin significantly enhanced differentiation of 3T3-L1 preadipocytes, accompanied with an increase in the accumulation of lipid droplets and TG through upregulating the expression of PPARγ and C/EBPα and their target genes, adipocyte-specific fatty acid-binding protein (aP2) and GLUT4.[88,89]

In vivo, ge gen supplementation has been reported to protect against obesity in DIO mice supported by decreasing HFD-induced body weight gain, white adipose tissue weight increase, blood lipid levels, increasing body temperatures and energy metabolism through activation of PGC-1α, and AMPK in skeletal muscles.[90] More recently, a water extract of *ge gen* was observed to increase energy expenditure by inducing brown adipocyte activity and formation in DIO mice. The mice treated with *ge gen* exhibited a higher metabolic rate with increased carbon dioxide production and oxygen uptake and lower body weight and circulating TG levels. Further mechanism studies reported that in a cell-autonomous manner, not autonomic nervous system regulation, *ge gen* could promote the thermogenic programme in brown adipose tissue shown by the increased expression of UCP1, and induced the formation of brown-like cells in inguinal white adipose tissue shown by the enhanced expression of markers of brown fat activity such as PPARα, PPARγ1, PPARγ2 and CIDEA. Interestedly, the two isoflavones, daidzein and genistein, were identified as direct active mediators for this regulation effect, but not as the most abundant flavonoid puerarin.[91]

Puerarin supplementation in DIO mice has been shown to affect the activities of hepatic lipid metabolism-related enzymes by suppressing fatty acid synthase activity and increasing activities of AMPK, carnitine acyltransferase and hormone-sensitive lipase. The enhancement of lipolysis and suppression of fat synthesis resulted in the decrease in serum TC and TG levels, body weight gain and intraperitoneal adipose tissue weight.[92]

Regulation of Gut Microbiota

It was reported that puerarin supplementation significantly altered the composition of the gut microbiota, evidenced by the increase in the abundance of *Akkermansia muciniphila*, which inversely correlates with obesity and diabetes in both mice and humans, through increasing the intestinal expression levels of the major goblet cell mucin-producing gene *Muc2* and antimicrobial gene *Reg3g* and protecting intestinal barrier function (normal permeability) by enhancing the expression of ZO-1 and occludin *in vivo* and *in vitro*.[93]

Summary of Pharmacological Actions of the Common Herbs

Each of these 10 herbs has attracted research attention in experimental models of relevance to obesity. The actions of anti-obesity were observed in all herbs. In particular, *chen pi, huang lian, dan shen, huang qi, da huang, he ye* and *ge gen* exerted very strong anti-obesity effects from many aspects of the pathogenesis of obesity through multiple mechanisms.

Regulation of gut microbiota was observed in most of the herbs, with the exception of *ban xia* and *chen pi*. All of them showed very powerful modulation of gut microbiota, mainly through increasing the B/F ratio and short-chain fatty acid-producing bacteria to exert a beneficial anti-obesity effect.

Of particular attention, modulation of the microbiota-gut-brain axis was observed in *huang lian* through AMPK-mediated neuropeptide expressions in the hypothalamus, and modulation of appetite-associated genes was observed in *huang qi* through leptin-medicated neuropeptide expressions in the hypothalamus to regulate food intake and body weight.

These *in vitro* and *in vivo* studies examined herb actions specific to obesity and provide potential explanations of the clinical benefits of all the common herbs. The findings highlight that herbal medicines have multiple components that can act on multiple pathways relevant to obesity.

References

1. Kleinert M, Clemmensen C, Hofmann SM, *et al.* (2018) Animal models of obesity and diabetes mellitus. *Nat Rev Endocrinol* **14(3):** 140–162.
2. Rios JL. (2011) Chemical constituents and pharmacological properties of Poria cocos. *Planta Med* **77(7):** 681–691.

3. Wang X, Liu H, Zhao L, *et al.* (2011) Effects of the crude polysaccharides from Poria cocos on the proliferation and differentiation of 3T3-L1 Cells. *Res J Biol Sci* **6(11):** 597–601.

4. Miao H, Zhao YH, Vaziri ND, *et al.* (2016) Lipidomics biomarkers of diet-induced hyperlipidemia and its treatment with Poria cocos. *J Agric Food Chem* **64(4):** 969–979.

5. Sato M, Tai T, Nunoura Y, *et al.* (2002) Dehydrotrametenolic acid induces preadipocyte differentiation and sensitizes animal models of noninsulin-dependent diabetes mellitus to insulin. *Biol Pharm Bull* **25(1):** 81–86.

6. Turnbaugh PJ, Ley RE, Mahowald MA, *et al.* (2006) An obesity-associated gut microbiome with increased capacity for energy harvest. *Nature* **444(7122):** 1027–1031.

7. Sun SS, Wang K, Ma K, *et al.* (2019) An insoluble polysaccharide from the sclerotium of Poria cocos improves hyperglycemia, hyperlipidemia and hepatic steatosis in ob/ob mice via modulation of gut microbiota. *Chin J Nat Med* **17(1):** 3–14.

8. Wang C, Yang S, Gao L, *et al.* (2018) Carboxymethyl pachyman (CMP) reduces intestinal mucositis and regulates the intestinal microflora in 5-fluorouracil-treated CT26 tumour-bearing mice. *Food Funct* **9(5):** 2695–2704.

9. Zhu B, Zhang QL, Hua JW, *et al.* (2018) The traditional uses, phytochemistry, and pharmacology of Atractylodes macrocephala Koidz.: A review. *J Ethnopharmacol* **226:** 143–167.

10. Kim CK, Kim M, Oh SD, *et al.* (2011) Effects of Atractylodes macrocephala Koidzumi rhizome on 3T3-L1 adipogenesis and an animal model of obesity. *J Ethnopharmacol* **137(1):** 396–402.

11. Wang JH, Bose S, Kim HG, *et al.* (2015) Fermented Rhizoma Atractylodis Macrocephalae alleviates high fat diet-induced obesity in association with regulation of intestinal permeability and microbiota in rats. *Sci Rep* **5:** 8391.

12. Song MY, Kang SY, Oh TW, *et al.* (2015) The roots of Atractylodes macrocephala Koidzumi enhanced glucose and lipid metabolism in C2C12 myotubes via mitochondrial regulation. *Evid Based Complement Alternat Med* **2015:** 643654.

13. Song MY, Jung HW, Kang SY, *et al.* (2017) Atractylenolide III enhances energy metabolism by increasing the SIRT-1 and PGC1alpha expression with AMPK phosphorylation in C2C12 mouse skeletal muscle cells. *Biol Pharm Bull* **40(3):** 339–344.

14. Song MY, Lim SK, Wang JH, *et al.* (2018) The root of Atractylodes macrocephala Koidzumi prevents obesity and glucose intolerance and increases energy metabolism in mice. *Int J Mol Sci* **19(1):** E278.

15. Wang R, Zhou G, Wang M, *et al.* (2014) The metabolism of polysaccharide from Atractylodes macrocephala Koidz and its effect on intestinal microflora. *Evid Based Complement Alternat Med* **2014:** 926381.

16. Ji X, Huang B, Wang G, *et al.* (2014) The ethnobotanical, phytochemical and pharmacological profile of the genus Pinellia. *Fitoterapia* **93:** 1–17.

17. Kim YJ, Shin YO, Ha YW, *et al.* (2006) Anti-obesity effect of Pinellia ternata extract in Zucker rats. *Biol Pharm Bull* **29(6):** 1278–1281.

18. Rozema E, Atanasov AG, Fakhrudin N, *et al.* (2012) Selected extracts of Chinese herbal medicines: Their effect on NF-kappaB, PPARalpha and PPARgamma and the respective bioactive compounds. *Evid Based Complement Alternat Med* **2012:** 983023.

19. Yu X, Sun S, Guo Y, *et al.* (2018) Citri Reticulatae Pericarpium (Chenpi): Botany, ethnopharmacology, phytochemistry, and pharmacology of a frequently used traditional Chinese medicine. *J Ethnopharmacol* **220:** 265–282.

20. Guo J, Tao H, Cao Y, *et al.* (2016) Prevention of obesity and type 2 diabetes with aged citrus peel (Chenpi) Extract. *J Agric Food Chem* **64(10):** 2053–2061.

21. Kanda K, Nishi K, Kadota A, *et al.* (2012) Nobiletin suppresses adipocyte differentiation of 3T3-L1 cells by an insulin and IBMX mixture induction. *Biochim Biophys Acta* **1820(4):** 461–468.

22. Lee YS, Cha BY, Choi SS, *et al.* (2013) Nobiletin improves obesity and insulin resistance in high-fat diet-induced obese mice. *J Nutr Biochem* **24(1):** 156–162.

23. Kurowska EM, Manthey JA, Casaschi A, *et al.* (2004) Modulation of HepG2 cell net apolipoprotein B secretion by the citrus polymethoxyflavone, tangeretin. *Lipids* **39(2):** 143–151.

24. Kurowska EM, Manthey JA. (2004) Hypolipidemic effects and absorption of citrus polymethoxylated flavones in hamsters with diet-induced hypercholesterolemia. *J Agric Food Chem* **52(10):** 2879–2886.

25. Lai CS, Ho MH, Tsai ML, *et al.* (2013) Suppression of adipogenesis and obesity in high-fat induced mouse model by hydroxylated polymethoxyflavones. *J Agric Food Chem* **61(43):** 10320–10328.

26. Feng K, Zhu X, Chen T, *et al.* (2019) Prevention of obesity and hyperlipidemia by Heptamethoxyflavone in high-fat diet-induced rats. *J Agric Food Chem* **67(9):** 2476–2489.

27. Chou YC, Ho CT, Pan MH. (2018) Immature citrus reticulata extract promotes browning of beige adipocytes in high-fat diet-induced C57BL/6 mice. *J Agric Food Chem* **66(37):** 9697–9703.

28. Wang J, Wang L, Lou GH, *et al.* (2019) Coptidis Rhizoma: A comprehensive review of its traditional uses, botany, phytochemistry, pharmacology and toxicology. *Pharm Biol* **57(1):** 193–225.

29. Choi JS, Kim JH, Ali MY, *et al.* (2014) Coptis chinensis alkaloids exert anti-adipogenic activity on 3T3-L1 adipocytes by downregulating C/EBP-alpha and PPAR-gamma. *Fitoterapia* **98:** 199–208.

30. Huang C, Zhang Y, Gong Z, *et al.* (2006) Berberine inhibits 3T3-L1 adipocyte differentiation through the PPARgamma pathway. *Biochem Biophys Res Commun* **348(2):** 571–578.

31. Zhang J, Tang H, Deng R, *et al.* (2015) Berberine suppresses adipocyte differentiation via decreasing CREB transcriptional activity. *PLoS One* **10(4):** e0125667.

32. Jiang D, Wang D, Zhuang X, *et al.* (2016) Berberine increases adipose triglyceride lipase in 3T3-L1 adipocytes through the AMPK pathway. *Lipids Health Dis* **15(1):** 214.

33. Xie W, Gu D, Li J, *et al.* (2011) Effects and action mechanisms of berberine and Rhizoma coptidis on gut microbes and obesity in high-fat diet-fed C57BL/6J mice *PLoS One* **6(9):** e24520.

34. He K, Kou S, Zou Z, *et al.* (2016) Hypolipidemic effects of alkaloids from Rhizoma Coptidis in diet-induced hyperlipidemic hamsters. *Planta Med* **82(8):** 690–697.

35. Yang W, She L, Yu K, *et al.* (2016) Jatrorrhizine hydrochloride attenuates hyperlipidemia in a high-fat diet-induced obesity mouse model. *Mol Med Rep* **14(4):** 3277–3284.

36. Xu JH, Liu XZ, Pan W, *et al.* (2017) Berberine protects against diet-induced obesity through regulating metabolic endotoxemia and gut hormone levels. *Mol Med Rep* **15(5):** 2765–2787.

37. Zhang Z, Zhang H, Li B, *et al.* (2014) Berberine activates thermogenesis in white and brown adipose tissue. *Nat Commun* **5:** 5493.

38. Hu X, Zhang Y, Xue Y, *et al.* (2018) Berberine is a potential therapeutic agent for metabolic syndrome via brown adipose tissue activation and metabolism regulation. *Am J Transl Res* **10(11):** 3322–3329.

39. Kahn BB, Alquier T, Carling D, *et al.* (2005) AMP-activated protein kinase: Ancient energy gauge provides clues to modern understanding of metabolism. *Cell Metab* **1(1):** 15–25.

40. Lee YS, Kim WS, Kim KH, *et al.* (2006) Berberine, a natural plant product, activates AMP-activated protein kinase with beneficial metabolic effects in diabetic and insulin-resistant states. *Diabetes* **55(8):** 2256–2264.

41. Kim WS, Lee YS, Cha SH, *et al.* (2009) Berberine improves lipid dysregulation in obesity by controlling central and peripheral AMPK activity. *Am J Physiol Endocrinol Metab* **296(4):** E812–9.

42. Huynh MK, Kinyua AW, Yang DJ, *et al.* (2016) Hypothalamic AMPK as a regulator of energy homeostasis. *Neural Plast* **2016:** 2754078.

43. Perry B, Wang Y. (2012) Appetite regulation and weight control: The role of gut hormones. *Nutr Diabetes* **2:** e26.

44. Sun H, Wang N, Cang Z, *et al.* (2016) Modulation of microbiota-gut-brain axis by berberine resulting in improved metabolic status in high-fat diet-fed rats. *Obes Facts* **9(6):** 365–378.

45. Li ZQ, Zuo DY, Qie XD, *et al.* (2012) Berberine acutely inhibits the digestion of maltose in the intestine. *J Ethnopharmacol* **142(2):** 474–480.

46. Liu L, Yu YL, Yang JS, *et al.* (2010) Berberine suppresses intestinal disaccharidases with beneficial metabolic effects in diabetic states, evidences from in vivo and in vitro study. *Naunyn Schmiedebergs Arch Pharmacol* **381(4):** 371–381.

47. He K, Hu Y, Ma H, *et al.* (2016) Rhizoma Coptidis alkaloids alleviate hyperlipidemia in B6 mice by modulating gut microbiota and bile acid pathways. *Biochim Biophys Acta* **1862(9):** 1696–1709.

48. Zhang X, Zhao Y, Xu J, *et al.* (2015) Modulation of gut microbiota by berberine and metformin during the treatment of high-fat diet-induced obesity in rats. *Sci Rep* **5:** 14405.

49. Zhang X, Zhao Y, Zhang M, *et al.* (2012) Structural changes of gut microbiota during berberine-mediated prevention of obesity and insulin resistance in high-fat diet-fed rats. *PLoS One* **7(8):** e42529.

50. Cao Y, Pan Q, Cai W, *et al.* (2016) Modulation of gut microbiota by berberine improves steatohepatitis in high-fat diet-fed BALB/C mice. *Arch Iran Med* **19(3):** 197–203.

51. Su CY, Ming QL, Rahman K, *et al.* (2015) Salvia miltiorrhiza: Traditional medicinal uses, chemistry, and pharmacology. *Chin J Nat Med* **13(3):** 163–182.

52. Gong Z, Huang C, Sheng X, *et al.* (2009) The role of tanshinone IIA in the treatment of obesity through peroxisome proliferator-activated receptor gamma antagonism. *Endocrinology* **150(1):** 104–113.

53. Park YK, Obiang-Obounou BW, Lee J, *et al.* (2017) Anti-adipogenic effects on 3T3-L1 cells and zebrafish by Tanshinone IIA. *Int J Mol Sci* **18(10):** 2065.

54. Pan Y, Zhao W, Zhao D, *et al.* (2018) Salvianolic acid B improves mitochondrial function in 3T3-L1 adipocytes through a pathway involving PPARgamma coactivator-1alpha (PGC-1alpha). *Front Pharmacol* **9:** 671.

55. Zhao D, Zuo J, Yu N, *et al.* (2017) Salvianolic acid B improves glucolipid metabolism by regulating adipogenic transcription factors in mice with diet-induced obesity. *J Tradit Chin Med Sci.* **4:** 280–289.

56. An T, Zhang J, Lv B, *et al.* (2019) Salvianolic acid B plays an anti-obesity role in high fat diet-induced obese mice by regulating the expression of mRNA, circRNA, and lncRNA. *PeerJ* **7:** e6506.

57. Gu JF, Su SL, Guo JM, *et al.* (2017) The aerial parts of Salvia miltiorrhiza Bge. strengthen intestinal barrier and modulate gut microbiota imbalance in streptozocin-induced diabetic mice. *J Funct Foods* **36:** 362–374.

58. Fu J, Wang Z, Huang L, *et al.* (2014) Review of the botanical characteristics, phytochemistry, and pharmacology of Astragalus membranaceus (Huangqi). *Phytother Res* **28(9):** 1275–1283.

59. Agyemang K, Han L, Liu E, *et al.* (2013) Recent advances in astragalus membranaceus anti-diabetic research: Pharmacological effects of its phytochemical constituents. *Evid Based Complement Alternat Med* **2013:** 654643.

60. Long Y, Zhang XX, Chen T, *et al.* (2014) Radix astragali improves dysregulated triglyceride metabolism and attenuates macrophage infiltration in adipose tissue in high-fat diet-induced obese male rats through activating mTORC1-PPAR gamma signaling pathway. *PPAR Res* **2014:** 189085.

61. Huang YC, Tsay HJ, Lu MK, *et al.* (2017) Astragalus membranaceus-polysaccharides ameliorates obesity, hepatic steatosis, neuroinflammation and cognition impairment without affecting amyloid deposition in metabolically stressed APPswe/PS1dE9 mice. *Int J Mol Sci* **18(12):** E2746.

62. Du Q, Zhang S, Li A, *et al.* (2018) Astragaloside IV inhibits adipose lipolysis and reduces hepatic glucose production via Akt dependent PDE3B expression in HFD-fed mice. *Front Physiol* **9:** 15.

63. Wu H, Gao Y, Shi HL, *et al.* (2016) Astragaloside IV improves lipid metabolism in obese mice by alleviation of leptin resistance and regulation of thermogenic network. *Sci Rep* **6:** 30190.

64. Nie T, Zhao S, Mao L, *et al.* (2018) The natural compound, formononetin, extracted from Astragalus membranaceus increases adipocyte thermogenesis by modulating PPARgamma activity. *Br J Pharmacol* **175(9):** 1439–1450.

65. Li XY, Shen L, Ji HF. (2019) Astragalus alters gut-microbiota composition in type 2 diabetes mice: Clues to its pharmacology. *Diabetes Metab Syndr Obes* **12:** 771–778.

66. Cao YJ, Pu ZJ, Tang YP, *et al.* (2017) Advances in bio-active constituents, pharmacology and clinical applications of rhubarb. *Chin Med* **12:** 36.

67. Liu Q, Zhang XL, Tao RY, *et al.* (2011) Rhein, an inhibitor of adipocyte differentiation and adipogenesis. *J Asian Nat Prod Res* **13(8):** 714–723.

68. Zhang Y, Fan S, Hu N, *et al.* (2012) Rhein reduces fat weight in db/db mouse and prevents diet-induced obesity in C57Bl/6 mouse through the inhibition of PPARgamma signaling. *PPAR Res* **2012:** 374936.

69. Sheng X, Zhu X, Zhang Y, *et al.* (2012) Rhein protects against obesity and related metabolic disorders through liver X receptor-mediated uncoupling protein 1 upregulation in brown adipose tissue. *Int J Biol Sci* **8(10):** 1375–1384.

70. Wang YJ, Huang SL, Feng Y, *et al.* (2012) Emodin, an 11beta-hydroxysteroid dehydrogenase type 1 inhibitor, regulates adipocyte function in vitro and exerts anti-diabetic effect in ob/ob mice. *Acta Pharmacol Sin* **33(9):** 1195–1203.

71. Li J, Ding L, Song B, *et al.* (2016) Emodin improves lipid and glucose metabolism in high fat diet-induced obese mice through regulating SREBP pathway. *Eur J Pharmacol* **770:** 99–109.

72. Lim H, Park J, Kim HL, *et al.* (2016) Chrysophanic acid suppresses adipogenesis and induces thermogenesis by activating AMP-activated protein kinase alpha in vivo and in vitro. *Front Pharmacol* **7:** 476.

73. Lee SJ, Cho SJ, Kwon EY, *et al.* (2019) Physcion reduces lipid accumulation and prevents the obesity in mice. *Nutr Metab* **16:** 31.

74. Zheng CD, Duan YQ, Gao JM, *et al.* (2010) Screening for anti-lipase properties of 37 traditional Chinese medicinal herbs. *J Chin Med Assoc* **73(6):** 319–324.

75. Wang R, Zang P, Chen J, *et al.* (2018) Gut microbiota play an essential role in the antidiabetic effects of rhein. *Evid Based Complement Alternat Med* **2018:** 6093282.

76. Cui HX, Zhang LS, Luo Y, *et al.* (2019) A purified anthraquinone-glycoside preparation from rhubarb ameliorates type 2 diabetes mellitus by modulating the gut microbiota and reducing inflammation. *Front Microbiol* **10:** 1423.

77. Kaur P, Kaur L, Kaur N, *et al.* (2019) A brief review on pharmaceutical uses of Nelumbo nucifera. *J Pharmacogn Phytochem.* **8(3):** 3966–3972.

78. Ma C, Li G, He Y, *et al.* (2015) Pronuciferine and nuciferine inhibit lipogenesis in 3T3-L1 adipocytes by activating the AMPK signaling pathway. *Life Sci* **136:** 120–125.

79. Lee B, Kwon M, Choi JS, *et al.* (2015) Kaempferol isolated from Nelumbo nucifera inhibits lipid accumulation and increases fatty acid oxidation signaling in adipocytes. *J Med Food* **18(12):** 1363–1370.

80. You JS, Lee YJ, Kim KS, *et al.* (2014) Anti-obesity and hypolipidaemic effects of Nelumbo nucifera seed ethanol extract in human pre-adipocytes and rats fed a high-fat diet. *J Sci Food Agric* **94(3):** 568–575.

81. Du H, You JS, Zhao X, *et al.* (2010) Antiobesity and hypolipidemic effects of lotus leaf hot water extract with taurine supplementation in rats fed a high fat diet. *J Biomed Sci* **17(Suppl 1):** S42.

82. Wu CH, Yang MY, Chan KC, *et al.* (2010) Improvement in high-fat diet-induced obesity and body fat accumulation by a Nelumbo nucifera leaf flavonoid-rich extract in mice. *J Agric Food Chem* **58(11):** 7075–7081.

83. Ahn JH, Kim ES, Lee C, *et al.* (2013) Chemical constituents from Nelumbo nucifera leaves and their anti-obesity effects. *Bioorg Med Chem Lett* **23(12):** 3604–3608.

84. Zeng H, Huang C, Lin S, *et al.* (2017) Lotus seed resistant starch regulates gut microbiota and increases short-chain fatty acids production and mineral absorption in mice. *J Agric Food Chem* **65(42):** 9217–9225.

85. Lu X, Zeng S, Zhang Y, *et al.* (2015) Effects of water-soluble oligosaccharides extracted from lotus (Nelumbo nucifera Gaertn.) seeds on growth ability of Bifidobacterium adolescentis. *Eur Food Res Technol* **241:** 459–467.

86. Zhang Z, Lam TN, Zuo Z. (2013) Radix Puerariae: An overview of its chemistry, pharmacology, pharmacokinetics, and clinical use. *J Clin Pharmacol* **53(8):** 787–811.
87. Wang N, Wang X, Cheng W, *et al.* (2013) Puerarin promotes osteogenesis and inhibits adipogenesis in vitro. *Chin Med* **8(1):** 17.
88. Lee OH, Seo DH, Park CS, *et al.* (2010) Puerarin enhances adipocyte differentiation, adiponectin expression, and antioxidant response in 3T3-L1 cells. *Biofactors* **36(6):** 459–467.
89. Yun J, Yu Y, Zhou G, *et al.* (2019) Effects of puerarin on the AKT signaling pathway in bovine preadipocyte differentiation. *Asian-Australas J Anim Sci* 4–11
90. Jung HW, Kang AN, Kang SY, *et al.* (2017) The root extract of Pueraria lobata and its main compound, puerarin, prevent obesity by increasing the energy metabolism in skeletal muscle. *Nutrients* **9(1):** E33.
91. Buhlmann E, Horvath C, Houriet J, *et al.* (2019) Puerariae lobatae root extracts and the regulation of brown fat activity. *Phytomedicine* **64:** 153075.
92. Zheng G, Lin L, Zhong S, *et al.* (2015) Effects of puerarin on lipid accumulation and metabolism in high-fat diet-fed mice. *PLoS One* **10(3):** e0122925.
93. Wang L, Wu Y, Zhuang L, *et al.* (2019) Puerarin prevents high-fat diet-induced obesity by enriching Akkermansia muciniphila in the gut microbiota of mice. *PLoS One* **14(6):** e0218490.

7

Clinical Evidence for Acupuncture and Related Therapies

OVERVIEW

Acupuncture for obesity has been widely researched, and 186 studies are presented in this chapter. More than half of the studies were controlled clinical trials (CCTs), and others were non-controlled studies. The CCTs were included in meta-analyses of outcome data to evaluate the efficacy of the acupuncture therapies for people who are overweight and obese. The non-controlled studies were evaluated to identify the intervention used and to explore their safety profiles. Results indicate that acupuncture can reduce weight, body mass index and waist circumference, compared to sham acupuncture, no treatment and other routine and lifestyle therapies.

Introduction

Acupuncture is part of a family of techniques that stimulates acupuncture points to correct imbalances of energy and restore health to the body. Methods of stimulating acupuncture points include:

- Acupuncture: Insertion of an acupuncture needle into acupuncture points.
- Electroacupuncture: Application of an electric current to the needle.
- Acupressure: Application of pressure to acupuncture points.
- Moxibustion: Burning of a herb (usually *ai ye*, 艾叶, *Artemesia vulgaris* L.) close to or on the skin to induce a warming sensation.

- Auricular (ear) acupuncture: Insertion of acupuncture needles on specific areas of the ear.
- Laser acupuncture: Application of laser irradiation to acupuncture points.
- Transcutaneous electrical nerve stimulation (TENS): Application of a transdermal electrical current to acupuncture points via conducting pads.

While many of these therapies have ancient roots, several have emerged as new techniques in the last century. This includes auricular (ear) acupuncture and laser acupuncture. Studies that evaluated acupuncture therapies not commonly used outside of China were excluded, for example, catgut embedding.

Previous Systematic Reviews

More than 15 systematic reviews of acupuncture for people who are overweight and obese have been published between 2003 and 2018. The more recent reviews include a meta-analysis of 27 randomised controlled trials (RCTs) published in 2018.[1] The authors concluded that a combination of auricular (ear) acupuncture and body acupuncture or pharmacopuncture with lifestyle modification in patients who were overweight (a body mass index (BMI) of between 25 to 30 kg/m^2) but not obese (BMI ≥ 30 kg/m^2) might be the most beneficial. Adverse events were few and mild in the included studies.

A network meta-analysis included 34 RCTs and compared the effectiveness of different acupuncture and related therapies.[2] Meta-analysis showed that acupuncture and related therapies were superior to lifestyle modifications and placebos in reducing weight and BMI. When the acupuncture therapies were combined with lifestyle modifications, there was slightly more weight loss. Despite the positive results, the included studies had an unclear risk of bias in terms of random sequence generation and a high risk of bias for blinding because intervention and control groups were open, and both participants and personnel knew the treatment they were receiving.

Acupuncture and lifestyle modification treatments were analysed by Fang and colleagues in 2017.[3] A total of 23 studies comprising 1,808 participants were included. The authors reported that acupuncture alone or combined with lifestyle modifications significantly reduced the BMI compared with no treatment, placebo control or lifestyle modification alone. However, the authors noted the risk of bias and methodological shortfalls in the included studies, and heterogeneity was high in the meta-analysis, leading to uncertainty in the results.

A systematic review of seven laser acupuncture RCTs showed positive effects in terms of reducing the body weight, BMI, waist and hip circumference, and waist–hip ratio (WHR).[4] However, the authors noted that despite some positive effects, there was a relative lack of well-designed studies.

In terms of auricular (ear) acupuncture, a recent systematic review published by Yeh and colleagues in 2017 included 18 RCTs of auricular acupoint stimulation.[5] The review reported a significantly reduced weight, BMI, body fat mass and waist circumference (WC) compared to sham acupuncture in overweight and obese adults. There was significant heterogeneity, and meta-regression indicated it might have been due to the total number of treatments and/or treatment duration. Treatments longer than six weeks also resulted in a further decrease in the BMI, WC and hip circumference. Another review published by Ruan and colleagues in 2016 was superseded by Yeh's review and included the same studies.[6]

Identification of Clinical Studies

Over 60,000 citations were identified through database searches, and 2,823 full-text articles were reviewed for eligibility. A total of 186 clinical studies (A1–186) met the inclusion criteria. A total of 107 RCTs, 4 controlled clinical trials (CCTs) and 75 non-controlled studies were included (Fig. 7.1). Interventions not commonly practised outside of China, for example, catgut embedding, are not included in the analysis.

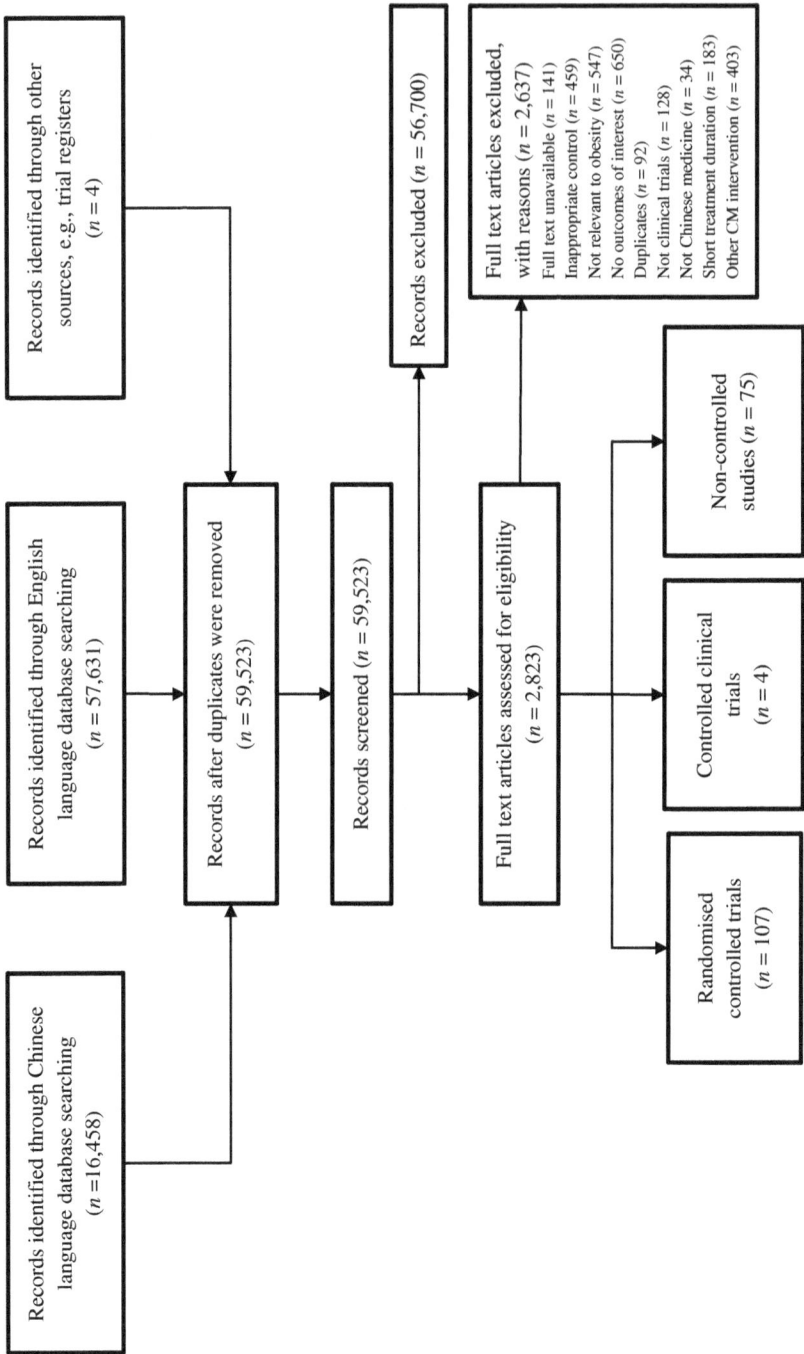

Fig. 7.1. Flow chart of the study selection process: Acupuncture and related therapies.

Records identified through other sources, e.g., trial registers (*n* = 4)

Records identified through English language database searching (*n* = 57,631)

Records identified through Chinese language database searching (*n* =16,458)

Records after duplicates were removed (*n* = 59,523)

Records screened (*n* = 59,523)

Records excluded (*n* = 56,700)

Full text articles assessed for eligibility (*n* = 2,823)

Full text articles excluded, with reasons (*n* = 2,637)
Full text unavailable (*n* = 141)
Inappropriate control (*n* = 459)
Not relevant to obesity (*n* = 547)
No outcomes of interest (*n* = 650)
Duplicates (*n* = 92)
Not clinical trials (*n* = 128)
Not Chinese medicine (*n* = 34)
Short treatment duration (*n* = 183)
Other CM intervention (*n* = 403)

Non-controlled studies (*n* = 75)

Controlled clinical trials (*n* = 4)

Randomised controlled trials (*n* = 107)

Over 18,000 people participated in the studies and their ages ranged from 18 to 72 years. Chinese medicine syndromes were reported in 107 studies (57.5%). The most common syndromes were Stomach heat, Spleen deficiency with dampness, Liver *qi* stagnation, and Spleen and Kidney *yang* deficiency. The treatment duration ranged from four weeks to six months. Acupuncture therapies included manual acupuncture, electroacupuncture, auricular (ear) acupuncture, moxibustion, laser acupuncture, TENS, electromagnetic pulse acupoint stimulation and plum-blossom needle therapy. Acupuncture therapies were administered alongside diet and exercise interventions in 69 studies (37.1%) or drug therapy in 15 studies. The remaining 102 studies evaluated acupuncture as a stand-alone therapy for obesity.

Outline of the Data Analyses

Studies are grouped by the type of study (i.e., RCTs, CCTs and non-controlled studies). They are also grouped by the type of acupuncture and related therapies (some studies included multiple treatment arms; therefore, the total number of interventions listed below is more than the overall number of included studies):

- Manual acupuncture and/or electroacupuncture: 75 RCTs, 2 CCTs, 33 non-controlled studies.
- Manual acupuncture and/or electroacupuncture plus ear acupuncture/acupressure: 12 RCTs, 28 non-controlled studies.
- Ear acupuncture/acupressure: 13 RCTs, 2 non-controlled studies.
- Moxibustion: 6 RCTs, 2 CCTs, 8 non-controlled studies.
- Laser acupuncture: 5 RCTs.
- Transcutaneous electrical nerve stimulation (TENS): 2 RCTs, 1 non-controlled study.
- Electromagnetic pulse acupoint stimulation: 2 RCTs.
- Plum-blossom needle therapy: 2 non-controlled studies.
- Photoelectric (light) therapy: 1 non-controlled study.

Meta-analysis results of RCTs are presented for each type of acupuncture therapy for the following outcomes (if available):

- Body weight or BMI: weight (kilograms) and BMI (kg/m^2).
- Reduction in waist circumference or WHR.
- Change in fat mass, abdominal fat, lean body mass, visceral fat and skinfold thickness.
- Total effective rate according to recognised standards.

Outcomes relevant to other health complications alongside obesity, such as diabetes mellitus and hypertension, were also analysed (if relevant); these outcomes included serum lipids, serum glucose, serum uric acid, blood pressure, glycated haemoglobin (HbA1c), fasting insulin, Homeostatic Model Assessment of Insulin Resistance (HOMA-IR), leptin and C-peptide excretion.

Randomised Controlled Trials of Acupuncture

A total of 107 RCTs (10,831 participants) were included in the analysis. Most studies were undertaken in China ($n = 85$), 7 in China-Taiwan, 6 in Iran, 2 each in South Korea and Egypt and 1 each in the United States, Austria, Australia, Turkey and Poland. Most of the studies had two arms (i.e., acupuncture *vs.* control, $n = 85$), 16 studies had three arms (i.e., acupuncture *vs.* control 1 or control 2), and 5 studies had four arms (i.e., acupuncture 1 or acupuncture 2 *vs.* control 1 or control 2).

Participants were recruited via outpatient and inpatient departments or through the community. The age range was from 18 to 70 years (mean 38 years). Females and males were exclusively included in 29 studies and 1 study, respectively, and the other studies included both genders. Participants were diagnosed with obesity based on established guidelines such as the:

- *Chinese adults body mass index classification recommendation by the Working Group on Obesity of China* (WGOC).[7]
- *Obesity report of the WHO consultation.*[8]
- *Diagnostic and therapeutic criteria for simple obesity modified at the national conference on obesity research in 1997 in China.*[9]
- BMI.

All participants had a BMI of at least 23 kg/m^2 or more, but most studies required participants to have a BMI of greater than or equal to 25 kg/m^2. Some studies also required participants to have a waist circumference of 80 cm or more. Most studies included participants with simple obesity without complications/comorbidities (n = 76, 71.0%). However, complications/comorbidities in other studies included diabetes mellitus/pre-diabetes — impaired fasting glucose/impaired glucose tolerance (11 studies), polycystic ovarian syndrome (PCOS) (8), metabolic syndrome (5), hyperlipidaemia (4), hypertension (2) and asymptomatic hyperuricemia (1).

Chinese medicine syndrome differentiation was performed in about half of the studies. Syndromes were used as an inclusion criterion in 22 studies and a basis for treatment selection in 32 studies. Common syndromes were Stomach heat, Spleen deficiency and dampness, Spleen and Kidney *yang* deficiency, Liver *qi* stagnation, and Spleen and Stomach *qi* deficiency.

Acupuncture therapies included manual acupuncture (33 studies), electroacupuncture (42), acupuncture plus auricular (ear) acupuncture/acupressure (13), ear acupuncture/acupressure (12), moxibustion (6), laser acupuncture (5), electromagnetic pulse acupoint stimulation (2) and TENS on acupuncture points (2). Note that some studies had multiple intervention arms.

The acupuncture points most frequently used in the RCTs were ST36 *Zusanli* 足三里, ST25 *Tianshu* 天枢, CV12 *Zhongwan* 中脘, SP6 *Sanyinjiao* 三阴交 and ST40 *Fenglong* 丰隆 (Table 7.1). The most common ear acupuncture points were Stomach 胃 (CO4), Hunger 饥点,

Table 7.1. Frequently Used Acupuncture Points in the Randomised Controlled Trials

Point Name	Frequency
ST36 *Zusanli* 足三里	72
ST25 *Tianshu* 天枢	64
CV12 *Zhongwan* 中脘	60
SP6 *Sanyinjiao* 三阴交	56
ST40 *Fenglong* 丰隆	49
CV4 *Guanyuan* 关元	47
LI11 *Quchi* 曲池	37
SP9 *Yinlingquan* 阴陵泉	35
CV6 *Qihai* 气海	34
CV9 *Shuifen* 水分	31
SP15 *Daheng* 大横	29
ST44 *Neiting* 内庭	28
BL20 *Pishu* 脾俞	24
ST28 *Shuidao* 水道	23
TE6 *Zhigou* 支沟	22
LR3 *Taichong* 太冲	21
ST37 *Shangjuxu* 上巨虚	21
LI4 *Hegu* 合谷	20
BL23 *Shenshu* 肾俞	19
GB26 *Daimai* 带脉	17

Acupuncture point names are referenced to the World Health Organization's *Standard Acupuncture Nomenclature*.[10]

Endocrine 内分泌 (CO18), *Shenmen* 神门 (TF4) and *San Jiao* 三焦 (CO12) (Table 7.2).

Risk of Bias

The 107 RCTs stated that they randomised participants; however, only 50 (46.7%) provided adequate details of sequence generation,

Table 7.2. Frequently Used Ear Acupuncture Points in the Randomised Controlled Trials

Point Name*	Frequency
Stomach 胃 (CO4)	22
Shenmen 神门 (TF4)	18
Hunger 饥点	18
Endocrine 内分泌 (CO18)	17
San Jiao 三焦 (CO12)	12
Sympathetic 交感 (AH6a)	10
Kidney 肾 (CO10)	9
Mouth 口 (CO1)	9
Large Intestine 大肠 (CO7)	8
Spleen 脾 (CO13)	8

Ear acupuncture point names are referenced to Wang's *Micro-Acupuncture in Practice*.[11]

and only 13 (12.1%) described an appropriate method for allocation concealment, such as concealed envelopes, and were judged to be at low risk of bias (Table 7.3). A total of 28 studies (26.2%) used a sham or placebo control and effectively blinded participants to the treatments. The other studies did not blind participants and were judged to be at high risk of bias. Blinding of personnel is difficult in acupuncture studies, and this was only done in one study that used a laser acupuncture device (A78). Assessor blinding was only implemented in five studies (A34, A50, A76, A78, A93); the others did not describe assessor blinding and were judged to be an unclear risk of bias. All studies provided detailed information on dropouts and their methods of data imputation where appropriate. Therefore, this domain was judged to be at low risk of bias for all studies. Study protocols could not be located, so all studies were judged to be at an unclear risk of bias for selective outcome reporting.

Table 7.3.   Risk of Bias of Randomised Controlled Trials: Acupuncture

Risk of Bias Domain	Low Risk n (%)	Unclear Risk n (%)	High Risk n (%)
Sequence generation	50 (46.7)	55 (51.4)	2 (1.9)
Allocation concealment	13 (12.1)	92 (86.0)	2 (1.9)
Blinding of participants	28 (26.2)	0	79 (73.8)
Blinding of personnel*	1 (0.9)	3 (1.9)	103 (97.2)
Blinding of outcome assessors	5 (4.7)	102 (95.3)	0
Incomplete outcome data	107 (100)	0	0
Selective outcome reporting	0	107 (100)	0

* Blinding of personnel (acupuncturists) is challenging in manual therapy studies.

Acupuncture

Acupuncture vs. Sham Acupuncture

Twelve RCTs (A28, A35, A39, A42, A43, A52, A71, A72, A84, A85, A90, A102) used sham control, including 1,011 participants. All studies evaluated participants with simple obesity except for three that evaluated polycystic ovarian syndrome (PCOS), and one included participants with metabolic syndrome. The treatment duration ranged from four weeks to six months.

Manual acupuncture or electroacupuncture was compared to sham acupuncture in eight studies (A20, A39, A42, A43, A52, A71, A72, A90). Weight was assessed in five of the studies comprising 258 participants and was found to be significantly reduced in the acupuncture group compared to the sham (mean difference [MD] −2.88 kg [95% confidence interval [CI] −5.20, −0.56], $I^2 = 0$%). The BMI was also significantly reduced in the acupuncture group compared to the sham (MD −1.73 kg/m^2 [95% CI −2.52, −0.95], $I^2 = 40$%, 8 studies and 423 participants). Furthermore, the WC and WHR were also significantly reduced after the treatment, when compared to the sham (MD −7.28 cm [95% CI −9.65, −4.92], $I^2 = 0$% and MD: −0.03 [95% CI −0.04, −0.01], $I^2 = 0$%).

Acupuncture vs. sham acupuncture plus metformin

One study (A102) compared acupuncture to sham acupuncture and metformin. The weight was not measured, and the BMI was not significantly reduced after acupuncture, compared to the sham and metformin (MD −0.10 kg/m^2 [95% CI −0.90, 0.70]. However, the WHR was significantly reduced after the treatment (MD −0.03 [95% CI −0.05, −0.01]).

Acupuncture plus metformin vs. sham acupuncture plus metformin

Acupuncture was administered alongside metformin, compared to sham acupuncture and metformin in two studies (A28, A102). The BMI and WHR were both significantly reduced after the acupuncture treatment, compared to the sham control (MD −1.74 kg/m^2 [95% CI −2.24, −1.24] I^2 = 0% and MD −0.11 [95% CI −0.14, −0.09], I^2 = 79%, respectively).

Acupuncture plus diet vs. sham acupuncture plus diet

Three studies (A35, A84–85) used acupuncture alongside diet therapy compared to sham acupuncture plus diet therapy (low-calorie diet) for six weeks. The outcome was that the weight and BMI were significantly reduced in the intervention group compared to the control in two of the studies (A84–85) comprising 247 participants (MD −1.58 [95% CI −2.12, −1.05], I^2 = 0%; BMI: MD −0.69 kg/m^2 [95% CI −0.87, −0.52], respectively). The WC and WHR were significantly reduced after the treatment in one study (A84) (MD −1.54 cm [95% CI −1.92, −1.16] and MD −0.01 [95% CI −0.013, −0.007], respectively).

Acupuncture vs. No Treatment

Six studies (A9, A37, A76, A77, A88, A99) compared acupuncture to no treatment. The BMI was significantly reduced in the acupuncture group compared to no treatment in four studies (A9, A37, A76, A99) (MD −1.67 kg/m^2 [95% CI −2.31, −1.03], I^2 = 0%). However, weight and WC were not significantly different between the groups after the treatment (MD −1.10 kg [95% CI −6.56, 4.37], I^2 = 50% (A88, A99) and MD −1.48 cm [95% CI −4.58, 1.61], I^2 = 59% (A88, A99), respectively).

Acupuncture vs. Lifestyle Therapies

Acupuncture/electroacupuncture was compared to lifestyle therapies, such as diet and exercise programs and behavioural therapy, in 10 studies (A17, A27, A32, A49, A55, A86, A99, A100, A101, A105). The treatment duration ranged from one to three months. Weight-related outcomes were significantly reduced in the acupuncture groups compared to the control:

- Weight: MD −3.19 kg [95% CI −4.79, −1.58], I^2 = 14%, 7 studies, 447 participants.
- BMI: MD −0.71 kg/m^2 [95% CI −1.08, −0.24], I^2 = 82%, 7 studies, 447 participants.
- WC: MD −2.77 cm [95% CI −4.42, −1.13], I^2 = 64%, 7 studies, 432 participants.
- WHR and fat mass percentage were not significantly different between the groups at the end of the treatment.

Acupuncture vs. Drug Therapy

Acupuncture vs. metformin

Six studies (A1, A4, A14, A24, A51, A103) compared acupuncture/electroacupuncture to metformin. In the six studies comprising 408 participants, the BMI was reduced in the acupuncture group, significantly more than in the metformin group (MD −0.71 kg/m^2 [95% CI −1.37, −0.05], I^2 = 46%). However, there was no difference in weight, WC, WHR or fat mass percentage between the groups at the end of the treatment.

Acupuncture plus metformin vs. metformin

Three studies (A3, A67, A103) comprising 216 participants compared acupuncture and metformin to metformin alone. The BMI was significantly reduced in the acupuncture group (MD −1.82 kg/m^2 [95% CI −2.32, −1.32], I^2 = 13%). One study (A103) comprising 28 participants reported a reduction in weight and WC after the treatment in the intervention group (MD −5.67 kg [95% CI −9.17, −2.17] and MD −10.77 cm [95% CI −14.03, −7.51], respectively).

Acupuncture plus metformin plus routine diabetic management vs. metformin plus routine diabetic management

Two studies (A18, A29) included participants with obesity and diabetes mellitus. Acupuncture plus metformin plus routine diabetic management was compared with metformin plus routine diabetic management. After two months of treatment, the weight, BMI and WC were not significantly different between the groups. There was no difference in other parameters, such as fasting blood glucose or fasting insulin.

Acupuncture plus Lifestyle Therapies vs. Lifestyle Therapies

A total of 30 studies (A8, A10–12, A15, A21, A23, A26, A31, A38, A40, A41, A45, A48, A54, A58, A60, A61, A64–66, A68–70, A73–75, A92, A101, A105) comprising 3,474 participants evaluated acupuncture/electroacupuncture plus lifestyle therapies. Lifestyle therapies included diet advice, structured or general exercise, education, etc. All types of lifestyle therapies were grouped together for meta-analysis. The treatment duration ranged from four weeks to six months.

Acupuncture plus lifestyle therapies were superior to lifestyle therapies alone in terms of weight reduction, BMI, WC and WHR (Table 7.4). Although heterogeneity was high, the fat mass percentage was not significantly different between the groups at the end of the

Table 7.4. Acupuncture plus Lifestyle Therapies vs. Lifestyle Therapies

Outcomes	No. of Studies (Participants)	Effect Size MD [95% CI], I^2%	Included Studies
Weight	15 (1,304)	−4.36 kg [−5.34, −3.19]*, 58	A8, A12, A23, A31, A40, A48, A54, A58, A60–61, A65, A70, A73, A92, A105
BMI	22 (2,820)	−2.06 kg/m^2 [−2.59, −1.54]*, 86	A8, A11–12, A15, A21, A23, A26, A31, A40, A48, A54, A58, A60–61, A64–66, A70, A73–74, A75, A105
WC	9 (1,065)	−3.95 cm [−6.37, −1.54]*, 90	A8, A23, A64, A60, A66, A70, A73, A75, A105
WHR	6 (891)	−0.07 [−0.14, 0.00], 98	A11, A21, A26, A31, A54, A69
Fat mass	8 (826)	−2.20 [−4.52, 0.12], 94	A8, A12, A23, A48, A61, A65–66, A105
Effective rate	11 (897)	RR 1.43 [1.27, 1.62]*, 58	A8, A10, A12, A21, A23, A41, A45, A61, A65, A68, A73

Abbreviations: BMI, body mass index; CI, confidence interval; MD, mean difference; RR, risk ratio; WC, waist circumference; WHR, waist–hip ratio.
* Statistically significant, see *Statistical Analysis* methods in Chapter 4.

treatment. Eleven studies evaluated benefits in terms of the total effective rate based on the *Chinese obesity efficacy evaluation criteria* (1997), and the acupuncture group was superior to the control.

Acupuncture plus Ear Acupressure

Acupuncture plus ear acupressure vs. sham acupuncture

Four RCTs (A53, A57, A82, A94) used acupuncture alongside ear acupressure compared to a sham control comprising 816 participants. In two studies (A53, A57), electroacupuncture plus ear acupressure did not significantly reduce weight or BMI when compared to sham acupuncture (MD 0.46 kg [95% CI −2.51, 3.44], I^2 = 0% and MD −0.46 kg/m^2 [95% CI −2.59, 1.66], I^2 = 0%, respectively). Acupuncture plus ear acupressure plus diet and lifestyle education compared to sham acupuncture plus diet and lifestyle education was assessed in two studies (A82, A94). Data from A94 could not be analysed. In study A82, the acupuncture treatments significantly reduced the BMI but not the WC, when compared to the control (MD -0.19 kg/m^2 [95% CI -0.35, -0.03] and MD -0.13 cm [95% CI -0.56, 0.30], respectively).

Acupuncture plus ear acupressure vs. drug therapy

One study (A19) compared acupuncture plus ear acupressure plus metformin plus routine diabetic management with metformin plus routine diabetic management. Participants in the study had obesity and diabetes mellitus. After 12 weeks of treatment, there were no significant differences between the groups in terms of weight, BMI, WC or WHR. However, the fasting blood glucose was reduced after the intervention, when compared to the control (MD -1.67 mmol/L [95% CI -2.44, -0.90].

One study (A36) compared body acupuncture plus ear acupuncture to tibolone (Livial™) hormone therapy in menopausal women. After three months of treatment, the weight, BMI and fat mass percentage were significantly reduced in women in the acupuncture group compared to the hormone therapy group (MD -4.05 kg [95% CI -7.79, -0.31], MD -3.02 kg/m^2 [95% CI -4.20, -1.84] and MD -6.51% [95% CI -9.84, -3.18], respectively).

Acupuncture plus ear acupressure vs. lifestyle therapies

Two studies (A46, A106) compared acupuncture plus ear acupressure to diet advice and behavioural therapy for weight loss. There was no statistically significant difference between the intervention and control groups in terms of weight and BMI.

Acupuncture plus ear acupressure plus lifestyle therapies vs. lifestyle therapies

Five studies (A5, A13, A50, A106, A107) assessed a combination of acupuncture plus ear acupuncture/acupressure with various lifestyle therapies such as diet and exercise advice. The weight and WC were not significantly different between the groups at the end of the treatment (weight: MD −3.37 kg [95% CI −8.96, 2.22], I^2 = 89%, 4 studies, 254 participants); and WC: MD −5.46 cm [95% CI −14.20, 3.28], I^2 = 91%, 3 studies, 264 participants). However, the BMI was significantly reduced after the treatment compared to the control (MD −2.28 kg/m^2 [95% CI −4.13, −0.42], I^2 = 91%, 5 studies, 390 participants).

Ear Acupuncture

Ear acupuncture vs. sham ear acupuncture

Eight studies (A6, A33, A35, A79, A80, A83, A93, A95) compared ear acupuncture/acupressure to the sham control. All studies assessed simple obesity in people with a BMI of over 23 kg/m^2. By using a small device that sits on the ear, ear points were stimulated by acupuncture needles, pressure or electro-stimulation. The treatment duration ranged from 6 to 12 weeks. Ear acupuncture plus lifestyle therapies such as diet and exercise advice compared to sham ear acupuncture plus lifestyle therapies showed a significant reduction in the BMI (change from baseline) in the intervention group compared to the control (MD −0.88 kg/m^2 [95% CI −0.50, −1.27], I^2 = 0%) (A6, A93). Other outcomes such as weight, WC and WHR could not be pooled in the analysis due to differences in the outcome units and some missing data.

Ear acupressure vs. no treatment

One study (A104) showed a significant reduction in weight and BMI after ear acupressure plus behavioural treatments, such as psychology, eating habits and exercise (MD −3.50 kg [95% CI −6.69, −0.31] and MD −2.50 kg/m^2 [95% CI −3.54, −1.46], respectively). Ear acupressure alone in two studies (A81, A104) reduced weight and BMI, compared to no treatment (MD −2.85 kg [95% CI −5.47, −0.24],

I^2 = 19% and MD −0.84 kg/m^2 [95% CI −1.64, −0.04], I^2 = 0%, respectively).

Ear acupressure vs. lifestyle therapies

One study (A104) compared ear acupressure to behavioural therapy for weight loss. There were no statistically significant differences between the intervention and control groups in terms of weight or BMI.

Ear acupuncture/acupressure plus lifestyle therapies vs. lifestyle therapies

Five studies (A34, A56, A63, A87, A104) used ear acupressure or ear acupuncture plus lifestyle therapies compared to the same lifestyle therapies alone. Weight was significantly reduced in the intervention group compared to the control after the treatment in four studies comprising 297 participants (MD −1.63 kg [95% CI −3.19, −0.07], I^2 = 0%). The BMI, WC, WHR and fat mass percentage were not significantly different between the groups after the treatment:

- BMI: MD −0.17 kg/m^2 [95% CI −1.14, 0.79], I^2 = 72%, 5 studies, 315 participants.
- WC: MD −1.81 cm [95% CI −6.56, 2.94], I^2 = 90%, 3 studies, 197 participants.
- WHR: MD −0.01 [95% CI −0.03, 0.01], 1 study, 49 participants.
- Fat mass percentage: MD 1.76% [95% CI −1.10, 4.62], I^2 = 51%, 2 studies, 106 participants.

Acupuncture plus Moxibustion Therapies

Acupuncture and moxibustion vs. drug therapy

One study (A25) evaluated six months of electroacupuncture plus moxibustion plus ear acupressure plus metformin compared to metformin in women with PCOS. Weight and BMI were significantly reduced in the intervention group compared to the control (MD −3.17 kg [95% CI −5.15, −1.19] and MD −1.13 kg/m^2 [95% CI −1.60, −0.66], respectively).

Acupuncture plus moxibustion vs. routine care

One study (A100) showed that moxibustion could reduce the WC in people with metabolic syndrome compared to routine treatments for metabolic syndrome such as antihypertensives, hypoglycaemics and lipid-lowering therapy (MD −4.60 cm [95% CI −5.66, −3.54]). Weight and BMI were not measured. Other outcomes such as fasting blood glucose, total triglycerides and blood pressure were not significantly improved in the intervention group compared to the control.

Acupuncture and moxibustion plus lifestyle therapies vs. lifestyle therapies

Three studies (A5, A22, A47) used warming needle style moxibustion along with acupuncture and lifestyle therapies. Lifestyle therapies included diet and exercise advice. Weight was reduced in the acupuncture group compared to the control (2 studies, 120 participants, MD −2.72 kg [95% CI −5.09, −0.35], I^2 = 20%). However, the BMI, WC, WHR and fat mass were not significantly different between the groups after the treatment:

- BMI: MD −1.58 kg/m^2 [95% CI −3.88, 0.72], I^2 = 83%, 3 studies, 180 participants.
- WC: MD −1.31 cm [95% CI −8.88, 6.26], I^2 = 87%, 2 studies, 140 participants.
- WHR: MD −0.03 [95% CI −0.08, 0.02], 1 study, 40 participants.
- Fat mass percentage: MD −2.06 % [95% CI −4.42, 0.30], 1 study, 60 participants.

Transcutaneous Electrical Stimulation on Acupoints

Transcutaneous electrical stimulation vs. no treatment

One study (A96) compared TENS on acupuncture points to no treatment in women with menopause. Weight and the WHR were not significantly different between the groups after 12 weeks of the treatment. However, the WC was significantly reduced in the intervention group compared to no treatment (MD −3.45 cm [95% CI −5.42, −1.48]).

Electromagnetic pulse acupoint stimulation vs. lifestyle therapies

One study (A16) used electromagnetic pulse acupoint stimulation (patches on acupoints) compared to exercise for six weeks. Weight and BMI were not reported. The fat mass percentage was not significantly different between the groups after the treatment.

Electromagnetic pulse acupoint stimulation plus lifestyle therapies vs. lifestyle therapies

The fat mass percentage was evaluated in two studies (A30, A89) comprising 118 participants using electromagnetic pulse acupoint stimulation plus exercise compared to exercise alone. The fat mass was significantly reduced in the intervention group, compared to the control (MD −1.35 % [95% CI −2.58, −0.12], $I^2 = 0\%$); other outcomes were not measured.

Laser Acupuncture

Laser acupuncture vs. sham laser acupuncture

Two studies (A78, A98) compared laser acupuncture (low-level laser light therapy) to sham laser acupuncture (no power output) for four and eight weeks. The BMI, weight, WC and WHR were not significantly different between the groups after the treatment.

Laser acupuncture plus lifestyle therapies vs. lifestyle therapies

Three studies (A91, A97, A107) compared lifestyle therapies (healthy/low-calorie diet and exercise program) to laser acupuncture plus diet and exercise therapies. There was no significant difference between the groups at the end of the treatment in terms of weight, BMI, WC and WHR.

Weight-related Complications and Comorbidities

Several studies included participants with specific conditions along with obesity. Comorbidities included diabetes mellitus, PCOS, hyperlipidaemia, hypertension and metabolic syndrome.

Diabetes Mellitus

Eleven studies (A3, A15, A18, A19, A27, A29, A51, A56, A63, A74, A75) included people with obesity and diabetes mellitus or pre-diabetes (impaired fasting glucose/impaired glucose tolerance). Acupuncture/electroacupuncture and ear acupressure were used alone or alongside metformin and/or other routine treatments for diabetes, such as diet and exercise advice. Comparators were routine treatments for diabetes. Weight, BMI, WC and WHR were all significantly reduced after the intervention when compared to the control, but fat mass was not (Table 7.5). Indices of related complications, such as fasting insulin, total cholesterol, total triglycerides and HbA1c, were also improved after the intervention, when compared to the control.

Polycystic Ovarian Syndrome

Eight studies (A4, A20, A24, A25, A28, A67, A102, A103) included women with PCOS and a BMI of at least 23 kg/m^2. Treatments

Table 7.5. Acupuncture for Obesity and Diabetes Mellitus

Outcome	No. of Studies (Participants)	Effect Size MD [95% CI], I²%	Included Studies
Weight	5 (355)	−3.04 [−4.73, −1.35]*, 0	A19, A27, A29, A56, A63
BMI	11 (1,067)	−1.47 [−2.19, −0.75]*, 83	A3, A15, A18–19, A27, A29, A51, A56, A63, A74–75
WC	7 (725)	−2.81 [−5.20, −0.42]*, 83	A18–19, A27, A29, A56, A63, A75
WHR	2 (109)	−0.01 [−0.02, −0.00], 0	A19, A63
Fat mass	1 (88)	0.46 [−2.02, 2.94]	A56
Fasting blood glucose	11 (1,127)	−0.12 [−0.72, 0.49], 96	A3, A15, A18–19, A27, A29, A51, A56, A63, A74–75
Fasting insulin	4 (256)	SMD −0.60 [−1.08, −0.12]*, 72	A18, A29, A51, A74
HOMA-IR	4 (392)	SMD −0.37 [−0.75, 0.02], 67	A15, A18, A51, A74
Total cholesterol	4 (507)	−0.23 [−0.41, −0.05]*, 16	A18, A56, A63, A75
Total triglycerides	5 (567)	−0.17 [−0.32, −0.03]*, 30	A18–19, A56, A63, A75
HbA1c	5 (448)	−0.96 [−1.57, −0.34]*, 84	A3, A15, A18–19, A74

Abbreviations: BMI, body mass index; CI, confidence interval; HbA1c, Hemoglobin A1c; HOMA-IR, Homeostatic Model Assessment of Insulin Resistance; MD, mean difference; WC, waist circumference; WHR, waist–hip ratio.

* Statistically significant, see *Statistical Analysis* methods in Chapter 4.

included acupuncture/electroacupuncture alone or with metformin compared to a sham or metformin. Compared to sham acupuncture, the BMI and WHR were significantly reduced in the acupuncture groups (4 studies, 394 participants, MD −1.36 kg/m² [95% CI −2.32, −0.41], I² = 78% and MD −0.07 [95% CI −0.12, −0.02], I² = 96%, respectively).

Hormone levels were also assessed in three studies (A20, A28, A102). Luteinising hormones (LH) and the follicle-stimulating hormone (FSH) ratio were significantly reduced in the intervention group compared to the control (MD −0.17 [95% CI −0.24, −0.10], $I^2 = 0$%). Androgens were also measured, but there was no significant difference between the groups after the treatment. Indices of risk factors including fasting blood glucose, total triglycerides and cholesterol were also measured, but there were no significant differences between the groups.

Compared to metformin, the BMI was reduced after acupuncture treatments alone or combined with metformin (MD −1.30 kg/m^2 [95% CI −1.72, −0.87], $I^2 = 29$%) (A4, A24, A25, A67, A103). In two studies, the weight was also significantly reduced in the intervention group (MD −3.96 kg [95% CI −6.37, −1.54], $I^2 = 38$%), as was the WC in one study (MD −10.77 cm [95% CI −14.03, −7.51]). Similar to the result from sham-controlled studies, LH/FHS was significantly reduced in the intervention group compared to the control (MD −0.29 [95% CI −0.39, −0.18], $I^2 = 35$%), but the indices of risk factors were not.

Metabolic Syndrome

Four studies (A2, A42, A62, A100) evaluated people with obesity and metabolic syndrome. Two studies (A2, A62) evaluated acupuncture/electroacupuncture plus drug therapy as compared to drug therapy alone. Drug therapies included the use of rosiglitazone, glipizide, felodipine and simvastatin, as well as other routine treatments for diabetes and healthy lifestyle education.

The BMI was significantly reduced in the acupuncture group compared to control therapies (MD −2.28 kg/m^2 [95% CI −2.83, −1.73], $I^2 = 0$%). Fasting blood glucose and fasting insulin were also significantly reduced in the acupuncture treatment group compared to the control (MD −0.96 mmol/L [95% CI −1.32, −0.61], $I^2 = 79$%, and SMD −0.62 [95% CI −1.00, −0.23], $I^2 = 22$%, respectively).

One study (A42) compared acupuncture to sham acupuncture, and the other (A100) compared acupuncture or moxibustion to conventional antihypertensives, hypoglycaemics and lipid-lowering therapy. Compared to the sham, the acupuncture study (A42) did not show any significant difference in terms of weight, BMI and WC. Compared to basic therapies for metabolic syndrome, acupuncture significantly reduced the WC (MD −3.72 cm [95% CI −4.77, −2.67]), fasting blood glucose (MD −0.90 mmol/L [95% CI −0.32, −1.48]), triglycerides (MD −0.06 mmol/L [95% CI −0.01, −0.11]), but not blood pressure (A100).

Hypertension

In two studies (A44, A59) of participants with obesity and hypertension, acupuncture was compared to angiotensin-converting enzyme (ACE) inhibitors or angiotensin receptor blockers. Study A44 also included other routine treatments for hypertension, but the details were not specified. After eight weeks of treatment, weight and BMI were significantly reduced in the acupuncture group, when compared to the control (MD −5.18 kg [95% CI −8.01, −2.34], $I^2 = 0\%$ and MD −2.55 kg/m^2 [95% CI −4.11, −1.00], $I^2 = 76\%$, respectively).

The WC was also significantly reduced in the intervention group compared to the control (MD −5.54 cm [95% CI −7.80, −3.27], $I^2 = 0\%$). The WHR showed no differences between the groups (MD −0.03 [95% CI −0.06, 0.00], $I^2 = 45\%$). Indices of related complications were also analysed — cholesterol and low/high-density lipoprotein were not different between the groups after the treatment. However, the total triglycerides were significantly reduced in the acupuncture group when compared to the control (MD −0.34 mmol/L [95% CI −0.55, −0.12]), as were the systolic and diastolic blood pressure (MD −8.72 mmHg [95% CI −11.28, −6.15], $I^2 = 0\%$, and MD −3.56 mmHg [95% CI −5.60, −1.52], $I^2 = 0\%$, respectively).

Hyperlipidaemia

Four studies (A8, A11, A17, A30) included people with obesity and hyperlipidaemia. Treatments included acupuncture/electroacupuncture or electromagnetic pulse acupoint stimulation alone or combined with diet and/or exercise advice, as compared to diet and/or exercise advice. The BMI was significantly reduced after the intervention compared to the control in two studies, but the fat mass was not (MD −1.34 kg/m^2 [95% CI −2.22, −0.45], I^2 = 0% and MD −3.78% [95% CI −7.56, 0.01], I^2 = 78%). In single studies, weight and WC were significantly reduced after the treatment compared to the control (MD 4.25 kg [95% CI −6.52, −1.98] and MD −10.12 cm [95% CI −12.26, −7.98], respectively). Indices of related complications, including total cholesterol and triglycerides, were also reduced after the acupuncture interventions as compared to the control in four studies (MD −0.89 mmol/L [−1.46, −0.32], I^2 = 92% and MD −0.60 mmol/L [95% CI −1.05, −0.14], I^2 = 96%, respectively).

Frequently Reported Acupuncture Points in Meta-analyses Showing Favourable Effect

The frequently reported acupuncture points in meta-analyses showing favourable effects were: ST36 *Zusanli* 足三里, ST25 *Tianshu* 天枢, CV12 *Zhongwan* 中脘, SP6 *Sanyinjiao* 三阴交, CV4 *Guanyuan* 关元, ST40 *Fenglong* 丰隆, CV6 *Qihai* 气海, CV9 *Shuifen* 水分, SP9 *Yinlingquan* 阴陵泉, SP15 *Daheng* 大横 and ST28 *Shuidao* 水道. The ear acupuncture points were Endocrine 内分泌 (CO18), Stomach 胃 (CO4), Hunger 饥点, *Shenmen* 神门 (TF4) and Spleen 脾 (CO13).

Assessment Using GRADE

An assessment of the strength and quality (certainty) of the evidence from RCTs was made using Grading of Recommendations Assessment, Development and Evaluation (GRADE). Interventions, comparators and outcomes to be included were selected based on a consensus process described in Chap. 4. Two GRADE tables were produced.

Acupuncture/electroacupuncture was compared to sham acupuncture in seven studies (A20, A39, A42, A43, A52, A71, A72), and acupuncture plus lifestyle therapies were compared to lifestyle therapies in 30 studies (A8, A10–12, A15, A21, A23, A26, A31, A38, A40–41, A45, A48, A54, A58, A60–61, A64–66, A68–70,

Table 7.6. GRADE: Acupuncture vs. Sham-acupuncture

Outcome	Absolute Effect		Relative Effect (95% CI) No. of Participants & Studies	Certainty of the Evidence GRADE
	With ACU	Without ACU		
Weight (kg) Treatment duration: range – 4 to 12 weeks	**74.29** Average difference: 2.88 kg lower (95% CI: 5.20 lower to 0.56 lower)	**77.17**	**MD −2.88** (−5.20, −0.56) Based on data from 258 patients in 5 studies	⊕⊕⊕◯ MODERATE[1]
BMI Treatment duration: range – 4 to 12 weeks	**27.27** Average difference: 1.73 kg/m² lower (95% CI: 2.52 lower to 0.95 lower)	**29.00**	**MD −1.73** (−2.52 to −0.95) Based on data from 423 patients in 8 studies	⊕⊕⊕◯ MODERATE[2]
Waist circumference Treatment duration: range – 4 to 12 weeks	**94.17** Average difference: 7.28 cm lower (95% CI: 9.65 lower to 4.92 lower)	**101.45**	**MD −7.28** (−9.65, −4.92) Based on data from 200 patients in 4 studies	⊕⊕⊕◯ MODERATE[1]

The risk in the intervention group (and its 95% CI) is based on the assumed risk in the comparison group and the relative effect of the intervention (and its 95% CI).

Abbreviations: ACU, acupuncture; BMI, body mass index; CI, confidence interval; cm, centimetres; kg, kilogram; MD, mean difference.

1. Small sample size.
2. Unclear sequence generation and allocation concealment.

References

Weight: A39, A42, A52, A71, A90
Body mass index: A20, A39, A42–43, A52, A71–72, A90
Waist circumference: A20, A39, A42, A72

A73–75, A92, A101, A105). Outcomes included weight, BMI and WC (Tables 7.6 and 7.7).

Controlled Clinical Trials of Acupuncture

Four studies (A108–A111) used a non-randomised CCT design to evaluate acupuncture therapies compared to lifestyle therapies, no

Table 7.7. GRADE: Acupuncture plus Lifestyle Therapies vs. Lifestyle Therapies

	Absolute Effect		Relative Effect (95% CI) No. of Participants & Studies	Certainty of the Evidence GRADE
Outcome	With ACU	Without ACU		
Weight (kg) Treatment duration: range – 4 to 12 weeks	**68.27** Average difference: 4.36 kg lower (95% CI: 5.34 lower to 3.19 lower)	**72.63**	**MD –4.36** (–5.34, –3.19) Based on data from 1,304 patients in 15 studies	⊕⊕○○ LOW[1,2]
BMI Treatment duration: range – 4 to 24 weeks	**25.82** Average difference: 2.06 kg/m² lower (95% CI: 2.59 lower to 1.54 lower)	**27.88**	**MD –2.06** (–2.59, –1.54) Based on data from 2,820 patients in 22 studies	⊕⊕○○ LOW[1,2]
Waist circumference reatment duration: range – 4 to 24 weeks	**85.63** Average difference: 3.95 cm lower (95% CI: 6.37 lower to 1.54 lower)	**89.58**	**MD –3.95** (–6.37, –1.54) Based on data from 1,065 patients in 9 studies	⊕⊕○○ LOW[1,2]

The risk in the intervention group (and its 95% confidence interval) is based on the assumed risk in the comparison group and the relative effect of the intervention (and its 95% CI). Abbreviations: ACU, acupuncture; BMI, body mass index; CI, confidence interval; cm, centimetres; kg, kilogram; MD, mean difference.

1. Unclear sequence generation and allocation concealment. Lack of blinding of participants and personnel.
2. Considerable statistical heterogeneity.

References
Weight: A8, A12, A23, A31, A40, A48, A54, A58, A60–61, A65, A70, A73, A92, A105
Body mass index: A8, A11–12, A15, A21, A23, A26, A31, A40, A48, A54, A58, A60–61, A64–66, A70, A73–75, A105
Waist circumference: A8, A23, A60, A64, A66, A70, A73, A105

treatment, or metformin. Two studies included three arms — A110 had two control groups (no treatment or exercise) and A111 had two intervention groups (acupuncture alone or acupuncture plus exercise). A total of 303 participants were included in the studies. They all had simple obesity and were aged between 18 and 56 years. Two studies (A110, A111) only included female participants. Acupuncture points used in multiple studies were: CV10 *Xiawan* 下脘, CV12

Zhongwan 中脘, CV4 *Guanyuan* 关元, CV5 *Shimen* 石门, CV6 *Qihai* 气海, GB26 *Daimai* 带脉, SP6 *Sanyinjiao* 三阴交, ST24 *Huaroumen* 滑肉门, ST25 *Tianshu* 天枢, ST26 *Wailing* 外陵 and ST36 *Zusanli* 足三里.

Acupuncture plus Exercise *vs.* No Treatment or Exercise

One study (A111) compared acupuncture plus exercise to no treatment or exercise for two months. The BMI was significantly reduced in the intervention group, when compared to the no treatment control (MD -6.65 kg/m^2 [95% CI -6.71, -6.59]). The WHR and fat mass were also reduced in the intervention group when compared to the control (MD -0.14 [95% CI -0.17, -0.11] and MD -8.80 % [95% CI -11.77, -5.83], respectively). When the results from the exercise control group were analysed, acupuncture plus exercise was superior to exercise alone in terms of BMI reduction (MD -1.92 kg/m^2 [95% CI -1.96, -1.88]) and WHR (MD -0.06 [95% CI -0.09, -0.03]), but not the fat mass percentage.

One study (A110) with three arms compared acupuncture to exercise or acupuncture plus exercise to acupuncture alone over eight weeks. Acupuncture was administered every second day in the intervention groups, and exercise was undertaken for 60 minutes, three times a week. Acupuncture alone or acupuncture plus exercise, when compared to exercise, did not show any significant differences between the groups in terms of weight, BMI, WC, WHR or fat mass.

Acupuncture, Moxibustion, Ear Acupressure

One study (A109) comprising 63 participants used a comprehensive treatment of acupuncture, moxibustion and ear acupressure plus weight loss education, including diet and exercise guidance, was compared to metformin plus weight loss education. After two months of treatment, the BMI and WC were reduced in the intervention group, compared to the control (MD -1.86 kg/m^2 [95% CI -3.34, -0.38] and MD -3.86 cm [95% CI -6.86, -0.86], respectively).

One study (A108) included 105 participants and compared acupuncture therapies (manual acupuncture, moxibustion and ear acupressure) plus group psychotherapy to diet advice for two months. Weight was significantly reduced in the intervention group, compared to the control (MD −4.20 kg [95% CI −3.17, −5.23]), as was fat mass (MD −2.10 % [95% CI −3.92, −0.28]). However, the BMI was not significantly different between the groups.

Non-controlled Studies of Acupuncture

Acupuncture therapies were evaluated in 75 non-controlled clinical studies with a total of 7,212 participants. Most studies included people with simple obesity (59 studies, 78.7%), hyperlipidaemia (8 studies), diabetes mellitus (3), hypertension (3), PCOS (1) and fatty liver disease (1). Chinese medicine syndrome differentiation was performed in most studies (54 studies, 72%). Syndromes were used as an inclusion criterion in 17 studies and as a basis for treatment selection in 37 studies. Common syndromes were the same as in the RCT studies, including Stomach and intestine heat, Spleen deficiency and dampness, Liver *qi* stagnation, and Spleen and Kidney *yang* deficiency.

Acupuncture therapies included manual acupuncture (23 studies), acupuncture plus ear acupuncture (19), electroacupuncture (10), electroacupuncture plus ear acupuncture (9), acupuncture plus moxa (4), acupuncture plus ear acupuncture plus moxa (3), ear acupuncture (2), acupuncture plus ear acupuncture plus plum needle (1), ear acupuncture plus moxa (1), acupuncture plus plum needle (1), TENS (1) and photoelectric acupuncture (1).

The acupuncture points most frequently used in the studies were ST36 *Zusanli* 足三里, SP6 *Sanyinjiao* 三阴交, CV12 *Zhongwan* 中脘, ST25 *Tianshu* 天枢 and ST40 *Fenglong* 丰隆. The most common ear acupuncture points were Endocrine 内分泌 (CO18), Stomach 胃 (CO4), Spleen 脾 (CO13), *San Jiao* 三焦 (CO12) and *Shenmen* 神门 (TF4).

Safety of Acupuncture

About one-third of the RCTs and CCTs reported adverse events (31 studies, 28.2%). Of these studies, 15 reported no adverse events.

In 16 studies (A12, A19, A24, A32, A39, A40, A42, A50, A56, A63, A86, A94–96, A99, A102), adverse events occurred.

Overall, the acupuncture therapies were well tolerated, and only mild and temporary adverse events occurred. There were 30 cases of bruising in 678 participants receiving acupuncture therapies (from 16 studies that reported adverse events), 4 cases of pain, 2 cases of abdominal discomfort after electroacupuncture and 1 case of swelling at the acupuncture points. There were also three cases of prolonged menstruation after acupuncture/electroacupuncture. One study (A94) reported slight pain upon needle insertion and mild bruising following acupuncture and ear acupuncture in about 10% of its participants. Metformin was used alongside acupuncture in one study (A102), and 18 participants reported nausea, vomiting, diarrhoea, dizziness and a loss of appetite. The symptoms lasted more than a week, and the authors indicated that the adverse events were likely related to the use of metformin.

A total of 50 adverse events were reported in 617 participants in the control groups (from 16 studies that reported adverse events). Most events (46 cases) related to the use of metformin, including nausea, vomiting, gastrointestinal upset, diarrhoea, dizziness and a loss of appetite. One study (A50) reported two cases of weakness in participants taking the diet therapy, and another study (A96) reported that two participants were hospitalised in the no treatment control group; details were not given.

In the non-controlled studies, three (A139, A154, A186) reported that no events occurred, and one study (A168) reported 13 adverse events in 45 participants. In all 13 cases, the participants reported bruising and slight tingling after the acupuncture.

Summary of Acupuncture and Related Therapies Clinical Evidence

Acupuncture for obesity has been widely researched in clinical trials. A comprehensive search of electronic databases found over 60,000 possible citations. After screening, 186 clinical trials met the inclusion criteria. RCTs accounted for the highest number ($n = 107$), followed by non-controlled studies ($n = 75$), and then CCTs ($n = 4$). Previous systematic reviews have indicated that acupuncture can reduce weight, BMI and waist circumference in overweight and obese people as compared to lifestyle modifications or sham acupuncture.[2–3] In a study of ear acupuncture, the authors indicated that the best results were related to the total number of treatments and/or a treatment duration of longer than six weeks.[5]

An analysis of 107 published RCTs showed that acupuncture alone or combined with lifestyle therapies significantly reduced weight, BMI and WC as compared with sham acupuncture or lifestyle therapies alone. More than 10,000 people with a BMI of at least 23 kg/m² and aged between 18 and 70 years were included in these studies. Some studies included people with obesity alongside other health conditions, such as pre-diabetes or diabetes, PCOS, metabolic syndrome, hyperlipidaemia, hypertension, etc. About half of the studies also used Chinese medicine syndrome differentiation as an inclusion criterion or as a basis for treatment. Common syndromes were Stomach heat, Spleen deficiency and dampness, Spleen and Kidney *yang* deficiency, Liver *qi* stagnation, and Spleen and Stomach *qi* deficiency. These syndromes are consistent with those mentioned in the clinical practice guidelines (Chapter 2).

Electroacupuncture was the most commonly evaluated form of acupuncture therapy. This was followed by manual acupuncture, acupuncture plus auricular (ear) acupuncture/acupressure, ear acupuncture/acupressure alone, moxibustion, laser acupuncture, electromagnetic pulse acupoint stimulation and TENS on acupuncture points. The Stomach, Spleen and Conception Vessel points were commonly used in the studies, especially ST36, ST25 and CV12, and ear points, Stomach, *Shenmen* and Hunger. Results were similar for all the acupuncture interventions, but the electroacupuncture and manual acupuncture results for the reduction in weight, BMI and WC were greater than the results from studies that assessed acupuncture combined with ear acupressure, ear acupressure alone, moxibustion or laser acupuncture.

In terms of obesity comorbidities, acupuncture reduced the BMI and WHR, when compared to sham acupuncture or metformin in women with PCOS, but hormone levels showed mixed results. For obesity complicated with pre-diabetes, diabetes and hyperlipidae-mia, weight, BMI and WC were significantly reduced when the intervention was compared to the control, as did other indices of related complications, such as fasting insulin, HbA1c, total choles-terol and total triglycerides. Reduction in weight, BMI and WC were also seen in studies of obesity and hypertension and metabolic syn-drome, but there were only a small number of studies assessing participants with this profile.

Acupuncture

- Compared to sham acupuncture, manual acupuncture or electroa-cupuncture reduced weight, BMI, WC and WHR (moderate certainty evidence).
- Acupuncture alongside lifestyle therapies reduced weight, BMI and WC, but not the WHR or fat mass percentage, as compared to lifestyle therapies (low certainty evidence).
- Acupuncture alongside diet therapy significantly reduced weight, BMI, WC and WHR, when compared to sham acupuncture plus diet (not graded).
- Acupuncture plus lifestyle therapies were superior to lifestyle therapies in terms of weight, BMI, WC and WHR reduction, but not body fat mass (not graded).

Acupuncture plus Ear Acupressure

- Results from the RCTs showed variable effects of acupuncture plus ear acupressure.
- When compared to lifestyle therapies, there was no difference in terms of weight and BMI with acupuncture plus ear acupressure groups compared to lifestyle therapies.

- There was a significant reduction in the BMI in acupuncture plus ear acupressure plus lifestyle therapies group (not graded).

Ear Acupuncture

- Compared to sham ear acupuncture alongside lifestyle therapies, ear acupuncture plus lifestyle therapies significantly reduced BMI (not graded).
- Ear acupuncture alone or alongside lifestyle therapies was superior to no treatment in reducing weight and BMI (not graded).

Acupuncture plus Moxibustion Therapies

- Electroacupuncture plus moxibustion plus ear acupressure plus metformin was superior to metformin in reducing weight and BMI (not graded).
- Moxibustion reduced the WC in people with metabolic syndrome, compared to routine treatments (not graded).
- Acupuncture and moxibustion plus lifestyle therapies made no difference in body composition except for body weight when compared to lifestyle therapies (not graded).

Transcutaneous Electrical Stimulation on Acupoints

- TENS reduced the WC when compared to no treatment (not graded).
- Compared to lifestyle therapies, there was no difference in terms of the fat mass percentage when using electromagnetic pulse acupoint stimulation alone. However, the fat mass percentage was significantly reduced when using this therapy plus lifestyle therapies (not graded).

Laser Acupuncture

- Laser acupuncture was not superior to sham laser acupuncture in reducing BMI, weight, WC or WHR (not graded).

- Laser acupuncture plus lifestyle therapies did not reduce BMI, weight, WC or WHR when compared to lifestyle therapies (not graded).

Safety

Acupuncture therapies appeared to be safe for overweight and obese adults. Adverse events relating to the site of acupuncture included pain, bleeding, bruising and local allergic reactions. These events were mild and self-resolving. Other events that may be related but were too few to determine included heavy/prolonged menstruation.

Limitations

Despite the positive results, there was a general lack of high-quality studies, and a risk of bias was identified in most of the RCTs. The main bias came from the lack of description of random sequence generation and allocation concealment, as well as most studies using an open design, whereby participants and personnel knew the treatment they were receiving. Furthermore, heterogeneity was high in some of the meta-analyses, leading to uncertainty of the results. Many of the studies only assessed the short-term effect of acupuncture therapies (up to 12 weeks), and the long-term benefit is unclear.

Best Available Evidence

The best available evidence comes from a group of eight studies (A20, A39, A42, A43, A52, A71, A72, A90) comprising 423 participants. They compared acupuncture to sham acupuncture for up to 12 weeks. An assessment using GRADE showed moderate certainty evidence that acupuncture could reduce more weight (by ~2.9 kg, about 4% of one's body weight), BMI (by 1.7 kg/m^2) and WC (by 7.3 cm) than sham acupuncture. In studies that evaluated acupuncture alongside lifestyle therapies, results showed a greater reduction in weight (by ~4.4 kg, about 6% of one's body weight), BMI (by 2.1 kg/m^2) and WC (by 4 cm) than lifestyle therapies alone in the short term (up to

12 weeks). However, the certainty of results from these studies was low due to the lack of blinding of participants and personnel and heterogeneity in pooled results. Taken together, it appears that acupuncture alongside lifestyle therapies may be better than acupuncture alone in reducing weight, BMI and WC. This is not surprising as lifestyle therapies, such as reduced-calorie diets and increased physical activity, are important interventions for weight loss.[12,13]

References

1. Kim SY, Shin IS, Park YJ. (2018) Effect of acupuncture and intervention types on weight loss: A systematic review and meta-analysis. *Obes Rev* **19(11):** 1585–1596.

2. Zhang Y, Li J, Mo G, *et al*. (2018) Acupuncture and related therapies for obesity: A network meta-analysis. *Evid Based Complement Altern Med* **2018:** 9569685.

3. Fang S, Wang M, Zheng Y, *et al*. (2017) Acupuncture and lifestyle modification treatment for obesity: A meta-analysis. *Am J Chin Med* **45(2):** 239–254.

4. Namazi N, Khodamoradi K, Larijani B, *et al*. (2017) Is laser acupuncture an effective complementary therapy for obesity management? A systematic review of clinical trials. *Acupunct Med* **35(6):** 452–459.

5. Yeh TL, Chen HH, Pai TP, *et al*. (2017) The effect of auricular acupoint stimulation in overweight and obese adults: A systematic review and meta-analysis of randomized controlled trials. *Evid Based Complement Alternat Med* **2017:** 3080547.

6. Ruan ZX, Li Y, Zhou J, Huang X, *et al*. (2016) Auricular acupuncture for obesity: A systematic review and meta-analysis. *Int J Clin Exp Med* **9(2):** 1772–1779.

7. 国际生命科学学会中国办事处中国肥胖问题工作组联合数据汇总分析协作组. (2001) 中国成人体质指数分类的推荐意见简介. 中华预防医学杂志 **35(05):** 62–63.

8. WHO Consultation on Obesity (1999: Geneva, Switzerland), World Health Organization. (2000) *Obesity: preventing and managing the global epidemic. Report of a WHO consultation.* World Health Organization Technical Report Series 894. World Health Organization; Geneva, Switzerland.

9. 危北海, 贾葆鹏. (1998) 单纯性肥胖病的诊断及疗效评定标准. *中国中西医结合杂志*, **18(05):** 317–319.

10. World Health Organization. (1993) *Standard acupuncture nomenclature*. 2nd edition. World Health Organization; Geneva, Switzerland.

11. Wang Y. (2009) Ear acupuncture. In *Micro-acupuncture in practice*. Churchill Livingstone; St Louis, Missouri.

12. Shaw KA, Gennat HC, O'Rourke P, *et al*. (2006) Exercise for overweight or obesity. *Cochrane Database Syst Rev*. Issue 4. DOI: 10.1002/14651858. CD003817.pub3

13. Dombrowski SU, Knittle K, Avenell A, *et al*. (2014) Long term maintenance of weight loss with non-surgical interventions in obese adults: Systematic review and meta-analyses of randomised controlled trials. *BMJ* **348:** g2646.

References for Included Acupuncture Therapies Clinical Studies

Study No.	Reference
A1	王玉婷. (2017) 通腑泻热法针刺治疗单纯性肥胖病的临床研究. 南京中医药大学.
A2	安静. (2010) 针药复合对代谢综合征患者胰岛素抵抗和胰岛细胞功能的影响. 北京中医药大学.
A3	包扬, 白玉, 吴巍. (2014) 针刺联合盐酸二甲双胍片治疗肥胖 2 型糖尿病患者 60 例临床观察. *中国医学工程*. **22(12):** 34–35.
A4	蔡贤兵, 李亚, 王俊玲, 曹健. (2016) 电针及穴位埋线治疗肥胖型多囊卵巢综合征的临床观察. *光明中医*. **31(4):** 538–541.
A5	曾小冬. (2016) 针灸治疗肝郁脾虚型单纯性肥胖病并发痛经的疗效观察. *中国民族民间医药*. **25(21):** 72–73.
A6	Yeh ML, Chu NF, Hsu MY, *et al*. (2015) Acupoint stimulation on weight reduction for obesity: A randomized sham-controlled study. *West J Nurs Res* **37(12):** 1517–1530.
A7	陈纪华. (2016) 针灸对单纯性肥胖症伴血尿酸增高影响的临床研究. 广西中医药大学.
A8	陈霞, 周仲瑜, 黄伟, *et al*. (2017) 针灸疗法配合饮食运动治疗单纯性肥胖并发高脂血症的临床研究. *针灸临床杂志*. **33(7):** 1–5.

(Continued)

(*Continued*)

Study No.	Reference
A9	陈晓, 罗馨, 雷红, *et al.* (2017) 磁共振 IDEAL-IQ 序列评价"接力赛"电针法对腹型肥胖女性肝脏脂肪含量的影响. 放射学实践. **32(5):** 471–474.
A10	陈雁英. (2013) 电针配合饮食疗法治疗单纯性肥胖 52 例疗效观察. 湖南中医杂志. **29(2):** 76–77.
A11	程玲, 黄冬梅, 黄艳, *et al.* (2018) 秦亮甫教授"从脾论治"针刺治疗中心型肥胖伴高脂血症的临床研究. 世界中医药. **13(5):** 1233–1237, 1241.
A12	党辉. (2012) 电针结合中频治疗胃热湿阻型单纯性肥胖症的临床观察. 湖北中医药大学.
A13	邓春兰. (2006) 电针结合耳穴贴压疗法治疗单纯性肥胖症临床疗效观察. 北京中医药大学.
A14	丁莉莉, 马其江, 马建华. (2016) 阳明五行针法治疗单纯性肥胖病 60 例临床观察. 中医临床研究. **8(23):** 123–125.
A15	丁浔, 涂萍, 吴和平, *et al.* (2013) 针刺对 2 型糖尿病患者胰岛素抵抗及脂肪细胞因子水平的影响. 中国全科医学. **16(13):** 1184–1186.
A16	杜小伟. (2014) 脉冲穴位刺激干预下有氧训练对肥胖症患者体脂和血脂含量的影响研究. 现代预防医学. **41(3):** 491–493.
A17	范月侠, 白玉昊, 桂花. (2005) 针刺治疗伴有高脂血症的单纯性肥胖患者的症疗效观察. 宁夏医学院学报. **27(2):** 144–145.
A18	高立霞. (2014) 低频脉冲电刺激治疗肥胖 2 型糖尿病（湿热困脾证）的临床观察. 长春中医药大学.
A19	古丽加娜·奴尔包拉提. (2014) 针药结合治疗维吾尔族 2 型糖尿病脾虚痰瘀型的临床观察. 新疆医科大学.
A20	郭乃君. (2014) 针刺治疗多囊卵巢综合征胰岛素抵抗患者的临床疗效评价. 南京中医药大学.
A21	贺旭艳, 潘希方, 邹剑平. (2011) 针刺结合社区干预治疗成人肥胖症疗效观察. 中国现代医生. **49(18):** 159–160.
A22	金瑛, 王爱君, 薛平, *et al.* (2009) 温针治疗脾虚湿阻型单纯性肥胖症临床观察. 上海针灸杂志. **28(10):** 565–567.
A23	孔月晴. (2018) 腹穴齐刺法治疗单纯性肥胖胃热湿阻证 50 例. 中国中医药科技. **25(02):** 282–284.
A24	赖毛华, 马红霞, 姚红, *et al.* (2010) 腹针对肥胖型多囊卵巢综合征患者内分泌及糖脂代谢的影响. 针刺研究. **35(4):** 298–302.
A25	兰思杨. (2018) 针灸加耳穴帖压联合二甲双胍治疗肥胖型多囊卵巢综合征的疗效观察. 河北医科大学.

(Continued)

Study No.	Reference
A26	李广周. (2016) 康复运动结合针灸治疗对老年肥胖患者肥胖指标、心血管功能及生活质量的影响. *中国老年学杂志*. **36(22):** 5677–5679.
A27	李凯, 周仲瑜. (2016) 电针对单纯性肥胖症伴葡萄糖耐量异常的疗效观察. *针灸临床杂志*. **32(7):** 40–42.
A28	李赛赛. (2015) 针灸辅助二甲双胍治疗肥胖型多囊卵巢综合征不孕症 75 例. *中国中医药现代远程教育*. **13(6):** 78–79.
A29	李永华, 崔淑玫, 徐洪涛, 马建. (2013) 针灸治疗糖尿病合并肥胖患者临床观察. *针灸临床杂志*. **29(9):** 30–32.
A30	栗岩. (2018) 低强度有氧训练并脉冲穴位刺激治疗中老年高脂血症的效果. *中国老年学杂志*. **38(9):** 2074–2075.
A31	梁媚. (2016) 针灸治疗对单纯性肥胖患者肠道菌群的调节效应. 广西中医药大学.
A32	林宴菱. (2012) 三种治疗单纯性肥胖方法的临床疗效研究. 广州中医药大学.
A33	Hsieh CH. (2007) Auricular acupressure for weight reduction in obese Asian young adults: A randomized controlled trial. *Med Acupunct* **19(4):** 181–184.
A34	He W, Zhou Z, Li J, *et al.* (2012) Auricular acupressure plus exercise for treating primary obese women: A randomized controlled clinical trial. *Med Acupunct* **24(4):** 227–232.
A35	Darbandi M, Darbandi S, Owji AA, *et al.* (2014) Auricular or body acupuncture: Which one is more effective in reducing abdominal fat mass in Iranian men with obesity: A randomized clinical trial. *J Diabetes Metab Disord* **13(1):** 92.
A36	刘志诚, 孙凤岷, 闫润虎, *et al.* (2004) 针灸治疗女性单纯性肥胖并发更年期综合征的疗效观察(英文). *中国临床康复*. **(06):** 1198–1200.
A37	罗华丽. (2006) 电针对单纯性肥胖症的治疗作用及机制研究. 重庆医科大学.
A38	罗树华. (2007) 针灸治疗单纯性肥胖 60 例临床观察. *针灸临床杂志*. **23(9):** 17–18.
A39	潘晓伟. (2017) 针刺疗法对腹型肥胖及相关并发症的防治研究. 北京中医药大学.
A40	邵艳霞. (2014) 针灸配合生活方式干预单纯性肥胖的研究. *按摩与康复医学*. **5(1):** 69–70.

(Continued)

Study No.	Reference
A41	施洁, 朱小娟, 郭海莲, 季蓉. (2018) 针灸对单纯性肥胖患者血脂状态、炎症指标及减肥疗效的影响. 河北中医药学报. **33(05):** 39–41.
A42	孙玉秀. (2016) 针灸干预腹型肥胖防治代谢综合征的探索性研究. 北京中医药大学.
A43	童娟, 姚红, 陈健雄, *et al.* (2006) 腹针疗法治疗单纯性肥胖临床疗效观察. 针刺研究. **31(3):** 176–178.
A44	汪春, 程志清. (2006) 针灸对高血压肥胖患者的临床疗效评价及机理分析. 辽宁中医杂志. **33(10):** 1327–1328.
A45	王佳捷. (2017) 电针及埋线对单纯性肥胖患者血清瘦素、胰岛素影响的研究. 湖北中医药大学.
A46	王江华, 陈晓谦, 盛奕, *et al.* (2012) 针刺"腹六针"为主治疗单纯性肥胖症临床研究. *湖北中医杂志.* **34(8):** 17–19.
A47	王冉冉. (2015) 针灸对单纯性肥胖病患者 CRP 的影响及临床疗效观察. 广州中医药大学.
A48	王武杰, 肖云跑. (2014) 电针疗法治疗肥胖症的疗效观察. *中国基层医药.* **21(12):** 1878–1879.
A49	魏玮, 陈全利, 汪元军, 李娟. (2015) 腹穴齐刺法治疗单纯性肥胖胃热湿阻证的临床研究. *南京中医药大学学报.* **31(2):** 190–193.
A50	吴昊赛. (2017) 排刺法加耳穴改善腹部脂肪堆积肥胖患者腹围的随机对照研究. 成都中医药大学.
A51	项琼瑶, 李国安, 沈小珩, 洪洁. (2013) 电针结合耳穴干预单纯性肥胖伴糖调节受损临床研究. *上海中医药杂志.* **47(5):** 31–33.
A52	Wu J, Li Q, Chen L, Tian D. (2014) Clinical research on using acupuncture to treat female adult abdominal obesity with spleen deficiency and exuberant dampness. *J Tradit Chin Med* **34(3):** 274–278.
A53	谢长才, 符文彬, 孙健, *et al.* (2011) 针刺治疗单纯性肥胖症的规范化方案. *中国老年学杂志.* **31(24):** 4751–4753.
A54	邢海娇. (2009) 针刺结合饮食调整及有氧运动治疗单纯性肥胖症的临床研究. 河北医科大学.
A55	熊炜, 袁弘洁, 罗诗雨, 盘艳辉. (2016) 针刺治疗单纯性肥胖 29 例疗效观察. 湖南中医杂志. **32(5):** 115–117.
A56	徐慧文. (2017) 耳穴埋针干预超重或肥胖 2 型糖尿病患者的相关临床指标研究. 南京中医药大学.
A57	许毅克. (2016) 针灸治疗单纯性肥胖症临床方案探讨. 亚太传统医药. **12(1):** 94–95.

(Continued)

Study No.	Reference
A58	薛维华, 尹清波, 刘玲, *et al.* (2018) 调和阳明针法联合综合干预治疗单纯性肥胖临床研究. *河北中医*. **40**(2): 280–283.
A59	闫爱珍, 车伟军. (2014) 针灸对高血压肥胖患者的临床疗效观察. *慢性病学杂志*. **15**(8): 637–639.
A60	颜晓蓉. (2015) 穴位埋线与电针治疗单纯性肥胖的临床对比研究. 湖北中医药大学.
A61	杨天颖. (2014) 穴位埋线疗法治疗单纯性肥胖症临床疗效观察. 湖北中医药大学.
A62	姚美美. (2016) 针刺干预对代谢综合征脾虚痰湿型糖代谢功能紊乱的影响. 河北医科大学.
A63	詹云, 单鸣, 袁艺, *et al.* (2009) 耳穴贴压治疗 2 型糖尿病肥胖患者的临床观察. *中国医学创新*. **6**(27): 10–11.
A64	张翠彦, 杨力. (2015) 针刺治疗对单纯性向心性肥胖内脏脂肪的影响. *针刺研究*. **40**(6): 484–488.
A65	张丽. (2011) 电针结合中频治疗单纯性肥胖症的临床观察. 湖北中医药大学.
A66	张圣淇, 吴景东. (2016) 针刺治疗脾虚痰湿型单纯性肥胖症 120 例临床观察. *中医药导报*. **22**(6): 101–102.
A67	张亚琴. (2017) 针灸对肥胖型多囊卵巢综合征患者脂联素、瘦素及胰岛素抵抗的影响. *中医学报*. **32**(11): 2259–2262.
A68	张琰, 崔海. (2007) 针刺治疗心脾两虚型单纯性肥胖的临床疗效观察. *四川中医*. **25**(9): 112–113.
A69	赵桂英, 邢海娇, 李梅, *et al.* (2011) 电针结合饮食、有氧运动对单纯性肥胖症患者腰臀比值及血清瘦素的影响. *河北中医*. **33**(10): 1520–1522.
A70	赵李清. (2009) 电针结合饮食和运动疗法治疗胃肠实热型单纯性肥胖症的临床研究. 上海中医药大学.
A71	赵煜, 刘军, 刘耀, 林敏琴. (2011) 健脾化湿涤痰针刺法治疗单纯性肥胖的临床研究. *四川中医*. **29**(4): 123–125.
A72	郑阳, 任媛媛. (2018) 电针治疗胃肠实热型肥胖饮食行为数据变化的相关性分析. *世界最新医学信息文摘*. **18**(16): 166–167, 169.
A73	郑易炜, 周仲瑜. (2018) 电针疗法配合饮食运动治疗腹型肥胖疗效观察. *中国民族民间医药*. **27**(6): 111–113.
A74	周平南, 彭鹏鸣, 王蓉娣. (2013) 针灸治疗新发肥胖 2 型糖尿病疗效观察. *针灸临床杂志*. **29**(1): 21–23.

(Continued)

(Continued)

Study No.	Reference
A75	朱艺平, 黄盛新, 黎玮, *et al.* (2016) 平衡针灸治疗成人肥胖型糖耐量减低的临床观察. *现代生物医学进展*. **16(34):** 6694–6697.
A76	Xu Z, Li R, Zhu C, *et al.* (2013) Effect of acupuncture treatment for weight loss on gut flora in patients with simple obesity. *Acupunct Med* **31(1):** 116–117.
A77	Lei H, Chen X, Liu S, *et al.* (2017) Effect of electroacupuncture on visceral and hepatic fat in women with abdominal obesity: A randomized controlled study based on magnetic resonance imaging. *J Altern Complement Med* **23(4):** 285–294.
A78	Tseng CC, Tseng A, Tseng J, *et al.* (2016) Effect of laser acupuncture on anthropometric measurements and appetite sensations in obese subjects. *Evid Based Complement Alternat Med* **2016:** 1–8.
A79	Darbandi M, Darbandi S, Mobarhan MG, *et al.* (2012) Effects of auricular acupressure combined with low-calorie diet on the leptin hormone in obese and overweight Iranian individuals. *Acupunct Med* **30(3):** 208–213.
A80	Hsieh CH. (2010) The effects of auricular acupressure on weight loss and serum lipid levels in overweight adolescents. *Am J Chin Med* **38(4):** 675–682.
A81	Kim D, Ham OK, Kang C, *et al.* (2014) Effects of auricular acupressure using Sinapsis alba seeds on obesity and self-efficacy in female college students. *J Altern Complement Med* **20(4):** 258–264.
A82	Abdi H, Abbasi-Parizad P, Zhao B, *et al.* (2012) Effects of auricular acupuncture on anthropometric, lipid profile, inflammatory, and immunologic markers: A randomized controlled trial study. *J Altern Complement Med* **18(7):** 668–677.
A83	Schukro RP, Heiserer C, Michalek-Sauberer A, *et al.* (2014) The effects of auricular electroacupuncture on obesity in female patients — A prospective randomized placebo-controlled pilot study. *Complement Ther Med* **22(1):** 21–25.
A84	Abdi H, Zhao B, Darbandi M, *et al.* (2012) The effects of body acupuncture on obesity: Anthropometric parameters, lipid profile, and inflammatory and immunologic markers. *Scientific World Journal* **2012(1–11):** 603539.

(Continued)

Study No.	Reference
A85	Darbandi S, Darbandi M, Mokarram P, *et al.* (2013) Effects of body electroacupuncture on plasma leptin concentrations in obese and overweight people in Iran: A randomized controlled trial. *Altern Ther Health Med* **19(2):** 24–31.
A86	Hsu CH, Hwang KC, Chao CL, *et al.* (2005) Effects of electroacupuncture in reducing weight and waist circumference in obese women: A randomized crossover trial. *Int J Obes* **29(11):** 1379–1384.
A87	Nourshahi M, Ahmadizad S, Nikbakht H, *et al.* (2009) The effects of triple therapy (acupuncture, diet and exercise) on body weight: A randomized, clinical trial. *Int J Obes* **33(5):** 583–587.
A88	Lin CH, Lin YM, Liu CF. (2010) Electrical acupoint stimulation changes body composition and the meridian systems in postmenopausal women with obesity. *Am J Chin Med* **38(4):** 683–694.
A89	Jiao C, Zhu X, Zhang H, *et al.* (2015) EMP acupoint stimulation conducive to increase the effect of weight reduction through aerobic exercise. *Int J Clin Exp Med* **8(7):** 11317–11321.
A90	Gucel F, Bahar B, Demirtas C, *et al.* (2012) Influence of acupuncture on leptin, ghrelin, insulin and cholecystokinin in obese women: A randomised, sham-controlled preliminary trial. *Acupunct Med* **30(3):** 203–207.
A91	Wozniak P, Stachowiak G, Pieta-Dolinska A, *et al.* (2003) Laser acupuncture and low-calorie diet during visceral obesity therapy after menopause. *Acta Obstet Gynecol Scand* **82(1):** 69–73.
A92	Guo Y, Xing M, Sun W, *et al.* (2014) Plasma nesfatin-1 level in obese patients after acupuncture: A randomised controlled trial. *Acupunct Med* **32(4):** 313–317.
A93	Yeo S, Kim KS, Lim S. (2014) Randomised clinical trial of five ear acupuncture points for the treatment of overweight people. *Acupunct Med* **32(2):** 132–138.
A94	Fogarty S, Stojanovska L, Harris D, *et al.* (2015) A randomised cross-over pilot study investigating the use of acupuncture to promote weight loss and mental health in overweight and obese individuals participating in a weight loss program. *Eat Weight Disord* **20(3):** 379–387.

(Continued)

(Continued)

Study No.	Reference
A95	Allison DB, Kreibich K, Heshka S, *et al.* (1995) A randomised placebo-controlled clinical trial of an acupressure device for weight loss. *Int J Obes Relat Metab Disord* **19(9)**: 653–658.
A96	Liu CF, Chien LW, Lin MH, *et al.* (2011) Transcutaneous electrical stimulation of acupoints changes body composition and heart rate variability in postmenopausal women with obesity. *Evid Based Complement Alternat Med* **2011**: 1–7.
A97	El-Mekawy HS, El Deeb AM, Ghareib HO. (2015) Effect of laser acupuncture combined with a diet-exercise intervention on metabolic syndrome in post-menopausal women. *J Adv Res* **6(5)**: 757–763.
A98	Liu XG, Zhang J, Lu JL, *et al.* Laser acupuncture reduces body fat in obese female undergraduate students. *Int J Photoenergy* **2012**: 1–4.
A99	Hsu CH, Hwang KC, Chao CL, *et al.* (2005) Electroacupuncture in obese women: A randomized, controlled pilot study. *J Womens Health* **14(5)**: 434–440.
A100	郝燕. (2008) 温针灸任脉穴治疗代谢综合征的临床观察. 广州中医药大学.
A101	李海燕, 马朝阳, 徐芬. (2018) "标本配穴"电针疗法配合行为疗法治疗单纯性肥胖疗效及对胰岛素抵抗, 血脂水平的影响. *中华中医药学刊.* **36(8)**: 1848–1851.
A102	李荔, 莫蕙, 文斌, *et al.* (2014) 针灸联合二甲双胍治疗肥胖型多囊卵巢综合征不孕症的临床研究. *中华中医药杂志.* **29(7)**: 2115–2119.
A103	李凝, 巩静, 华川. (2016) 腹针联合二甲双胍治疗肥胖型多囊卵巢综合征患者的临床研究. *中西医结合研究.* **8(1)**: 11–13.
A104	李云燕. (2008) 耳穴磁珠贴压配合行为疗法治疗肥胖症 50 例. 针灸临床杂志. **(5)**: 29–30.
A105	裴海寅 (Bae Hae In). (2016) 电针结合饮食控制治疗单纯性肥胖的临床研究. 南京中医药大学.
A106	张安仁, 王文春, 胡斌, *et al.* (2007) 针灸结合行为疗法治疗老年单纯性肥胖病的临床研究. *西南军医.* **9(3)**: 1–4.
A107	Hassan NE, El-Masry SA, Elshebini SM, *et al.* (2014) Comparison of three protocols: Dietary therapy and physical activity, acupuncture, or laser acupuncture in management of obese females. *Maced J Med Sc* **7(2)**: 191–197.

(Continued)

Study No.	Reference
A108	Buevich V, Bozhko A, Vtorova L, *et al.* (2010) Acupuncture and psychotherapy in the complex treatment of obesity. *Med Acupunct* **22(3):** 187–190.
A109	刘鹏, 谷海鹰. (2010) 温针配合耳穴贴压治疗脾虚湿阻型单纯性肥胖 63 例临床观察. *四川中医.* **28(7):** 112–113.
A110	葛瀛. (2013) 有氧运动与针刺对中年肥胖女性脂代谢的影响研究. 河南大学.
A111	刘新荣. (2016) 中频电治疗结合有氧运动对青年女性肥胖者的影响. *河南科技大学学报 · 医学版.* **34(2):** 121–123.
A112	武君丽. (2000) Treatment of 150 cases of simple obesity with body acupuncture and otopoint pellet-pressing therapy. *世界针灸杂志: 英文版.* **10(4):** 39–41.
A113	安军明. (2007) 电针治疗单纯性肥胖症 72 例. *现代中医药.* **27(6):** 44–45.
A114	蔡敬宙. (2002) 针刺治疗单纯性肥胖症 50 例疗效观察. *中国临床康复.* **6(7):** 1037.
A115	曹新, 刘志诚, 徐斌. (2011) 针灸治疗单纯性肥胖病并发高血压病 731 例疗效观察. *天津中医药大学学报.* **30(4):** 207–211.
A116	曾士林, 胡建芳, 金丽珍. (2009) 针刺配合贴耳穴治疗突尼斯女性肥胖 68 例疗效观察. *实用中西医结合临床.* **9(6):** 25–26.
A117	陈彬沁, 李玉兰, 刘晓茹, *et al.* (2016) 脐全息隔姜灸配合耳穴贴压法治疗痰湿质单纯性肥胖 56 例. *中医外治杂志.* **25(5):** 9–10.
A118	陈锋, 吴凡, 张艳. (2005) 针刺对单纯性肥胖症患者 TNF-α 和 Resistin 水平的影响. *针刺研究.* **30(4):** 243–245.
A119	陈鎏香. (2006) 针刺治疗单纯性肥胖 85 例的临床研究. 成都中医药大学.
A120	陈天芳. (2012) 体针加耳穴贴压治疗单纯性肥胖症 46 例. *实用中医内科杂志.* **26(6):** 72–73.
A121	陈玉笋, 李如良, 牛秀莲. (2014) 针灸治疗女性肥胖伴发更年期综合征的临床研究. *微创医学.* **9(6):** 700–701, 688.
A122	徐斌, 袁锦虹, 刘志诚, *et al.* (2006) 脂联素在针刺抑制脂毒性中作用的临床观察. *上海针灸杂志.* **4(2):** 7–10.
A123	冯虹, 刘志诚, 徐斌. (2013) 温针灸治疗痰湿壅盛型原发性高血压并发肥胖 36 例. *安徽中医学院学报.* **32(1):** 47–50.

(Continued)

(Continued)

Study No.	Reference
A124	冯骅, 李健, 周欣, 杨帆. (2009) 针灸减肥 56 例疗效观察. *辽宁中医药大学学报*. **11(08):** 182–183.
A125	高秀领. (2004) 针刺治疗单纯性肥胖症的临床研究. 河北医科大学.
A126	郝燕, 王鹏. (2010) 针灸治疗痰湿内盛型单纯性肥胖 69 例. *中医研究*. **23(8):** 68–69.
A127	洪承铉. (2002) 针灸治疗单纯性肥胖病并发痛经的临床研究. 南京中医药大学.
A128	胡葵, 李嘉, 刘志诚. (2001) 针灸治疗肥胖型 NIDDM 的临床研究. *上海针灸杂志*. **20(4):** 8–10.
A129	黄黎珊, 陈友义, 纪峰. (2015) 通调任脉针刺法治疗腹型肥胖临床研究. 实用中医药杂志. **31(10):** 950–951.
A130	焦琳. (2006) 电针治疗单纯性肥胖病并发脂肪肝的临床研究. 南京中医药大学.
A131	金来星. (2005) 针刺减肥的临床研究. 湖北中医药大学; 湖北中医学院.
A132	居诗如, 尹晶, 徐芸, *et al.* (2018) 电针调节胃肠腑热型单纯性肥胖症患者肠道菌群临床观察. *湖北中医杂志*. **40(10):** 37–40.
A133	孔月晴, 杨常青. (2010) 针刺联合耳穴治疗单纯性肥胖 35 例疗效观察. *新中医*. **42(5):** 91–92.
A134	李尚安, 李佩佩, 阮骊韬, *et al.* (2017) 超声在针灸减肥对腹部脂肪影响研究中的应用价值. 临床医学研究与实践. **2(7):** 5–7.
A135	李思康, 张正龙, 丁定明, 马岚. (2012) 针刺治疗单纯性肥胖临床观察. *上海针灸杂志*. **31(8):** 548–549.
A136	李晓宁, 孙晓玲. (2011) 针刺结合耳穴法治疗 II 度单纯性肥胖症患者 50 例体会. *中医药信息*. **28(2):** 86–87.
A137	梁承凡. (2006) 电针治疗腹型肥胖的临床研究. 南京中医药大学.
A138	梁翠梅, 胡慧, 李媛媛. (2012) 通调带脉法针刺治疗腹型肥胖疗效观察. 针刺研究. **37(6):** 493–496.
A139	梁炜. (2014) 用针刺腹部腧穴配合饮食调节治疗单纯肥胖症的临床疗效观察. 当代医药论丛. **12(7):** 51–52.
A140	刘志诚, 孙凤岷, 赵东红, *et al.* (2004) 针灸对单纯性肥胖症瘦素和胰岛素抵抗的影响. *中国临床康复*. **8(3):** 562–565.
A141	陆春霞, 刘志诚, 徐斌. (2015) 温针灸治疗女性痰湿内阻型肥胖并发高脂血症患者疗效分析. 针灸临床杂志. **31(3):** 21–24.

(Continued)

Study No.	Reference
A142	吕雅妮, 刘志诚. (2015) 针灸调整单纯性肥胖病患者免疫功能 30 例. *中医研究*. **28(7)**: 31–33.
A143	马文明, 泰黎虹. (2008) 辨证配穴针刺治疗单纯性肥胖症 40 例. *中国医药指南*. **6(23)**: 346–347.
A144	庞婷婷, 刘志诚, 徐斌. (2015) 温针灸治疗女性脾肾阳虚型肥胖并发高脂血症患者疗效分析. *针灸临床杂志*. **31(10)**: 4–7.
A145	任彬彬, 刘志诚, 徐斌. (2012) 针灸治疗女性肥胖伴发更年期综合征疗效观察. *中国针灸*. **32(10)**: 871–876.
A146	施茵, 虞莉青, 尹小君. (2010) 针灸治疗肥胖型多囊卵巢综合征的临床疗效观察. *中华中医药学刊*. **28(4)**: 805–807.
A147	苏静, 沈素娥. (2005) 针刺治疗单纯性肥胖 32 例. *南京中医药大学学报*. **21(4)**: 262–263.
A148	唐其, 崔翔, 马冉, *et al.* (2014) 针刺治疗单纯性肥胖症 30 例临床观察. *光明中医*. **29(07)**: 1467–1468.
A149	陶善平, 王峰, 黄美芳, *et al.* (2007) 耳穴贴压治疗单纯性肥胖症临床观察. *北京中医*. **26(8)**: 514–515.
A150	田德润, 李晓东, 石玉顺, *et al.* (2003) 经皮神经电刺激治疗超重和肥胖症的初步研究. *北京大学学报(医学版)*. **35(3)**: 277–279.
A151	田华张, 王永兰. (2005) 针灸治疗单纯性肥胖症 80 例. *新疆中医药*. **23(5)**: 31–33.
A152	汪泓, 秦黎虹, 马文明. (2011) 俞募配穴针刺治疗单纯性肥胖症 35 例. *中国医药指南*. **9(13)**: 301–302.
A153	王凯悦, 刘志诚, 徐斌. (2015) 电针治疗女性胃肠腑热型肥胖并发高脂血症患者疗效分析. *针灸临床杂志*. **31(4)**: 22–25.
A154	王凌鸿, 陈爱武. (2014) 针灸治疗单纯性肥胖症 63 例. *中国中医药科技*. **21(2)**: 208–209.
A155	王鸣, 刘志诚, 徐斌. (2016b) 针灸治疗 1330 例单纯性肥胖病并发高脂血症的疗效. *世界华人消化杂志*. **24(05)**: 815–820.
A156	王鸣, 刘志诚, 徐斌. (2016a) 针刺加叩刺治疗阴虚夹瘀型肥胖并发高脂血症患者疗效分析. *中华中医药杂志*. **31(8)**: 3348–3351.
A157	王森, 黄根兰, 王培艳, *et al.* (2005) 针刺水穴治疗单纯性肥胖病疗效观察. *针灸临床杂志*. **21(10)**: 41–42.
A158	王铁云, 周志强. (2012) 腹针治疗单纯性肥胖临床疗效观察及其机制探讨. *基层医学论坛*. **16(2)**: 244–245.

(Continued)

(*Continued*)

Study No.	Reference
A159	王婷, 陈邦国. (2014) 电针治疗单纯性肥胖症 46 例. *湖北中医杂志*. **36(1):** 63–63.
A160	王燕珍. (2010) 针刺胃脘下俞等穴治疗单纯性肥胖临床观察. *山西中医学院学报*. **11(4):** 35–37.
A161	文漫红. (2007) 针灸对单纯性肥胖患者血浆环核苷酸含量的影响. *中医药导报*. **13(10):** 50–51, 71.
A162	谢莉, 刘志诚. (2009) 针灸对59例超重者临床疗效及相关指标的影响. *中国中医药信息杂志*. **16(10):** 75–76.
A163	谢新才, 周杰, 李彬, *et al.* (2012) 针刺治疗单纯性肥胖 60 例. *江西中医药*. **43(1):** 47–49.
A164	徐斌, 袁锦虹, 刘志诚, *et al.* (2005) 针刺影响单纯肥胖病患者血浆酪酪肽水平观察. *中国针灸*. **25(12):** 837–840.
A165	徐炳国, 刘志诚. (2005) 针灸对肥胖并发高血压瘦素胰岛素抵抗的影响. *上海中医药杂志*. **39(10):** 37–39.
A166	徐放明, 刘志诚, 宋琬北. (2002) 针灸治疗肥胖型 II 型糖尿病 45 例疗效观察. *天津中医*. **19(1):** 55–57.
A167	徐佳, 丘冰. (2007) 针刺配合耳压对中心型肥胖病患者血清胰岛素及睾酮的影响. *深圳中西医结合杂志*. **17(5):** 314–315.
A168	徐明明. (2008) 薄氏腹针为主治疗单纯性肥胖症的临床观察. 南方医科大学.
A169	闫利敏. (2017) 患者针感与临床疗效关系初步探究. 南京中医药大学.
A170	闫利敏, 刘志诚, 袁锦虹, 徐斌. (2016) 电针对胃肠腑热型单纯性肥胖病患者内脏脂肪的作用. *中国针灸*. **36(9):** 897–900.
A171	闫利敏, 袁锦虹, 刘志诚, 徐斌. (2017) 温针灸对痰湿内阻型单纯性肥胖病患者内脏脂肪作用. *辽宁中医药大学学报*. **19(03):** 57–59.
A172	殷茵, 刘志诚, 徐斌, 卢圣峰. (2016) 针刺联合耳针治疗肝郁脾虚型肥胖并发高脂血症患者疗效分析. *时珍国医国药*. **27(6):** 1411–1413.
A173	于雪婷. (2012) 针灸治疗肥胖症 60 例临床疗效分析. *中国民族民间医药*. **21(18):** 109–109.
A174	何玉. (2010) 针刺祛脂塑身疗效观察. *海南医学院学报*. **16(10):** 1353–1359.
A175	原萌谦, 刘志诚, 徐斌, 卢圣锋. (2016b) 针刺加叩刺联合耳针治疗肝郁脾虚型肥胖并发高脂血症患者疗效分析. *世界科学技术–中医药现代化*. **18(2):** 250–255.

(Continued)

Study No.	Reference
A176	原萌谦, 刘志诚, 徐斌, 卢圣锋. (2016a) 温针灸联合耳针治疗脾虚湿阻型肥胖并发高脂血症患者疗效分析. *辽宁中医杂志*. **43(12):** 2614–2617.
A177	张娜, 刘志诚, 徐斌. (2014) 电针治疗T2DM伴肥胖 203 例研究. *世界科学技术–中医药现代化*. **16(8):** 1809–1813.
A178	张少芸, 王玲, 杨卓欣, *et al.* (2015) 调任通督针刺法治疗单纯性肥胖 80 例临床观察. *新中医*. **47(2):** 191–192.
A179	张艳丽, 夏鸿清, 黄安. (2014) 电针治疗单纯性肥胖 56 例临床疗效观察. *世界中西医结合杂志*. **9(1):** 74–75, 85.
A180	张中成, 王嘉莉, 康钦凌. (2007) 针刺治疗单纯性肥胖病并发月经失调疗效观察. *四川中医*. **25(2):** 103–104.
A181	赵会玲. (2007) 体针结合耳穴贴压治疗单纯性肥胖病 80 例. *四川中医*. **25(5):** 103–104.
A182	周莉萍. (2011) 针灸治疗单纯性肥胖的肠道菌群调节机理探讨. *成都中医药大学*.
A183	周仲瑜, 何伟. (2009) 辨证选穴配合耳压治疗单纯性肥胖症. *针灸临床杂志*. **25(6):** 27–28.
A184	孙红, 陈正秋. (2008) Relation between treatment course and therapeutic effects of acupuncture for female obesity of different types. *中医杂志 · 英文版*. **28(4):** 258–261.
A185	Tür FT, Aksay E, Kiliç TY, *et al.* (2015) Therapeutic effects of acupuncture on obesity and HbA1c. *Eur J Integr Med* **7(2):** 88–93.
A186	Huang MH, Yang RC, Hu SH. (1996) Preliminary results of triple therapy for obesity. *Int J Obes Relat Metab Disord* **20(9):** 830–836.

8

Clinical Evidence for Other Chinese Medicine Therapies

OVERVIEW

Other Chinese medicine therapies for people who are overweight and obese include Chinese diet therapy, cupping therapy, *tuina* massage, *qigong* and *tai chi*. Only a small number of clinical trials have evaluated these therapies. However, there are some promising results that indicate they may be effective for weight loss.

Introduction

Apart from herbal medicine and acupuncture, Chinese medicine (CM) treatments include other therapies. For people who are overweight and obese, there are several therapies that have been evaluated in clinical trials, including diet therapy, cupping therapy, *tuina* massage, *qigong* and *tai chi*.

Previous Systematic Reviews

No systematic reviews were identified in either English or Chinese literature.

Identification of Clinical Studies

A search of Chinese and English literature found over 60,000 potentially relevant citations, and 2,823 full-text articles were evaluated.

A total of 28 clinical trials, including 3,080 participants, evaluated other CM therapies for overweight and obesity (O1–28). There were 21 randomised controlled trials (RCTs), two controlled clinical trials (CCTs) and five non-controlled studies included (Fig. 8.1). Evidence from the RCTs was evaluated to establish the efficacy and safety of other CM therapies for overweight and obesity. All studies were conducted in China, except for three from the United States, two from Italy, one from Iran and one from Australia.

Risk of Bias

The risk of bias of the 21 RCTs was analysed (O1–21). Overall, there was an unclear risk of bias for sequence generation, and only seven studies (O5, O6, O9, O10, O15, O18, O21) provided adequate information for this domain. Only two (O1, O18) provided details of allocation concealment. Blinding domains were judged to be at high risk of bias in all studies. This is not surprising as it is very difficult to blind participants and personnel undertaking physical activities or manual therapies. All studies provided detailed information on dropouts. Therefore, this domain was judged to be at low risk of bias for all studies. Study protocols could not be located, so all studies were judged to be at an unclear risk of bias for selective outcome reporting.

Qigong Therapies

Six RCTs (O4, O10–14) assessed *qigong* exercise in 399 people. Uncomplicated obesity participants were included in one study and the other studies included people with metabolic syndrome, diabetes mellitus or hypertension. Three different styles of *qigong* were evaluated: *ba duan jin* (4 studies), *dao yin* (1 study) and *yi jin jing* (1 study).

Three studies (O10, O11, O14) compared *qigong* to health education. One study (O10) evaluated people with hypertension and obesity and administered *dao yin* style *qigong* that incorporated squatting exercises, abdominal breathing and acupressure point massage twice a day for five minutes each time over 12 weeks. Compared

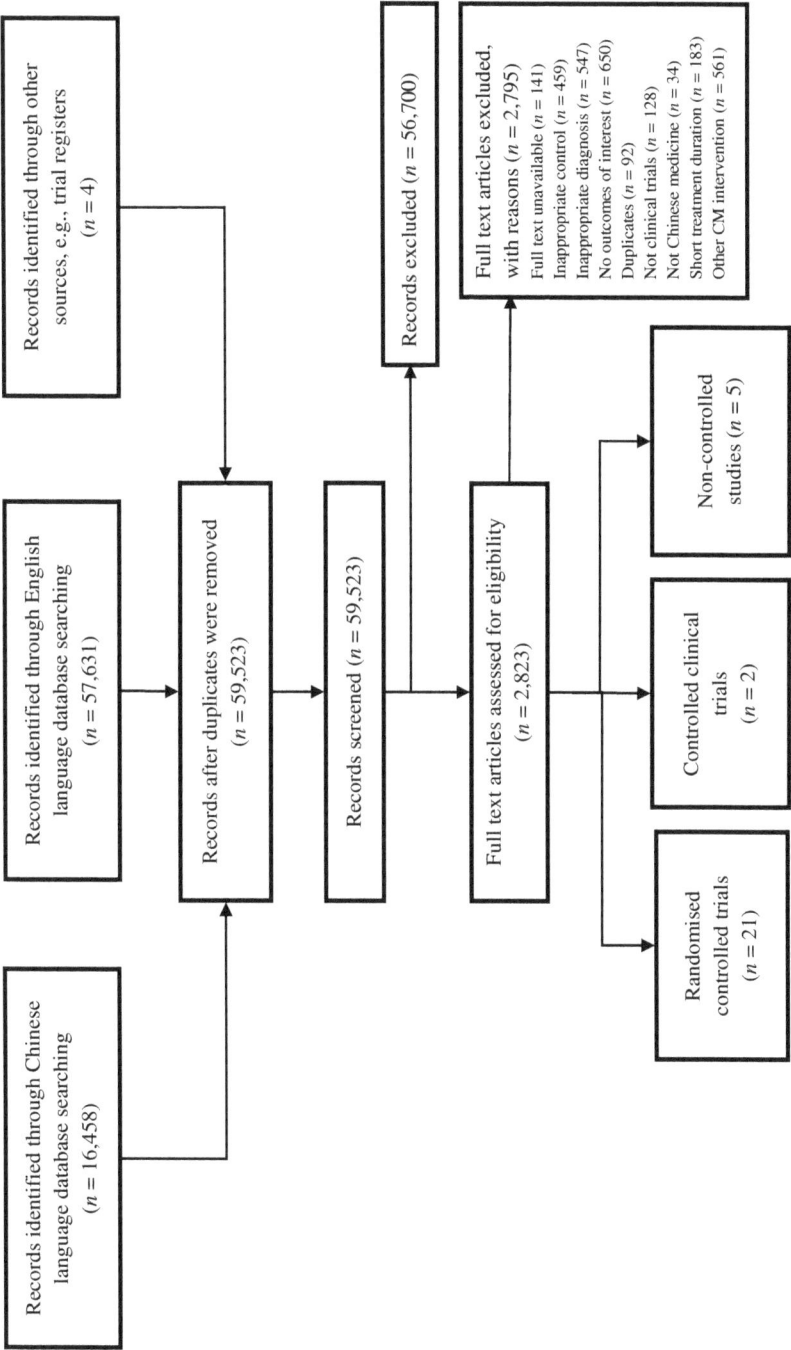

Fig. 8.1. Flow chart of the study selection process: Other Chinese medicine therapies.

Records identified through other sources, e.g., trial registers (*n* = 4)

Records identified through English language database searching (*n* = 57,631)

Records identified through Chinese language database searching (*n* = 16,458)

Records after duplicates were removed (*n* = 59,523)

Records screened (*n* = 59,523)

Records excluded (*n* = 56,700)

Full text articles assessed for eligibility (*n* = 2,823)

Full text articles excluded, with reasons (*n* = 2,795)
Full text unavailable (*n* = 141)
Inappropriate control (*n* = 459)
Inappropriate diagnosis (*n* = 547)
No outcomes of interest (*n* = 650)
Duplicates (*n* = 92)
Not clinical trials (*n* = 128)
Not Chinese medicine (*n* = 34)
Short treatment duration (*n* = 183)
Other CM intervention (*n* = 561)

Non-controlled studies (*n* = 5)

Controlled clinical trials (*n* = 2)

Randomised controlled trials (*n* = 21)

to health education alone, *qigong* did not significantly reduce weight or waist-hip ratio (WHR). In another study (O11) that evaluated people with hypertension and obesity, *ba duan jin* and health education were compared to health education alone over 12 months. Results showed no significant differences between the groups at the end of the treatment.

Yi jin jing style *qigong* plus health education were compared to health education alone in people with metabolic syndrome over six months. Outcomes were significantly reduced in the *qigong* group as compared to the control (O14):

- Weight: mean difference (MD) −4.47 kg [95% confidence interval (CI) −6.97, −1.97].
- Body mass index (BMI): MD −1.63 kg/m^2 [95% CI −2.01, −1.25].
- Waist circumference (WC): MD −3.09 cm [95% CI −4.64, −1.54].
- Fasting blood glucose: MD −0.81 mmol/L [95% CI −0.90, −0.72].

Ba duan jin was compared to no treatment in two studies (O12, O13) that assessed females with obesity. Both studies instructed participants to perform one hour of *ba duan jin* five days a week for 10 or 16 weeks. Weight and WC were not significantly reduced when the two studies were pooled; however, weight and WHR were significantly reduced in the *qigong* group as compared to the control in one study (O12) (MD −3.16 kg [95% CI −4.18, −2.14], and MD −0.03 [95% CI −0.04, −0.02], respectively).

In one study (O4), *qigong* was practised every day for 90 minutes in addition to participants taking the diabetes drug glipizide as compared to glipizide alone for 24 weeks. Weight and BMI did not decrease after the treatment, but the WC and WHR were significantly reduced in the *qigong* group as compared to the control (MD −3.95 cm [95% CI −7.51, −0.39] and MD −0.04 [95% CI −0.06, −0.02], respectively). Other outcomes such as blood glucose, cholesterol and triglycerides were not significantly different between the groups after the treatment.

None of the *qigong* studies reported whether any adverse events occurred.

Tai Chi

Seven studies evaluated *tai chi* for overweight and obesity. Four RCTs (O16–19) included 425 participants with different comorbidities. One study (O16) enrolled people with central obesity and metabolic syndrome and compared 12 weeks of *tai chi* to no treatment or a generic fitness program. Two studies (O17, O18) enrolled postmenopausal women to *tai chi* plus diet and weight loss meetings as compared to the diet and weight loss meetings or no treatment. Finally, one study (O19) enrolled people with obesity and depression and compared *tai chi* to no treatment. Results could not be pooled in meta-analysis but appeared mixed, with some studies showing a reduction in WC but no changes in key outcomes in others. Adverse events were not reported in the studies, except for one (O19) that reported two deaths in the control group and one case of worsening depression.

Two CCTs (O22, O23) evaluated *tai chi* plus lifestyle therapies, such as diet, exercise and education, as compared to no treatment. One study (O22) enrolled 54 female participants with simple obesity and a BMI of greater than 30 kg/m². *Yang style tai chi* was performed twice a week (45 minutes per session) for 16 weeks. The other study (O23) enrolled 33 postmenopausal women with obesity and a BMI of greater than 30 kg/m². *Tai chi* was undertaken three times per week for 12 weeks. Results from both studies were presented as a reduction in weight, BMI, WC and WHR. However, there were no significant differences between the *tai chi* intervention groups and controls. Adverse events were reported in the *tai chi* groups, but the events were unrelated to the intervention.

Tai chi was also evaluated in one non-controlled study (O28) comprising seven women with obesity and a BMI of greater than or equal to 40 kg/m². They undertook a weekly group *tai chi* session and two DVD-guided sessions at home for eight weeks. However, there was no significant weight loss after eight weeks. Adverse events were not reported in this study.

Tuina (Massage)

Tuina massage was evaluated in seven RCTs (O1–3, O6–8, O15), comprising 608 participants. All studies included participants with simple obesity and a BMI of greater than or equal to 25 kg/m². In the studies that mentioned CM syndromes, Spleen deficiency and dampness were common. Most studies evaluated *tuina* alongside a diet and exercise program as compared to the diet and exercise program alone, except for one study (O6), which enrolled participants with diabetes and compared *tuina* plus metformin to metformin alone. *Tuina* techniques, such as rolling and pushing, were applied to the abdomen, arms and legs, and acupuncture points were pressed. Points included ST25 *Tianshu* 天枢, CV4 *Guanyuan* 关元, PC6 *Neiguan* 内关, SP6 *Sanyinjiao* 三阴交, ST36 *Zusanli* 足三里, ST40 *Fenglong* 丰隆, etc. *Tuina* was self-administered after exercise in one study (O2).

Weight, BMI and WC were significantly reduced in the *tuina* intervention groups, compared to the control:

- Weight: MD −4.22 kg [95% CI −6.34, −2.10], $I^2 = 60\%$ (5 studies, O1–O3, O8, O15).
- BMI: MD −1.88 kg/m² [95% CI −3.27, −0.50], $I^2 = 96\%$ (5 studies, O1–O3, O8, O15).
- WC: MD −3.32 cm [95% CI −4.85, −1.78], $I^2 = 0\%$ (3 studies, O3, O8, O15).

In the study (O6) that compared *tuina* plus metformin to metformin alone in people with obesity and diabetes, weight, BMI and WC reduction were not significantly different between the groups.

Four non-controlled studies (O24–27) evaluated *tuina* in 166 people with simple obesity. All studies used an abdomen massage with or without pressing on acupuncture points, such as ST25 *Tianshu* 天枢, CV4 *Guanyuan* 关元, CV8 *Shenque* 神阙, etc. Most treatments lasted 30 minutes, three to seven times per week for four to six weeks.

Cupping Therapy

Two RCTs (O5, O9) evaluated cupping therapy in 124 people with obesity. One study compared cupping plus diabetes routine treatments to metformin and routine treatments in people with a BMI greater than or equal to 28 kg/m^2 and diagnosed with diabetes. Cupping was applied to the abdomen, upper arms and thighs every day in the first week, every second day for three weeks and twice a week for two months (total treatment duration: three months). Results showed that weight, BMI, WC and blood glucose were not reduced in the treatment group, compared to the control (O5).

In the other study (O9), mobile cupping was applied to the abdomen for five minutes, followed by stationary cupping on ST25 *Tianshu* 天枢 and CV4 *Guanyuan* 关元 for 10 minutes. The BMI was reduced in the cupping group as compared to the no treatment control (MD −1.76 kg/m^2 [95% CI −3.20, −0.32]), but other outcomes, such as weight and WC, were similar between the groups at the end of the treatment.

Chinese Diet Therapy

Two studies (O20, O21) compared a Chinese diet therapy of approximately 1,200 Kcal per day to a Western diet with the same number of calories. The Chinese diet included traditional staples such as soybeans, black beans, fish and green vegetables. The Western diet consisted of bread, potatoes, red meat, beans, fruit, etc. A total of 978 participants were enrolled in the studies for six weeks. The authors indicated that the BMI was reduced more in the Chinese diet groups as compared to the Western diet, but the results could not be pooled in a meta-analysis.

Summary of Other Chinese Medicine Clinical Evidence

Various other CM therapies have been evaluated for overweight and obesity, including *qigong, tai chi, tuina* massage, cupping therapy and diet therapy. *Qigong* styles included *ba duan jin, dao yin* and *yi jin jing*. Only six studies evaluated *qigong*, and the results were mixed. *Qigong* plus health education significantly reduced weight, BMI and WHR in one study, but two studies showed no difference between the groups. The other three studies showed no difference between *qigong* and no treatment or diabetes medication. The treatment duration ranged from 10 weeks to 12 months. Participants undertook one to seven *qigong* sessions per week, for approximately 5 to 90 minutes each time. The study with the largest benefit instructed participants to undertake *qigong* twice daily for 30 minutes each time alongside a health education program at a community health centre. Overall, the small number of studies (in older participants) does not allow for firm conclusions, but *qigong* may not be effective for weight loss. Similar to *qigong*, there was insufficient evidence to draw conclusions about the potential benefit of *tai chi* due to the small number of studies and methodological shortfalls. Results could not be pooled in meta-analysis but appeared mixed, with some studies showing a reduction in waist measures and no changes in others.

Tuina massage focused on the abdomen and meridian acupressure on the Stomach and Conception Vessel points. Most studies required three treatment sessions per week, and participant self-massage was also used to supplement the in-clinic treatments. *Tuina*, alongside a diet and exercise program, when compared to the diet and exercise program alone, reduced weight, BMI and WC. Cupping therapy was only evaluated in two studies, and results were mixed, but the small number of studies does not allow for a firm conclusion to be drawn.

A traditional Chinese diet reduced weight and BMI more than a Western diet in two studies. However, like the other therapies, the small number of studies does not allow for a firm conclusion to be drawn.

Overall, despite a comprehensive search of the available literature, only a small number of studies evaluated other CM therapies for overweight and obesity. Therefore, there is insufficient evidence to support the use of these therapies in routine clinical practice. Further research on the most promising therapies, such as *tuina* massage and Chinese diet therapy, is needed.

References for Included Other Chinese Medicine Therapies Clinical Studies

Study No.	Reference
O1	陈勇志. (2014) 健脾利湿手法治疗产后肥胖症（痰湿证）的临床研究. 长春中医药大学.
O2	江声策. (2014) 有氧运动与穴位按摩对肥胖女性身体成分和血脂水平的影响. 长春师范大学学报(自然科学版). **33**(4): 98–101.
O3	李慧梅, 于娟. (2010) 推拿点穴治疗脾虚湿阻型单纯性肥胖 67 例临床观察. 山东中医药大学学报. **34**(6): 508–509.
O4	刘涛, 白石, 张荣超. (2018) 健身气功八段锦对肥胖中年女性糖尿病患者相关指标的影响. 中国应用生理学杂志. **34**(1): 19–22.
O5	么焕新, 柴颖, 王文双. (2011) 拔罐辅助治疗肥胖型 2 型糖尿病临床疗效观察. 中国全科医学. **14**(15): 1723–1725.
O6	宋柏林, 朴春丽, 陈曦, 齐伟, 于淼, 王之虹. (2011) 推拿配合二甲双胍治疗肥胖Ⅱ型糖尿病患者 80 例临床观察. 成都中医药大学学报. **34**(3): 9–11.
O7	王本玲, 于娟. (2010) 健脾祛湿推拿法治疗单纯性肥胖症血脂变化临床观察. 吉林中医药. **30**(9): 786–788.
O8	王莉, 于娟, 于敏. (2015) 通腑深按推腹法治疗脾虚湿阻型单纯性肥胖症临床研究. 四川中医. **33**(8): 149–150.
O9	王晓曼. (2017) 药罐疗法对腹型肥胖人群内脏脂肪代谢影响的临床研究. 北京中医药大学.
O10	严培晶. (2015) 312 经络锻炼法对肥胖性高血压患者干预效果的研究. 福建中医药大学.

(Continued)

Study No.	Reference
O11	于海兰. (2013) 八段锦运动疗法干预高血压肥胖患者 104 例临床观察. *中国临床医生*. **41(8)**: 47–48.
O12	余忠舜, 喻治达, 沈建丽. (2017) 健身气功·八段锦对肥胖女大学生脂代谢的影响. *当代体育科技*. **7(04)**: 25–26.
O13	张晓强. (2008) 健身气功·八段锦对超重或肥胖中年女性代谢综合征相关指标的影响. 北京体育大学.
O14	邹忠, 施晓芬, 张宏. (2013) 易筋经干预代谢综合征 100 例临床研究. *长春中医药大学学报*. **29(3)**: 398–399.
O15	阎博华, 彭趣思, 魏启华, 丰芬. (2014) 经穴推拿对单纯性肥胖患者体质量、体质量指数, 腰围及臀围的影响: 随机对照研究(英文). *World J Acupunct Moxibustion*. **24(01)**: 6–9, 50.
O16	Siu PM, Yu AP, Yu DS, *et al.* (2017) Effectiveness of tai chi training to alleviate metabolic syndrome in abdominal obese older adults: A randomised controlled trial. *The Lancet* **390(Spec. Iss. 1)**: 11.
O17	Bekke J, Letendre J, Beebe N, *et al.* (2013) Effects of a dietary and tai chi intervention on body composition in obese older women. *FASEB Journal* **27**: 1068–1072.
O18	Beebe N, Magnanti S, Katkowski L, *et al.* (2013) Effects of the addition of t'ai chi to a dietary weight loss program on lipoprotein atherogenicity in obese older women. *J Altern Complement Med* **19(9)**: 759–766.
O19	Liu X, Vitetta L, Kostner K, *et al.* (2015) The effects of tai chi in centrally obese adults with depression symptoms. *Evid Based Complement Alternat Med*. **2015**: 879712.
O20	Liguori A, Petti F, Rughini S, *et al.* (2013) Effect of a basic Chinese traditional diet in overweight patients. *J Tradit Chin Med* **33(3)**: 322–324.
O21	Leonetti F, Liguori A, Petti F, *et al.* (2016) Effects of basic traditional Chinese diet on body mass index, lean body mass, and eating and hunger behaviours in overweight or obese individuals. *J Tradit Chin Med* **36(4)**: 456–463.
O22	Xu F, Letendre J, Bekke J, *et al.* (2015) Impact of a program of tai chi plus behaviorally based dietary weight loss on physical functioning and coronary heart disease risk factors: A community-based study in obese older women. *J Nutr Gerontol Geriatr.* **34(1)**: 50–65.

(Continued)

Study No.	Reference
O23	Maris S A, Quintanilla D, Taetzsch A, *et al.* (2014) The combined effects of tai chi, resistance training, and diet on physical function and body composition in obese older women. *J Aging Res* **2014:** 657851.
O24	尚蓉, 马七一. (2006) 腹部精油八法推拿治疗单纯性肥胖 37 例. *中华实用中西医杂志*. **19(8):** 911–912.
O25	许一鹤. (2016) 基于 fMRI 技术研究按摩治疗单纯性肥胖中枢机制的脑功能连接网络响应特征. 贵阳中医学院.
O26	张欣, 刘明军, 李冬梅, 卓越. (2009) 运腹推经法治疗单纯性肥胖症疗效观察. *吉林中医药*. **29(12):** 1050–1051.
O27	卓越, 周杨, 张欣, 陈邵涛, *et al.* (2014) 运腹通经推拿法治疗产后肥胖症的临床观察. *中国妇幼保健*. **29(35):** 5939–5940.
O28	Siegel SG, Stucker CL, Del Vecchio MS, *et al.* (2018) Tai Chi as an intervention to promote quality of life and mobility for women who are morbidly obese: A pilot study. *J Womens Health Phys Therap.* **42(1):** 2.

.

9

Clinical Evidence for Combination Therapies

OVERVIEW

In clinical practice, Chinese medicine therapies are often used together to improve treatment outcomes. Commonly, Chinese herbal medicine is used alongside acupuncture, as well as other therapies, such as cupping, *tuina* massage and *qigong*. This chapter includes clinical studies that use a combination of two or three treatments in people who are overweight or obese.

Introduction

Combination Chinese medicine (CM) therapies are defined as two or more CM interventions from different categories administered together; for example, herbal medicine plus acupuncture, or herbal medicine plus *tuina* massage. This approach is common in clinical practice.

Previous Systematic Reviews

Herbal medicine and acupuncture for the treatment of obesity were reviewed by Nam and colleagues in 2016.[1] The review included 4 clinical studies and 16 animal studies, and results indicated that pharmacopuncture (herbal medicine delivered via injection at acupuncture points) might be beneficial for treating obesity. However, further well-designed, randomised clinical trials are needed. Results from the animal studies indicated that the mechanisms of action include anti-inflammation, anti-oxidation and modulating lipid metabolism, etc. There were no other systematic reviews on combination CM therapies for obesity.

Identification of Clinical Studies

A search of electronic Chinese and English literature found over 60,000 potentially relevant citations. After screening, 2,823 full-text articles were evaluated, and 30 clinical trials (C1–30) were included. There were 18 randomised controlled trials (RCTs), 3 controlled clinical trials (CCTs) and 9 non-controlled studies (Fig. 9.1). Evidence from the RCTs was evaluated to establish the efficacy and safety of combination therapies. All studies were conducted in China, except for one that was from Italy. Combination therapies varied but mostly included Chinese herbal medicine (CHM) and acupuncture (Table 9.1).

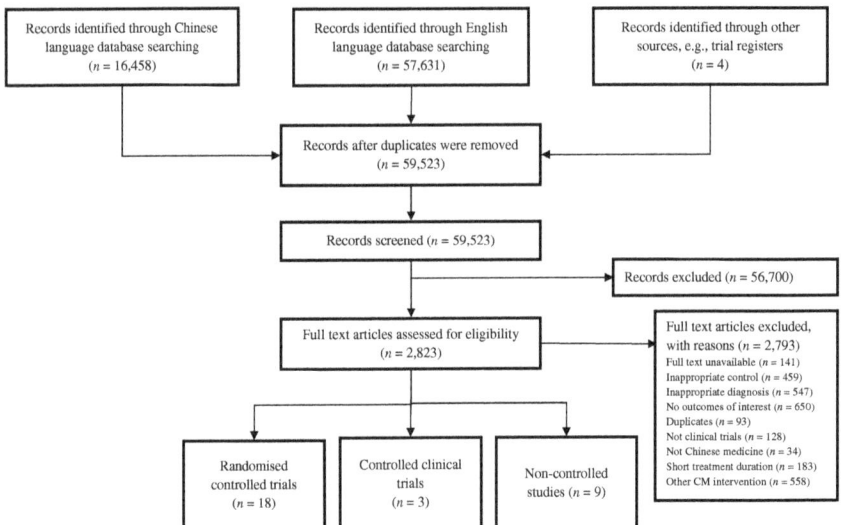

Fig. 9.1. Flow chart of the study selection process: Combination therapies.

Table 9.1. Summary of Interventions in Combination Therapies

Combination Therapies	No. of Studies	Included Studies
CHM and acupuncture	19	C3–9, C11–12, C16–19, C20, C24–26, C29–30
Acupuncture and cupping	4	C2, C21, C27–28
Acupuncture and *tuina* massage	3	C10, C14, C22
CHM and *tuina* massage	1	C23
CHM, acupuncture and *tuina* massage	1	C15
CHM, acupuncture and *qigong*	1	C13
Cupping and *tuina* massage	1	C1

Risk of Bias

The risk of bias of the 18 RCTs was analysed (C1–18). Due to the nature of the studies, including multiple interventions and the lack of blinding, there was a high risk of bias identified in the studies. All studies were described as randomised, and 10 (C1, C2, C4, C5, C7, C8, C11, C13, C16, C18) provided adequate information, such as a random number table, about sequence generation (Table 9.2). One study (C6) was at high risk of bias for sequence generation and allocation concealment because they used the time of diagnosis to randomise participants to the groups. Details about allocation concealment were not provided in any of the studies. Blinding domains were judged to be at high risk of bias in all studies. This is not surprising as it is very difficult to blind participants and personnel undertaking manual therapies and combination treatments. One study (C14) used a sham acupuncture control and mentioned that the personnel who assessed the results were unaware of the treatments each patient had received. This study was judged to be at low risk of bias for these blinding domains. Incomplete outcome data was judged to be a low risk of bias in all studies because there was information on dropouts and balance between groups. Study protocols could not be located, so all studies were judged to be at an unclear risk of bias for selective outcome reporting.

Table 9.2.   Risk of Bias of Randomised Controlled Trials: Combination Therapies

Risk of Bias Domain	Low Risk n (%)	Unclear Risk n (%)	High Risk n (%)
Sequence generation	10 (55.6)	7 (38.9)	1 (5.6)
Allocation concealment	0	17 (94.4)	1 (5.6)
Blinding of participants	1 (5.6)	0	17 (94.4)
Blinding of personnel	0	0	18 (100)
Blinding of outcome assessors	1 (5.6)	0	17 (94.4)
Incomplete outcome data	18 (100)	0	0
Selective outcome reporting	0	18 (100)	0

Clinical Evidence for Combination Therapies from Randomised Controlled Trials

A total of 18 RCTs (C1–18) assessed combination therapies for obesity in 1,242 participants. The participants had a body mass index (BMI) of greater than or equal to 24 kg/m^2, and four studies (C1, C4, C5, C14) included participants with simple obesity. The other studies included people with obesity and related complications, such as polycystic ovarian syndrome (PCOS) (6 studies), pre-diabetes or diabetes (4 studies), obesity-related nephropathy (1 study), non-alcoholic fatty liver disease (1 study), hypertension (1 study) and metabolic syndrome (1 study). Participants' mean age was 37.8 years, and the duration of obesity ranged from 2 to 12 years. Females made up the majority of participants (n = 900, 72.5%).

Seven studies included a CM syndrome differentiation as part of the inclusion criteria. Syndromes described in multiple studies were Spleen deficiency with dampness (3 studies) and Kidney deficiency and dampness (2 studies). CHM was given alongside acupuncture in 12 studies, acupuncture plus *tuina* massage in two studies, and one study each for acupuncture plus cupping, CHM plus acupuncture plus *tuina* massage, CHM plus ear acupressure plus *qigong*, and cupping plus *tuina* massage. The treatment duration ranged from one to three months.

CHM plus Acupuncture

In the 12 RCTs that evaluated CHM plus acupuncture, five (C4, C6, C12, C16–17) were compared to drug therapies, such as metformin or orlistat or hormone therapy. Two (C8, C11) assessed the combination CM therapies alongside drug therapies compared to drug therapies alone, and four (C3, C5, C7, C9) compared lifestyle therapies and drug therapies to the combination CM therapies with lifestyle therapies. One study (C18) had three arms and compared hormone therapy to CHM plus acupuncture alone or with hormone therapy.

In people with simple obesity, the CHM formula *Ping wei san* 平胃散 plus ear acupuncture was not superior to orlistat (lipase inhibitor) in terms of weight, BMI, waist circumference (WC) or fat mass reduction after four weeks of treatment (C4). CHM plus body acupuncture plus ear acupressure plus diet advice and exercise (60 minutes, three times per week) was superior to diet and exercise alone after eight weeks of treatment in terms of weight, WC and WHR reduction, but not the BMI (Table 9.3).

Polycystic Ovarian Syndrome

Women with obesity and PCOS were evaluated in six studies (C6, C9, C12, C16–18). CHM plus acupuncture was compared to metformin in four studies (C9, C12, C16–17) over three months, and results showed that the BMI was reduced in the CM group (MD -1.68 kg/m^2 [95% CI -3.00, -0.37], $I^2 = 78\%$. The WHR also was reduced in two studies (C12, C16) (MD -0.03 [95% CI -0.05, -0.01]). One study (C6) compared CHM and acupuncture to metformin and cyproterone acetate/ethinyloestradiol (progestogen and oestrogen hormones) for six months. The BMI was significantly reduced in the CM group compared to the control in terms of the BMI and WHR (MD -2.31 kg/m^2 [95% CI -4.08, -0.54] and MD -0.11 [95% CI -0.19, -0.03], respectively). In another study (C18) with three arms, CHM plus acupuncture alone or alongside acetate/

Table 9.3. Evidence for Combination Therapies from Randomised Controlled Trials

Intervention	Comparator	Outcome	No. of Studies (Participants)	Effect Estimate (MD, 95% CI)	Included Studies
CHM plus acupuncture	Orlistat	Weight	1 (64)	1.05 [−2.89, 4.99]	C4
		BMI	1 (64)	−0.40 [−0.97, 0.17]	C4
		WHR	1 (64)	−0.01 [−0.02, 0.00]	C4
		Fat mass	1 (64)	−1.26 [−2.84, 0.32]	C4
CHM, acupuncture, diet advice, plus exercise	Diet advice plus exercise	Weight	1 (60)	−3.46 [−6.75, −0.17]*	C5
		BMI	1 (60)	−1.11 [−2.25, 0.03]	C5
		WC	1 (60)	−3.44 [−6.77, −0.11]*	C5
		WHR	1 (60)	−0.05 [−0.09, −0.01]*	C5

Abbreviations: BMI, body mass index; CHM, Chinese herbal medicine; CI, confidence interval; MD, mean difference; WC, waist circumference; WHR, waist–hip ratio.
*Statistically significant, see *Statistical Analysis* methods in Chapter 4.

ethinyloestradiol was superior to acetate/ethinyloestradiol in terms of the BMI:

- CM therapies *vs.* acetate/ethinyloestradiol; MD −5.00 kg/m^2 [95% CI −6.14, −3.86].
- CM therapies plus acetate/ethinyloestradiol *vs.* acetate/ethinyloestradiol; MD −5.80 kg/m^2 [95% CI −6.95, −4.65].
- Other outcomes, such as weight and WC, were not reported.

Pre-diabetes and Diabetes

Two studies (C7, C11) evaluated people with obesity and pre-diabetes or diabetes. CHM plus acupuncture plus basic treatments for

diabetes, such as diet advice and exercise, were compared to metformin and diet advice and exercise for 8 or 12 weeks. One study
(C11) also used moxibustion on acupuncture points alongside needle
acupuncture. Weight was significantly reduced in one study (MD
−4.14 kg [95% CI −8.00, −0.28]), but the BMI and WC were not
significantly reduced when studies were pooled. Indices of diabetes
disease, such as blood glucose and insulin, were also not significantly different between groups after treatment. However, the total
cholesterol was significantly reduced in the intervention group compared to the control (MD −0.29 mmol/L [95% CI −0.52, −0.05], $I^2 =$
0%), as was the total triglycerides (MD −0.42 mmol/L [95% CI
−0.52, −0.32], $I^2 = 0$%).

Metabolic Syndrome

One study (C3) compared CHM plus acupuncture plus ear acupuncture plus lifestyle health education to fenofibrate (for
hypertriglyceridaemia) and health education in participants with
metabolic syndrome over eight weeks. The WC was significantly
reduced (MD −7.30 cm [95% CI −13.96, −0.64]). However, weight
was not significantly reduced in the intervention group as compared
to the control, nor were cholesterol or triglycerides.

Obesity-related Nephropathy

One study (C8) evaluated participants with obesity and nephropathy.
A high BMI is one of the key risk factors for new-onset chronic kidney
disease. This is due to hyperfiltration and an increase in intraglo-
merular pressure to meet the metabolic demands of the increased
body weight. CHM plus acupuncture plus candesartan cilexetil
(angiotensin II receptor antagonist used to treat high blood pressure)
plus health education, diet control and moderate aerobic exercise
was compared to the same treatments without the CM therapies. The
BMI was not different between groups, but the WHR was significantly reduced in the intervention group as compared to the control
(MD −0.07 [−0.09, −0.05]). Other indices of related complications

showed mixed results — blood glucose was not significantly different between the groups after the treatment; however, the fasting insulin was significantly reduced (MD −7.25 mIU/L [95% CI −10.92, −3.58]), as was Homeostatic Model Assessment of Insulin Resistance (HOMA-IR) (MD −2.40 [95% CI −2.53, −2.27]), total cholesterol (MD −1.75 mmol/L [95% CI −1.96, −1.54]) and total triglycerides (MD −1.82 mmol/L [95% CI −2.04, −1.60]).

Acupuncture Plus Cupping

One study (C2) compared acupuncture plus cupping plus metformin to metformin alone in 63 participants with obesity and diabetes for three months. All outcomes, including WC, blood glucose and triglycerides, showed no significant difference between the groups at the end of the treatment except for HOMA-IR (MD −1.62 [95% CI −2.41, −0.83]).

Acupuncture plus *Tuina* Massage

Two studies (C10, C14) assessed acupuncture plus massage. One study (C10) enrolled people with diabetes and obesity and compared acupuncture plus massage plus metformin plus routine diabetic interventions (such as diet advice and exercise) to the metformin plus routine diabetic interventions. After acupuncture, the therapist pressed and grasped the acupuncture points on the abdomen for 30 minutes. The acupuncture plus massage group showed a significant reduction in all reported outcomes as compared to the control:

- Weight: MD −6.24 kg [95% CI −10.19, −2.29].
- BMI: MD −2.56 kg/m² [95% CI −3.69, −1.43].
- WC: MD −4.13 cm [95% CI −8.15, −0.11].
- Fasting blood glucose: MD −0.93 mmol/L [95% CI −1.56, −0.30].
- Postprandial blood glucose: MD −1.32 mmol/L [95% CI −2.14, −0.50].

In another study (C14), 60 participants with a BMI of over 30 kg/m^2 were given acupuncture, moxibustion and ear acupuncture alongside daily abdominal self-massage plus diet advice and exercise advice. Compared to sham acupuncture, abdominal self-massage plus diet advice and exercise advice, the BMI was not significantly reduced in the acupuncture group.

Cupping plus *Tuina* Massage

Mobile cupping on the back and abdomen combined with *tuina* on the same areas plus diet advice was compared to diet advice alone for one month (C1). Weight and BMI were not measured, but the WC was significantly reduced in the intervention group compared to the control (MD −7.60 cm [95% CI −10.17, −5.03]).

Chinese Herbal Medicine plus Acupuncture plus *Tuina* Massage

CHM was combined with acupuncture and *tuina* for three months in obese people with non-alcoholic fatty liver disease (C15). After acupuncture, *tuina* massage was applied to the abdomen and limbs using pushing, rubbing, patting and pressing techniques for 20 minutes every second day. Compared to metformin, the combination of CM therapies significantly improved all outcomes:

- Weight: MD −4.80 kg [95% CI −8.15, −1.45].
- BMI: MD −2.12 kg/m^2 [95% CI −3.07, −1.17].
- WC: MD −3.18 cm [95% CI −5.89, −0.47].
- Fasting blood glucose: MD −0.64 mmol/L [95% CI −1.27, −0.01].
- Postprandial blood glucose: MD −1.82 mmol/L [95% CI −2.22, −1.42].
- Fasting insulin: MD −3.40 mIU/L [95% CI −4.11, −2.69].
- Total triglycerides: MD −0.72 mmol/L [95% CI −1.07, −0.37]).

Chinese Herbal Medicine plus Ear Acupressure plus *Qigong*

One study (C13) evaluated people with obesity and hypertension. The study combined CHM plus ear acupressure plus *wu qin xi* style *qigong* plus routine treatments for hypertension and health education for three months. The BMI and blood pressure were significantly reduced in the intervention group, compared to the control. However, weight, WC, blood glucose, insulin, cholesterol and triglycerides were not significantly different between the groups:

- BMI: MD −1.87 kg/m^2 [95% CI −3.09, −0.65].
- Systolic blood pressure: MD −4.33 mmHg [95% CI −8.11, −0.55].
- Diastolic blood pressure: MD −4.06 mmHg [95% CI −7.38, −0.74].

Clinical Evidence for Combination Therapies from Controlled Clinical Trials

Three controlled clinical trials (CCTs) (C19-21) were evaluated. One combined CHM with acupuncture, one combined ear acupressure with CHM and the other combined acupuncture with cupping. The comparators differed in all studies; therefore, the results were analysed separately.

In 48 women with PCOS and a BMI of over 25 kg/m^2, CHM plus ear acupressure plus ethinyloestradiol (progestogen and oestrogen hormones) plus lifestyle education were compared to hormone therapy and lifestyle education (C19). The BMI and WHR were significantly reduced in the intervention group as compared to the control after three months of treatment (MD −0.80 kg/m^2 [95% CI −1.38, −0.22] and MD −0.03 [95% CI −0.05, −0.01], respectively). Other indices of risk factor control showed mixed results — fasting blood glucose and total cholesterol were not significantly different between the groups; however, fasting insulin, HOMA-IR and total triglycerides were significantly reduced in the intervention group (fasting insulin: MD −1.50 mmol/L [95% CI −2.63, −0.37]; HOMA-IR: MD −0.11 [95% CI −0.20, −0.02]; total triglycerides: MD −0.17 mmol/L [95% CI −0.32, −0.02]).

In people with hyperlipidaemia and a BMI of greater than or equal to 26 kg/m^2, electroacupuncture plus ear acupressure plus CHM plus a lipid-lowering medication plus lifestyle education was assessed in one study (C20). The control group received orlistat plus lipid-lowering medication plus lifestyle education. After 56 days of treatment, the BMI and total triglycerides were not significantly different between the groups; however, the WC and total cholesterol were (MD −3.56 cm [95% CI −6.18, −0.94] and MD −0.36 mmol/L [95% CI −0.58, −0.14], respectively).

One study (C21) assessed 70 people with a BMI of over 24 kg/m^2. Acupuncture plus mobile cupping on the back, abdomen and thighs plus diet advice (eating vegetables and fruits as much as possible, less meat, no alcohol and eating seven small meals a day) was compared to diet advice alone for 36 days. Weight was significantly reduced in the intervention group as compared to the control (MD −8.63 kg/m^2 [95% CI −9.85, −7.41]. However, the WC and WHR were not significantly different between the groups.

Clinical Evidence for Combination Therapies from Non-controlled Studies

Nine non-controlled studies (C22–30) evaluated different combinations of CM therapies, including 443 participants. Therapies included:

- Acupuncture plus ear acupressure plus *tuina* massage for four months (C22).
- CHM external application plus *tuina* massage plus TDP lamp plus cupping and weight loss instrument (over the abdomen) for 50 days (C23).
- CHM plus electroacupuncture plus ear acupressure for two months (C24).
- CHM plus electroacupuncture plus moxibustion for three months (C25).
- CHM plus acupuncture for 72 days (C26).
- Ear acupuncture and acupressure plus cupping for three months (C27).
- Electroacupuncture plus cupping for three months (C28).

- CHM plus ear acupuncture plus TENS for two months (C29).
- CHM plus electroacupuncture for two months (C30).

Most of the studies included people with simple obesity; however, one study included women with PCOS, and another included people diagnosed with non-alcoholic fatty liver disease. Results indicated that weight and BMI reduced after the combination therapies.

Safety of Combination Therapies

Only seven studies (23.3%) (C3, C7, C11, C14–16, C19) included information about adverse events. Four of the studies stated that no adverse events occurred. One study (C14) reported a case of tibial fracture in the intervention group receiving acupuncture, massage, diet and exercise advice. Another study (C11) reported a case of abdominal discomfort and nausea and a subsequent withdrawal from the study in the control group that was receiving metformin, a low-calorie diet and exercise. Finally, four cases of mild gastrointestinal upset were reported in the intervention group receiving CHM plus ear acupressure plus ethinyloestradiol (progestogen and oestrogen hormones) plus lifestyle education, and three cases were reported in the control group receiving ethinyloestradiol (progestogen and oestrogen hormones) plus lifestyle education (C19).

Summary of Combination Therapies Evidence

Combination CM therapies are commonly used in clinical practice and have been evaluated in 30 clinical trials of overweight and obesity. By far, the most common combination was CHM and acupuncture; however, there were also multiple studies of acupuncture and cupping or acupuncture and *tuina* massage. These results are not surprising as manual therapies are often used in clinical practice in combination with herbal medicine to produce an improved clinical effect. Two studies used a very comprehensive treatment approach, including a triple therapy of CHM plus acupuncture plus *tuina* massage, or CHM plus acupuncture plus *qigong*.

CHM formulae and acupuncture points were similar to the individual therapies alone (Chapters 5 and 7), such as the herbs *fu ling* 茯苓 and *chen pi* 陈皮, acupuncture points CV12 *Zhongwan* 中脘, ST25 *Tianshu* 天枢 and CV4 *Guanyuan* 关元, and ear points, Endocrine 内分泌 (CO18) and Spleen 脾 (CO13). CM syndromes were not commonly used as an inclusion criterion. However, in the studies that reported syndromes, Spleen deficiency with dampness and Kidney deficiency and dampness were the most common. Treatment duration ranged from four weeks to six months, but most studies assessed participants after three months of treatment.

Overall, due to the varying nature of the interventions and controls, they could not be pooled in a meta-analysis, and results were drawn from single studies. Furthermore, due to the complex nature of the interventions and small sample sizes, there was a risk of bias and methodological shortfalls. Therefore, there was insufficient evidence to make a firm conclusion. Yet CM combination therapies, used for more than one month, appeared to reduce weight and waist-hip measures in some studies.

Reference

1. Nam MH, Lee SW, Na HY, *et al.* (2016) Herbal acupuncture for the treatment of obesity. *J Acupunct Meridian Stud* **9(2):** 49–57.

References for Included Combination Therapies Clinical Studies

Study No.	Reference
C1	陈秋帆, 文幸, 洪文扬. (2012) 游走罐配合腹部捏脂治疗女性腹型肥胖 40 例. *中医研究*. **25(12):** 60–62.
C2	陈员秀. (2013) 针药并用对2型糖尿病合并肥胖患者胰岛素抵抗及生化代谢的影响. *上海针灸杂志*. **32(11):** 911–913.
C3	陈月娥. (2017) 针药结合干预痰湿质代谢综合征血脂异常患者的临床研究. 广州中医药大学.

(Continued)

(*Continued*)

Study No.	Reference
C4	邓聪, 张艳红, 岑美婷, 蔡敬宙, 赖艳娴, 杨志敏. (2018) 平胃散联合耳穴对单纯性肥胖的临床疗效及对血清 NPY 和 Leptin 的影响. *广州医药*. **49(3):** 19–22.
C5	古青. (2008) 综合疗法治疗单纯性肥胖症的临床研究. *时珍国医国药*. **19(8):** 2033–2034.
C6	赖毛华, 马红霞, 宋兴华, 刘华. (2015) 针药结合治疗青春期肥胖型多囊卵巢综合征30例疗效观察. *云南中医中药杂志*. **36(10):** 42–44.
C7	林红坤. (2013) 针刺结合中药治疗肥胖2型糖尿病患者（湿热困脾证）胰岛素抵抗及微炎症状态的临床观察. 长春中医药大学.
C8	宁志春, 张淑红, 韩明. (2017) 加味升降散联合针灸治疗肥胖相关性肾病62例临床观察. *四川中医*. **35(7):** 135–137.
C9	徐传花, 曹佩霞, 李淑萍. (2017) 补肾化痰汤结合针灸疗法治疗肥胖型多囊卵巢综合征临床分析. *按摩与康复医学*. **8(10):** 23–26.
C10	张阳. (2015) 指针配合针刺联合盐酸二甲双胍治疗初期2型糖尿病肥胖症的临床研究. 长春中医药大学.
C11	张元花. (2016) 中药内服配合隔姜灸干预肥胖症合并IGR的临床研究. 山东中医药大学.
C12	周凌云, 徐传花, 李淑萍. (2016) 针药结合治疗肥胖型多囊卵巢综合征肾虚痰湿证临床观察. *上海针灸杂志*. **35(10):** 1213–1215.
C13	周训杰, 桂明泰, 姚磊, 芦波, 李建华, 韩亚楠, *et al.* (2018) 治未病理念在肥胖高血压患者早期肾损害中的应用. *成都中医药大学学报*. **41(2):** 41–44.
C14	Mazzoni R, Mannucci E, Rizzello SM, *et al.* (1999) Failure of acupuncture in the treatment of obesity: A pilot study. *Eat Weight Disord.* **4(4):** 198–202.
C15	董晗硕. (2015) "通经调脏"治疗代谢综合征(肝胃郁热证)的临床疗效观察. 长春中医药大学.
C16	庞颖. (2018) 基于斡旋中州法针药联合治疗肥胖型 PCOS-IR 的临床研究. 北京中医药大学.
C17	王晨晖, 孙忻, 丁彩飞, 沈瑛红. (2016) 苍附导痰汤加减联合针刺对肥胖型多囊卵巢综合征患者糖脂代谢及排卵率的影响. *现代中西医结合杂志*. **25(36):** 4056–4058.
C18	王亚校. (2013) 针刺配合中药治疗肥胖型多囊卵巢综合征不孕症 56 例. *福建中医药*. **44(2):** 6–7, 9.

(Continued)

Study No.	Reference
C19	徐树梅, 潘晓红. (2017) 耳穴贴压联合中药对肥胖型多囊卵巢综合征糖脂代谢影响的临床研究. *现代诊断与治疗*. **28(1):** 50–52.
C20	朱红霞, 肖晓华. (2013) 电针、耳穴加中药治疗单纯性肥胖病并高脂血症 45 例. *江西中医学院学报*. **25(3):** 29–31.
C21	张智芳, 蔡琛, 王海明. (2010) 针刺走罐配合科学饮食与单纯科学饮食治疗超重者临床疗效对比观察. *四川中医*. **28(6):** 114–116.
C22	曹淑刚. (2015) 针灸推拿结合治疗单纯性肥胖 39 例临床观察.医药. **6(12):** 21.
C23	陈素华. (2008) 中药外治结合理疗治疗中心型肥胖临床观察. *现代中西医结合杂志*. **17(3):** 331–332.
C24	樊红霞, 吴牵峰. (2010) 中医综合治疗脾虚湿阻型单纯性肥胖 48 例. *中医临床研究*. **2(9):** 78–79.
C25	房彩平, 管素芬, 陈琰, 王赛莉, 王华. (2018) 补肾化痰法联合针灸治疗超重型 PCOS 的临床研究. *临床医药文献电子杂志*. **5(40):** 15, 18.
C26	付京云. (2016) 针药并用治疗单纯性肥胖病脾虚湿阻型 40 例观察. *实用中医药杂志*. **32(6):** 529–529.
C27	孔月晴. (2013) 拔罐合耳穴贴压治疗单纯性肥胖 62 例. *科技创新导报*. **(22):** 254.
C28	张齐娟, 曹庭欣, 段婉娥, 李妮, 訾璐. (2014) 夹脊穴电针配合走罐治疗单纯性肥胖症疗效观察. *上海针灸杂志*. **33(9):** 807–808.
C29	赵东英, 陈路燕, 徐进广. (2002) 中医综合治疗单纯性肥胖 30 例. *河南中医*. **22(2):** 37.
C30	楼美红, 王超, 陈利芳, 高宏. (2014) 方剑乔教授针药并用治疗中青年腹型肥胖的临床经验撷要. *浙江中医药大学学报*. **38(6):** 792–794.

10

Summary and Conclusions

OVERVIEW

This chapter provides a summary and conclusions relating to the main findings of the previous chapters, including the efficacy and safety of Chinese herbal medicine, acupuncture and related therapies for the treatment of overweight and obesity. The quality and limitations of the evidence are discussed, and implications for clinical practice and future research are also proposed in this chapter.

Introduction

Weight gain and obesity are increasing worldwide.[1] Diet (calorie restriction), physical activity and lifestyle modifications are the cornerstones of conventional management for weight loss and maintaining a healthy weight. Pharmacotherapy and surgery are indicated in some groups of people with obesity and at risk of cardiovascular disease.[1-3] Chinese medicine (CM) therapies are increasingly used to treat people who are overweight and obese, usually alongside diet, physical activity and lifestyle modifications. Evidence taken from the previous chapters indicates that CM treatments may be of value for these people.

This monograph provides a 'whole evidence' analysis of the potential role of CM treatments for overweight and obesity in adults. Clinical practice guidelines and textbooks have recommended traditional CHM formulae and manufactured products, acupuncture and related therapies, CM diet therapy, cupping therapy, *tuina* and *qigong* (Chapter 2). An analysis of classical CM literature has determined that CHM has been used over hundreds of years to aid people to lose weight (Chapter 3). The methods used to evaluate the evidence from clinical trials are described in Chapter 4, and evidence indicates that CHM combined with lifestyle therapies and/or drug therapies offer promising benefits for reducing weight and improving metabolic parameters (Chapter 5). Experimental evidence of the most commonly used herbs is provided in Chapter 6. Findings from acupuncture clinical studies have revealed potential benefits and improved clinical outcomes (Chapter 7). Clinical trials of other therapies, including Chinese diet therapy, cupping therapy, *tuina* massage, *qigong* and *tai chi*, indicate some promising benefits, but the number of studies is small, and further research is needed to draw a firm conclusion (Chapter 8). An analysis of combination CM therapies shows that there may be additional benefits of combining therapies for people who are overweight and obese (Chapter 9).

Chinese Medicine Syndrome Differentiation

Syndrome differentiation is one of the features of CM. Four main syndromes were suggested according to the CM clinical practice guidelines and textbooks: Stomach heat with dampness obstruction, Spleen deficiency with dampness, Spleen and Kidney *yang* deficiency, and Liver depression and *qi* stagnation (Chapter 2). Formulae were also recommended for each syndrome. Most of the classical literature citations mentioned the pathogenesis, and the syndromes of obesity (Chapter 3) and phlegm (dampness) and *qi* deficiency were commonly described.

Chinese medicine syndrome differentiation was reported in over half of the CHM clinical studies (Chapter 5). The most common syndromes were Spleen deficiency with dampness obstruction, dampness-heat in the Spleen and Stomach, and phlegm-dampness. These syndromes were generally consistent with those described in clinical practice guidelines and textbooks. Similarly, in the acupuncture studies, about half of the studies used CM syndrome differentiation as an inclusion criterion or for treatment selection

(Chapter 7). Common syndromes were Stomach heat, Spleen deficiency and dampness, Spleen and Kidney *yang* deficiency, Liver *qi* stagnation, and Spleen and Stomach *qi* deficiency. Fewer studies that evaluated other CM therapies or combined therapies reported CM syndromes (Chapters 8 and 9). Common syndromes were Spleen deficiency and dampness, and Kidney deficiency and dampness.

While many studies reported using CM syndromes to allocate treatment, results for clinical outcomes were typically reported in aggregate for all participants, regardless of the syndrome. It is difficult to conduct further analysis on syndromes since they varied across studies and could not be standardised. However, key syndromes were clearly identified for people who are overweight and obese and should be the basis for CM differentiation and diagnosis.

Chinese Herbal Medicine

This section summarises the evidence from Chapters 2, 3 and 5. In Chapter 2, the CHM treatments are described based on clinical practice guidelines and textbooks. These treatments are recommended according to patients' syndrome differentiation. In clinical trials (Chapter 5), most of the participants were included based on CM syndromes.

Chinese herbal medicine treatment experience of obesity from classical literature is limited due to environmental influences, and people in ancient times were often underweight owing to a lack of food, but there were still reported cases of people who were obese. In classical literature, the commonly used herbs were those that tonify *qi* and eliminate phlegm, which is consistent with the functions of the herbs used nowadays. The high-frequency herbs in classical literature included *ban xia* 半夏, *cang zhu* 苍术, *bai zhu* 白术, *fu ling* 茯苓 and *chen pi* 陈皮. These herbs are still widely used in clinical practice and have been evaluated in clinical trials (Chapter 5). A number of typical formulae for weight-related complications and comorbidities are also commonly used today, such as *Cang fu dao tan wan* 苍附导痰丸 and *Qi gong wan* 启宫丸 for polycystic ovarian syndrome (PCOS) and *Liu wei di huang wan* 六味地黃丸 for diabetes.

There have been developments and changes in modern CHM use for treating weight gain and obesity. For example, *ren shen* 人参 was one of the most commonly prescribed herbs in ancient records. However, due to its limited yields and high price nowadays, *dang shen* 党参 is more commonly used as a substitute. Some herbs, such as *tian nan xing* 天南星, were frequently used in the past, but due to advances in knowledge, it was revealed that it has some toxic side effects;[4] thus, it is seldom used nowadays.

In Chapter 5, the clinical evidence for the efficacy and safety of CHM are synthesised. Weight-related complications that are either caused or exacerbated by people being overweight or obese (based on the complications listed in the 2016 AACE/ACE Guidelines)[1] were also included, such as pre-diabetes or diabetes, PCOS, metabolic syndrome, etc. In total, 232 clinical studies were included, and most of the studies (195 studies) were randomised controlled trials (RCTs). All CHM treatments were orally administrated. Comparators included placebo, no treatment, diet, physical exercise, health education and drug therapies.

Two main categories of outcomes were evaluated, including body composition and indices of cardiovascular risk factors. Body composition included changes in body weight, body mass index (BMI), waist circumference (WC), waist–hip ratio (WHR) and body fat mass. Indices of cardiovascular risk factors were based on complications, such as serum glucose, serum lipids, blood pressure, etc. Treatment durations ranged from 4 weeks to 12 months.

In terms of treatment efficacy and safety, evidence from RCTs suggests that:

Chinese Herbal Medicine Alone

- Compared to the placebo, CHM was not superior in terms of body composition, such as weight, BMI and WC (low certainty evidence).

- CHM significantly reduced BMI, but not WHR when compared to treatment (not graded).
- CHM was not superior to diet therapy in terms of BMI and WC (not graded).
- Compared to metformin, CHM could further reduce weight, BMI and WC, but not WHR (not graded).
- There is not enough data to prove the efficacy of CHM compared to orlistat drug therapy.

Chinese Herbal Medicine plus Lifestyle Therapies

- Compared to placebo plus lifestyle therapies, CHM plus lifestyle therapies reduced BMI (moderate certainty evidence) and WC (low certainty evidence), but there was no significant difference in weight (low certainty evidence) or WHR (not graded).
- Compared to lifestyle therapies alone, CHM plus lifestyle therapies produced greater reductions in weight (moderate certainty evidence), BMI (very low certainty evidence), WC (moderate certainty evidence), WHR (not graded) and fat mass percentage (not graded).
- Chinese herbal medicine plus lifestyle therapies was not superior to orlistat or metformin plus lifestyle therapies in terms of reducing weight, BMI, WC and WHR (not graded).

Chinese Herbal Medicine plus Drug Therapies

Compared to metformin alone, CHM plus metformin significantly reduced BMI, WC and glucometabolic outcomes, such as serum glucose and insulin; however, weight and WHR were not significantly reduced.

Chinese Herbal Medicine plus Drug Therapies and Lifestyle Therapies

Compared to metformin and lifestyle therapies, CHM alongside metformin and lifestyle therapies showed a positive effect, not only in body composition, including weight, BMI, WC and WHR, but also in serum glucose and serum lipid level.

Safety

No serious adverse events were reported in the included studies. Chinese herbal medicine treatments appeared to have fewer adverse events than non-CHM treatment. Gastrointestinal symptoms, such as nausea, vomiting, diarrhoea and stomachache, were the most frequent adverse events. These symptoms were usually mild and resolved without intervention.

Although evidence generated from clinical trials indicated that CHM plus lifestyle therapies were superior to lifestyle therapies alone or a placebo plus lifestyle therapies in treating overweight and obesity, confidence in these results was compromised because of heterogeneity in meta-analyses and the poor methodological quality of included studies. Heterogeneity may be partially explained by diverse CHM interventions, different populations and small sample sizes. The methodological quality was poor due to the inadequacy of allocation concealment and lack of blinding. As a result, the quality of evidence from RCTs was mostly judged to be at high risk of bias and low certainty.

Chinese Herbal Medicine Formulae in Key Clinical Guidelines and Textbooks, Classical Literature and Clinical Studies

Broadly similar CHM formulae are reported in clinical guidelines and textbooks (Chapter 2), classical literature (Chapter 3), and clinical studies (Chapter 5) (Table 10.1). Formulae with different names often had the same or similar herb ingredients. Similarity assessment of formulae is complex and was not undertaken; the actual number for each listed formula may be higher than reported below.

Based on CM syndrome differentiation, eight formulae were recommended in clinical practice guidelines in Chapter 2. Typical

Table 10.1. Summary of Chinese Herbal Medicine Formulae

Formula Name	Included in Clinical Guidelines and Textbooks	Included in Classical Literature (No. of Citations)	Included in Clinical Studies (Chap. 5)			Included in Combination Therapies (Chap. 9)
			RCTs (No. of Studies)	CCTs (No. of Studies)	Non-controlled Studies (No. of Studies)	
Bai zhu tang 白术汤	No	1	0	0	0	0
Bao he wan 保和丸	Yes	0	0	0	0	0
Bu qi xiao tan yin 补气消痰饮	No	1	0	0	0	0
Dao tan tang 导痰汤	Yes	0	3	0	0	0
Fang feng tong sheng san/wan 防风通圣散/丸	No	0	3	0	1	0
Fang ji huang qi tang 防己黄芪汤	Yes	0	0	0	1	1
Huang lian jie du tang 黄连解毒汤	No	0	6	0	1	0
Huang lian wen dan tang 黄连温胆汤	No	0	3	0	0	0
Huo tu liang pei dan 火土两培丹	No	1	0	0	0	0
Jue ming zi cha 决明子茶	No	0	3	0	0	0
Lin gui zhu gan tang 苓桂术甘汤	Yes	0	4	0	1	0
Liu jun zi tang 六君子汤	No	1	0	0	0	0
Pei lian ma huang fang 佩连麻黄方	No	0	4	0	0	0

(Continued)

265

Table 10.1. (*Continued*)

Formula Name	Included in Clinical Guidelines and Textbooks	Included in Classical Literature (No. of Citations)	Included in Clinical Studies (Chap. 5)			Included in Combination Therapies (Chap. 9)
			RCTs (No. of Studies)	CCTs (No. of Studies)	Non-controlled Studies (No. of Studies)	
Qi gong wan 启宫丸	No	0	0	0	2	0
Shan zha xiao zhi jiao capsule 山楂消脂胶囊	No	0	3	0	0	1
Shen ling bai zhu san 参苓白术散	Yes	0	4	1	1	1
Wu ling san 五苓散	No	0	8	1	1	0
Xiao cheng qi tang 小承气汤	Yes	0	0	0	0	0
Xiao yao san 逍遥散	Yes	0	0	0	0	0
Xiao zhi tang 消脂汤	No	0	0	2	0	0
Yi qi hua tan wan 益气化痰丸	No	1	0	0	0	0
Zhen wu tang 真武汤	Yes	0	0	0	0	0

Abbreviations: CCTs, controlled clinical trials; RCTs, randomised controlled trials.

formulae in clinical practice include *Dao tan tang* 导痰汤, *Lin gui zhu gan tang* 苓桂术甘汤 and *Shen ling bai zhu san* 参苓白术散. Some formulae, such as *Bao he wan* 保和丸, *Xiao cheng qi tang* 小承气汤, *Xiao yao san* 逍遥散 and *Zhen wu tang* 真武汤, are recommended in the guidelines but were not commonly found in classical literature or clinical trials. This may be due to changes in CM syndromes over time and a better understanding of obesity patients in the modern era. For example, Stomach heat combined with dampness is more common nowadays, compared with Stomach heat alone in the past. Therefore, the formulae gradually changed to those having heat-clearing and dampness-removing functions, such as *Huang lian jie du tang* 黄连解毒汤 and *Pei lian ma huang fang* 佩连麻黄方. In addition, clinical trials often used treatments that focused on obesity syndromes, such as Spleen deficiency and dampness; therefore, underlying syndromes or those indirectly related to obesity, such as Liver *qi* stagnation and the use of *Xiao yao san* 逍遥散, were not investigated in clinical trials despite being recommended in guidelines.

Only a few named formulae were found in classical literature (Chapter 3). Although none of these formulae were included in clinical guidelines and textbooks or tested in clinical trials, the herbal ingredients were common, such as *fu ling* 茯苓, *ban xia* 半夏 and *bai zhu* 白术.

In the included clinical trials (Chapter 5), *Wu ling san* 五苓散, *Huang lian jie du tang* 黄连解毒汤, *Pei lian ma huang fang* 佩连麻黄方, *Shen ling bai zhu san* 参苓白术散 and *Ling gui zhu gan tang* 苓桂术甘汤 were the most common formulae evaluated. Both *Shen ling bai zhu san* 参苓白术散 and *Ling gui zhu gan tang* 苓桂术甘汤 were recommended in textbooks.

Wu ling san 五苓散 ranked the highest frequency in the 232 included clinical studies. When compared to diet and exercise therapies, *Wu ling san*, alongside diet and exercise therapies, significantly reduced the BMI. *Wu ling san* plus anti-diabetic drugs and diabetes routine therapies also showed positive benefits in terms of reducing the BMI and WHR for overweight and obese people with diabetes when compared to anti-diabetic drugs and diabetes routine therapies.

However, *Wu ling san* was neither recommended in the textbooks nor found in the classical literature for obese people. The reason may be that *Wu ling san* was traditionally used for oedema, not obesity, according to classical literature records (*Shang Han Lun* 伤寒论), but it has been somewhat repurposed for obesity nowadays.

Huang lian jie du tang 黄连解毒汤 was also one of the most common formulae evaluated in clinical trials. All of these studies assessed obese people with pre-diabetes or diabetes, using metformin alone or metformin alongside diabetes routine therapies as the control. However, both the *Huang lian jie du tang* group and the integrative medicine group were not significantly better than the control in terms of the BMI. However, some serum glucose outcomes were improved in the *Huang lian jie du tang* group, and it appeared to be better at regulating glucometabolic disorders than reducing body weight. This may also account for the fact that *Huang lian jie du tang* is not primarily used or recommended for obesity in clinical guidelines and textbooks or classical literature citations. A few clinical trials have been conducted for CHM commercial products such as *Fang feng tong sheng san/wan* 防风通圣散/丸 and *Jiu zhi da duang pian* 九制大黄片. However, more high-quality clinical studies are needed to assess the efficacy and safety of these products.

In summary, CHM has been used for a long period of time for weight loss. Herbal treatments are broadly similar between classical literature citations, modern clinical practice and clinical trials. Yet there have been some refinements of treatment practices and herbs to incorporate the modern presentation of people who are overweight and obese. CHM appears to be effective and safe for this group of people. However, it is difficult to draw a firm conclusion due to the poor methodological quality of clinical trials, such as small sample sizes, lack of blinding and high heterogeneity.

Acupuncture and Related Therapies

This section summarises the evidence from clinical practice guidelines and textbooks, classical literature, and clinical trials (Chapters 2, 3 and 7). Filiform needle therapy, electroacupuncture and ear acupuncture are recommended in CM guidelines and textbooks. These forms of acupuncture therapies were also the most commonly evaluated acupuncture therapies in clinical studies. A basic acupuncture prescription was suggested in Chapter 2, and points included CV12 *Zhongwan* 中脘, ST25 *Tianshu* 天枢, ST28 *Shuidao* 水道, LI11 *Quchi* 曲池, ST37 *Shangjuxu* 上巨虚 and SP6 *Sanyinjiao* 三阴交. Most of the acupoints are on the Conception Vessel meridian, Spleen meridian and Stomach meridian to tonify *qi*, invigorate Spleen and eliminate phlegm. It is also suggested to add some points according to CM syndrome differentiation. As for auricular acupuncture prescription, three to five points can be selected from the following points: Mouth 口 (CO1), Stomach 胃 (CO4), Endocrine 内分泌 (CO18), *San Jiao* 三焦 (CO17), Spleen 脾 (CO13), Hunger 饥点 and Subcortex 皮质下 (AT4). Filiform needles or seeds can be used on the ear points.

In terms of evidence from classical literature (Chapter 3), no citations mentioned the use of acupuncture for the treatment of overweight and obesity. This is not surprising as obesity was rare in ancient times due to environmental factors and a shortage of food. Nowadays, acupuncture is a popular option for obesity treatment, especially in China. Evidence from clinical trials indicates that acupuncture has potential benefits in terms of reducing weight and WC. After a comprehensive search and analysis of clinical trials, 186 studies were eligible for inclusion in the systematic reviews and meta-analyses (Chapter 7). Over 18,000 people participated in the studies. Treatment duration ranged from four weeks to six months.

Various acupuncture therapies were assessed for obesity treatment, and the most common were manual acupuncture, electroacupuncture and auricular (ear) acupuncture. Most of the studies (62.9%) used acupuncture alone, while the remaining 84 studies evaluated acupuncture alongside diet and exercise interventions or drug therapies. Comparators included no treatment, sham acupuncture, lifestyle therapies or drug therapies, used alone or in combination. Despite positive results, the included RCTs had methodological shortfalls, including a lack of description of random sequence generation and allocation concealment, as well as a lack of blinding. Results of the acupuncture studies are summarised in Table 10.2.

Table 10.2. **Key Results from the Acupuncture Clinical Trials**

Acupuncture Therapy	Comparator	Results
Acupuncture/ electroacupuncture	Sham acupuncture	Reduced weight, BMI, WC and WHR (moderate certainty evidence).
Acupuncture/ electroacupuncture plus lifestyle therapies	Lifestyle therapies	Reduced weight, BMI, WC but not WHR or fat mass percentage (low certainty evidence).
Acupuncture plus ear acupressure plus lifestyle therapies	Lifestyle therapies	No difference between intervention and control in terms of weight and BMI (not graded).
Ear acupuncture plus lifestyle therapies	Sham ear acupuncture plus lifestyle therapies	Ear acupuncture group significantly reduced the BMI (not graded)

Abbreviations: BMI, body mass index; WC, waist circumference; WHR, waist–hip ratio.

Safety

Acupuncture therapies appeared to be safe for adults who are over-weight and obese. Common adverse events related to the site of acupuncture include pain, bleeding, bruising and local allergic reactions. These symptoms were usually mild and self-resolving.

Acupuncture Therapies in Key Clinical Guidelines and Textbooks, Classical Literature and Clinical Studies

This section summarises and compares the acupuncture therapies and commonly used acupoints provided in clinical guidelines, text-books (Chapter 2) and clinical studies (Chapters 7 and 9). All acupoints were standardised based on the WHO International Standard Terminologies on Traditional Medicine in the Western Pacific Region,[5] and the frequency of each point was calculated. The points that appeared in guidelines and textbooks, as well as clinical trials, are shown in Table 10.3.

Table 10.3.   Summary of Acupuncture and Related Therapies

Intervention	Included in Clinical Guidelines and Textbooks (Chap. 2)	Included in Classical Literature (Chap. 3) (No. of Citations)	Included in Clinical Studies (Chap. 7)*			Included in Combination Therapies (Chap. 9)
			RCTs (No. of Studies)	CCTs (No. of Studies)	Non-controlled Studies (No. of Studies)	
Acupuncture points						
CV12 Zhongwan 中脘	Yes	No	60	2	57	20
ST25 Tianshu 天枢	Yes	No	64	3	55	16
ST28 Shuidao 水道	Yes	No	23	0	17	4
LI11 Quchi 曲池	Yes	No	37	0	38	5
ST37 Shangjuxu 上巨虚	Yes	No	21	0	27	1
SP6 Sanyinjiao 三阴交	Yes	No	56	2	62	11
ST36 Zusanli 足三里	No	No	72	2	63	14
ST40 Fenglong 丰隆	No	No	49	1	52	14
CV4 Guanyuan 关元	No	No	47	2	37	13
SP9 Yinlingquan 阴陵泉	No	No	35	1	45	4
CV6 Qihai 气海	No	No	34	2	34	13
CV9 Shuifen 水分	No	No	31	1	18	4
Ear acupuncture points						
Mouth 口 (CO1)	Yes	No	9	0	7	1
Stomach 胃 (CO4)	Yes	No	22	1	27	5
Endocrine 内分 (CO18)	Yes	No	17	1	28	7

(Continued)

Table 10.3.   *(Continued)*

Intervention	Included in Clinical Guidelines and Textbooks (Chap. 2)	Included in Classical Literature (Chap. 3) (No. of Citations)	Included in Clinical Studies (Chap. 7)*			Included in Combination Therapies (Chap. 9)
			RCTs (No. of Studies)	CCTs (No. of Studies)	Non-controlled Studies (No. of Studies)	
San Jiao 三焦 (CO17)	Yes	No	12	1	21	4
Spleen 脾 (CO13)	Yes	No	8	1	26	5
Hunger 饥点	Yes	No	18	0	10	1
Subcortex 皮质下 (AT4)	Yes	No	0	1	10	4
Shenmen 神门 (TF4)	No	No	18	0	18	3
Sympathetic 交感 (AH6a)	No	No	10	1	6	3
Kidney 肾 (CO10)	No	No	9	0	14	2
Large Intestine 大肠 (CO7)	No	No	8	0	12	1

* Some studies used more than one intervention, e.g., acupuncture plus moxibustion. These are counted separately in this table. Abbreviations: CCTs, controlled clinical trials; RCTs, randomised controlled trials.

As presented in Table 10.3, the commonly used acupoints were mainly located on the meridians of the Spleen, Stomach and Conception Vessel. The function of these meridians and acupoints is to tonify *qi*, eliminate phlegm and remove dampness. ST36 *Zusanli* 足三里 is commonly used in clinical trials but is not included in the basic prescription in current guidelines and textbooks (Chapter 2). It is unclear why this point is not recommended as it is commonly used in clinical practice for phlegm-dampness obstruction, a common syndrome of obesity. In terms of ear acupoints, the points recommended in current textbooks were frequently used in clinical trials. Not surprisingly, Stomach 胃 (CO4) and Endocrine 内分泌 (CO18) were the top two points, which are believed to suppress appetite and regulate endocrine disorders.

Other Chinese Medicine Therapies

This section summarises the evidence relating to other CM therapies in Chapters 2, 3 and 8. In guidelines and textbooks, diet therapy, cupping therapy, *tuina* massage and *qigong* are recommended for treating obesity. These therapies were also examined in clinical trials. In the classical literature, these therapies were not specifically mentioned for treating obesity. However, there were a few citations that described diet therapy using herbs or foods for obesity, such as *dong gua* 冬瓜, *shan zha* 山楂 and *kun bu* 海带. In addition, a medical history book (*Zhong Guo Yi Xue Yuan Liu Lun* 中国医学源流论) published during the Republic of China (1912–1949) recorded that *tuina* massage therapy could be used for obese people who eat too much greasy food and seldom exercise.

In clinical trials, *tuina* massage was the most common therapy among other CM therapies. *Tuina* massage techniques, such as rolling and pushing, were usually applied to the abdomen, arms and legs, as well as pressing on acupuncture points. Compared to lifestyle therapies, *tuina* alongside lifestyle therapies appears to reduce weight, BMI and WC. *Qigong* therapies included different types and styles, such as *tai chi, wu qin xi, yi jin jing*, etc. However, there were only a limited number of studies with small sample sizes. Overall, it is difficult to conclude whether these therapies can assist people to lose weight. Further research is needed in the future.

Other Chinese Medicine Therapies in Key Clinical Guidelines and Textbooks, Classical Literature and Clinical Studies

This section summarises and compares the other CM therapies provided in clinical guidelines and textbooks (Chapter 2), classical literature (Chapter 3), and clinical studies (Chapters 8 and 9). The therapies are shown in Table 10.4.

Limitations of Evidence

Despite considerable efforts being made to collect and organise data from a wide range of sources, omissions from each of the data sets were possible. In order to present the overview of current CM clinical practice, authoritative clinical practice guidelines and textbooks at the time of writing were consulted in Chapter 2. However, the previous CM guideline for obesity was published in 1998, and it has not been updated, which may impede guidance.[6] Only CM syndromes and

Table 10.4 Summary of Other Chinese Medicine Therapies

Intervention	Included in Clinical Guidelines and Textbooks (Chap. 2)	Included in Classical Literature (Chap. 3) (No. of Citations)	Included in Clinical Studies (Chap. 8)			Included in Combination Therapies (Chap. 9)
			RCTs (No. of Studies)	CCTs (No. of Studies)	Non-controlled Studies (No. of Studies)	
Diet therapy	Yes	0	2	0	0	0
Cupping therapy	Yes	0	2	0	0	4
Tuina massage	Yes	0	7	0	4	6
Qigong therapy	Yes	0	10	2	1	1

Abbreviations: CCTs, controlled clinical trials; RCTs, randomised controlled trials.

treatments recommended in different guidelines and textbooks were presented. Therefore, some unusual CM syndromes and potentially effective CM treatments that are not widely acknowledged were not provided in Chapter 2.

In the classical literature evidence, the *Encyclopaedia of Chinese Medicine* (*Zhong Hua Yi Dian*, ZHYD, version 5) was used to source CM books published in the pre-modern era. Although the ZHYD is considered to be the largest searchable resource of books in CM, it does not contain every historical reference. Thus, some books and citations may have been missed. After expert consensus, over 20 search terms were determined, but they may not have been broad enough to capture all possible obesity citations. Furthermore, the fact that obesity was not always regarded as an independent disease in ancient China (closely related to *Tanyin* or *Tanshi*) and thus weight and height were not recorded, it is unclear if the citations referred to obesity or another disease. Moreover, citations that described the co-treatment for obesity and related complications, such as a stroke, menstrual disorders, diabetes, etc., were also included. The treatments may be beneficial for obesity, but the evidence was indirect and unclear. On the other hand, single herbs added for obesity were also selected. Besides CHM treatment, we could only find a few citations recording acupuncture treatment or other therapies. In addition, considering the notion that pre-modern CM books were written by sundry authors and have been passed down over thousands of years, linguistic changes and artificial errors when copying the manuscripts led to the likely misinterpretation and/or mistranslation of the meaning of some records. Likewise, during the standardised process of herb naming, regularisation errors could have been made due to the changes of herb names and species over time.

Evidence from clinical trials may also have limitations. For example, overlooking or misclassifying may happen during the screening process of study records. In order to focus on the efficacy and safety of CM interventions compared to conventional therapies in overweight and obese populations, strict criteria were applied to include and exclude studies. Consequently, some eligible studies may have been excluded due to the lack of detailed information to make judgements. The best available evidence regarding the effects of CM interventions is generated from RCTs. The reliability of the estimated effect increases when the same CM intervention that has been tested in multiple RCTs shows consistent treatment effects. However, this was not common in the included literature.

When appropriate, meta-analysis was conducted to provide aggregate data from multiple studies. Of studies included in the meta-analysis, variations such as demographic features, condition severity, different BMI criteria for obesity from diverse regions and populations, comorbidities, and outcome measurements were considerable. Consequently, substantial statistical heterogeneities were observed in pooled results. Subgroup analyses based on complications and comorbidity, as well as CM formulae, were conducted when appropriate to investigate the sources of heterogeneity and give a more focused evaluation of the treatment effects. Part of the heterogeneity can be explained by the above factors, but some remain unknown. Thus, a random effects model was used in all meta-analyses to take into account the clinical heterogeneity and the variation in treatment effects in order to provide conservative estimations of effect sizes.

In the majority of the included studies, methodological details of trial design and performance were not adequately reported. Random allocation procedures were not fully described in most of the studies, and neither participants nor investigators were always blinded in the trials. In addition, the reporting quality of adverse events was unsatisfactory, and more detailed information was needed. These defects in methodology and reporting compromised confidence in the accuracy of the estimated results, leading to the downgrading of the evidence certainty.

Due to the large number of eligible studies, it was not feasible to present all details of interventions used in each trial. Thus, the most commonly used CM interventions in the clinical trials, including herbal formulae and their ingredients, acupuncture therapies, and acupoints, are summarised in the form of frequency tables for each category of evidence. A similar method was used to summarise the high-frequency CM interventions applied in the studies included in the meta-analysis that showed favourable effects. The downside is that the potentially effective CM interventions with low frequency may be submerged under the large volume of data. In order to inform practitioners and researchers, the original sources are provided for those with a particular interest. Also, it should be noted that the most frequently used CM interventions were not necessarily the same as the most effective interventions.

Further analysis based on the BMI degree, disease course, participants' age and gender, as well as treatment duration, were not conducted due to insufficient original information. In terms of treatment duration, only studies conducted for over four weeks were included, according to guideline recommendations and expert consensus. Thus, studies that were conducted for less than four weeks may not have been included. In addition, lifestyle therapies such as diet, physical exercise and behavioural regulation are vital interventions for overweight and obesity. However, the details were not provided in most of the studies. As for obesity complications and comorbidities, only the common diseases listed in the 2016 AACE/ACE guidelines[1] and with data from more than two clinical trials were included in subgroup analysis. Therefore, evidence may not be comprehensive for other weight-related complications and comorbidity.

Participants of all included studies were adults over 18 years old. Thus, results cannot be generalised to children or adolescents. Likewise, most of the clinical trials were conducted in China, and most of the participants were Chinese. It is unclear whether treatment effects are applicable to other ethnicities or regions. Moreover, the pooled estimations of effect size are based on comparisons at the end of treatment. For those meta-analysis results showing significant group differences, it should be carefully examined whether the differences are large enough to suggest clinical importance. The limitations discussed above should be taken into consideration when interpreting the results in this book.

Implications for Practice

The summary of guidelines and textbooks provides consensus-based expert guidance for syndrome differentiation and CM treatments for overweight and obese people. Among the meta-analyses derived from RCTs, the most common herbs used in clinical trials to reduce weight and BMI included *fu ling* 茯苓, *bai zhu* 白术, *chen pi* 陈皮, *huang lian* 黄连 and *shan zha* 山楂. *Huang lian, shan zha, fu ling, bai zhu* and *ze xie* 泽泻 were the top five herbs in reducing the WC and WHR. In terms of the acupuncture treatment, the frequently reported acupuncture points in meta-analyses showing favourable effects were ST36 *Zusanli* 足三里, ST25 *Tianshu* 天枢, CV12 *Zhongwan* 中脘, SP6 *Sanyinjiao* 三阴交 and CV4 *Guanyuan* 关元. The common ear acupuncture points were Endocrine 内分泌 (CO18), Stomach 胃 (CO4), Hunger 饥点, *Shenmen* 神门 (TF4) and Spleen 脾 (CO13).

In terms of efficacy, the available clinical evidence of CM treatments for overweight and obesity indicates that:

- CHM alongside lifestyle therapies may reduce BMI and WC.
- Acupuncture alone or alongside lifestyle therapies may be beneficial for weight, BMI and WC reduction.
- There is not enough evidence to show if other CM therapies such as *qigong, tuina* massage, cupping therapy or Chinese diet therapies are beneficial for people who are overweight or obese.

Generally, adverse events of CM treatments appeared to be few in number, mild and well tolerated. As for CHM treatments, gastrointestinal symptoms, like nausea, vomiting and diarrhoea, were the most frequent symptoms, while localised pain, bleeding and bruising of the acupoints were common after acupuncture treatment. However, the safety of other CM therapies or combination therapies is unknown, as original information was not provided.

In summary, CM treatments appear to be effective and safe for people who are overweight and obese, especially CHM alongside lifestyle therapies or acupuncture alongside lifestyle therapies, which gives some implications for clinical practice.

Implications for Research

Up to now, many CM clinical trials have been conducted to investigate the efficacy and safety of CM in treating overweight and obesity. Chinese herbal medicine and acupuncture therapies showed promising clinical benefits for overweight and obesity, according to current evidence. However, the evidence is not strong enough to draw a firm conclusion. Thus, further research is still needed.

Herbs in positive meta-analyses, such as *chen pi* 陈皮 and *huang lian* 黄连, have been found to have strong anti-obesity effects from many aspects of the pathogenesis of obesity through multiple mechanisms. However, research about other potential anti-obesity herbs, like *fu ling* 茯苓 and *bai zhu* 白术, are yet to be determined. Further pharmacological studies of herbs could improve understanding of the mechanism of CHM in treating people who are overweight and obese, which will help to promote effective treatments in the future.

Clinical Trial Design

Despite a great number of trials evaluating CM interventions, well-designed clinical trials based on a clear hypothesis with long-term follow-up are still needed. Based on the limitations of previous studies, further clinical studies should focus on the following areas:

Clinical Questions

- For different CM interventions, such as CHM, acupuncture, *qigong*, etc., what are the optimal treatment duration of each kind of intervention?
- For baseline BMI, what is the optimal population to receive CM treatments?
- Which kinds of people can get the optimal benefit of CM treatments, for example, men or women, young people or older people, simple obesity or obesity with complications?

- Are CM interventions able to prevent weight regain? Does longer treatment duration help to maintain weight?

Methods

- Once the study design is completed, researchers should register their trials with detailed protocols in a public clinical trial registry.
- Methodological experts and statisticians should be involved from an early stage.
- Risk of bias should be minimised through proper and considered clinical trial design, including random sequence generation and allocation concealment and blinding of participants and investigators whenever possible.
- In order to evaluate the efficacy of CM treatment comprehensively, some clinical outcomes, such as body fat mass and basal metabolic rate, should also be included in the study design.
- Studies with sufficient sample sizes and long-term follow-up are required.
- Cost-effectiveness analysis should also be undertaken to provide data for health policy.

Intervention

- Lifestyle therapies, including diet, physical exercise and behavioural regulation, are fundamental interventions of obesity treatment. A clear, specific and quantified program is essential in future trials.
- CM treatments based on syndrome differentiation are favourable to verify the efficacy of CM interventions in treating people who are overweight and obese.

Reporting

Generally, the published CM study reports were too brief to provide sufficient information on methodological design, implementation processes, and efficacy and safety outcomes. The absence of this information affects the certainty of the results. Thus, for future clinical trials, researchers should be aware of study reporting guidelines and improve the reporting of CM interventions; for example, the CARE statement to report case reports,[7] STROBE statement to report observational studies[8] and the CONSORT statement to report RCTs.[9] Given the increasing number of clinical studies of CM interventions, the CONSORT extensions for acupuncture and CHM should also be used.[10–11] Statements can be obtained from the following website: http://www.equator-network.org.

References

1. Garvey WT, Mechanick JI, Brett EM, *et al.* (2016) American Association of Clinical Endocrinologists and American College of Endocrinology comprehensive clinical practice guidelines for medical care of patients with obesity. *Endocr Pract* **22**(Suppl 3): 1–203.

2. Jensen MD, Ryan DH, Apovian CM, *et al.* (2014) 2013 AHA/ACC/TOS Guideline for the management of overweight and obesity in adults: A report of the American College of Cardiology/American Heart Association Task Force on Practice Guidelines and The Obesity Society. *Circulation.* **129**(25 suppl 2): S102–S138.

3. 中华医学会内分泌学分会肥胖学组. (2011) 中国成人肥胖症防治专家共识. 中华内分泌代谢杂志. **27**(9): 711–717.

4. 国家药典委员会. (2015) 中华人民共和国药典. 中国医药科技出版社.

5. World Health Organization Regional Office for the Western Pacific. (2007) WHO international standard terminologies on traditional medicine in the Western Pacific Region.

6. 危北海, 贾葆鹏. (1998) 单纯性肥胖病的诊断及疗效评定标准. *中国中西医结合杂志.* **18**(5): 317–319.

7. Gagnier JJ, Kienle G, Altman DG, *et al.* (2013) The CARE Guidelines: Consensus-based clinical case reporting guideline development. *Glob Adv Health Med* **2**(5): 38–43.

8. Von Elm E, Altman DG, Egger M, *et al.* (2014) The Strengthening the Reporting of Observational Studies in Epidemiology (STROBE) statement: Guidelines for reporting observational studies. *Int J Surg* **12**(12): 1495–1499.

9. Schulz KF, Altman DG, Moher D, *et al.* (2010) CONSORT 2010 statement: Updated guidelines for reporting parallel group randomized trials. *Obstet Gynecol.* **115**(5): 1063–1070.

10. MacPherson H, Altman DG, Hammerschlag R, *et al.* (2010) Revised standards for reporting interventions in clinical trials of acupuncture (STRICTA): Extending the CONSORT statement. *J Evid Based Med* **3**(3): 140–155.

11. Cheng CW, Wu TX, Shang HC, *et al.* (2017) CONSORT extension for Chinese herbal medicine formulas 2017: Recommendations, explanation, and elaboration. *Ann Intern Med* **167**(2): 112–121.

Glossary

Terms	Acronym	Definition	Reference
95% confidence interval	95% CI	A measure of the uncertainty around the main finding of a statistical analysis. Estimates of unknown quantities, such as the odds ratio comparing an experimental intervention with a control, are usually presented as a point estimate and a 95% confidence interval. This means that if someone were to keep repeating a study in other samples from the same population, 95% of the confidence intervals from those studies would contain the true value of the unknown quantity. Alternatives to 95%, such as 90% and 99% confidence intervals, are sometimes used. Wider intervals indicate lower precision; narrow intervals, greater precision.	https://training. cochrane.org/ handbook
Acupressure	—	Application of pressure on acupuncture points.	—

(*Continued*)

(*Continued*)

Terms	Acronym	Definition	Reference
Acupuncture	—	The insertion of needles into humans or animals for remedial purposes.	World Health Organization. Regional Office for the Western Pacific. (2007) WHO international standard terminologies on traditional medicine in the Western Pacific Region. Manila: WHO Regional Office for the Western Pacific.
Allied and Complementary Medicine Database	AMED	Alternative medicine bibliographic database.	https://www.ebsco.com/ products/research-databases/ allied-and-complementary-medicine-database-amed
Australian New Zealand Clinical Trial Registry	ANZCTR	Clinical trial registry based in Australia.	http://www.anzctr.org.au/
Body Mass Index	BMI	An individual's body mass in kilograms divided by the square of their height in meters. The BMI is highly correlated in the general population with the proportion of body fat. The following BMIs are used to classify individuals; underweight <20 kg/m², acceptable weight, 20–25 kg/m²; overweight, 25–30 kg/m²; obese, >30 kg/m². High BMI is considered a risk factor for diabetes, cardiovascular and cerebrovascular diseases.	Harris P, Nagy S, Vardaxis N. (2019) *Mosby's Dictionary of Medicine, Nursing and Health Professions.* 3rd revised Australian and New Zealand edition. Elsevier, Australia
China National Knowledge Infrastructure	CNKI	Chinese language bibliographic database.	https://www.cnki.net/

(*Continued*)

Terms	Acronym	Definition	Reference
Chinese Biomedical Literature Database	CBM	Chinese language bibliographic database.	http://www.imicams.ac.cn/
Chinese Clinical Trial Registry	ChiCTR	Chinese clinical trial registry.	http://www.chictr.org.cn/
Chinese herbal medicine	CHM	Chinese herbal medicine.	—
Chinese medicine	CM	Chinese medicine.	—
Chongqing VIP Information Company	CQVIP	Chinese language bibliographic database.	http://www.cqvip.com/
ClinicalTrials.gov	—	Clinical trial registry based in the United States of America.	https://clinicaltrials.gov/
Cochrane Central Register of Controlled Trials	CENTRAL	Bibliographic database that provides a highly concentrated source of reports of controlled trials.	https://community.cochrane.org/editorial-and-publishing-policy-resource/overview-cochrane-library-and-related-content/databases-included-cochrane-library/cochrane-central-register-controlled-trials-central
Combination therapies	—	Two or more Chinese medicines from different therapy groups (e.g., Chinese herbal medicine, acupuncture therapies or other Chinese medicine therapies) administered together.	—
Controlled clinical trials	CCT	A study in which people are allocated to different interventions using methods that are not random.	https://training.cochrane.org/handbook

(*Continued*)

(Continued)

Terms	Acronym	Definition	Reference
Convention on International Trade in Endangered Species of Wild Fauna and Flora	CITES	International convention aimed at preventing or regulating trade in threatened and endangered species of plants and animals.	https://www.cites.org/eng/disc/text.php
Cumulative Index of Nursing and Allied Health Literature	CINAHL	Bibliographic database.	https://www.ebscohost.com/nursing/products/cinahl-databases
Cupping therapy	—	Suction by using a vaccumised cup or jar.	World Health Organization. Regional Office for the Western Pacific. (2007) WHO international standard terminologies on traditional medicine in the Western Pacific Region. Manila: WHO Regional Office for the Western Pacific.
Effect size	—	A generic term for the estimate of the effect of a treatment in a study.	https://training.cochrane.org/handbook
Effective rate	—	A measure of the proportion of participants who achieved an improvement, as outlined in Chap, 4.	—
Electroacupuncture	—	Electric stimulation of the acupuncture needle following insertion.	World Health Organization. Regional Office for the Western Pacific. (2007) WHO international standard terminologies on traditional medicine in the Western Pacific Region. Manila: WHO Regional Office for the Western Pacific.

Terms	Acronym	Definition	Reference
EU Clinical Trials Register	EU-CTR	European clinical trial registry.	https://www.clinicaltrialsregister.eu/
Excerpta Medica database	Embase	Bibliographic database.	http://www.elsevier.com/solutions/embase
Grading of Recommendations Assessment, Development and Evaluation	GRADE	Approach used to grade quality of evidence and strength of recommendations.	http://www.gradeworkinggroup.org/
Heterogeneity	—	Used in a general sense to describe the variation in, or diversity of, participants, interventions, and measurement of outcomes across a set of studies, or the variation in internal validity of those studies. Used specifically, as statistical heterogeneity, to describe the degree of variation in the effect estimates from a set of studies. Also used to indicate the presence of variability among studies beyond the amount expected due solely to the play of chance.	https://training.cochrane.org/handbook
Homogeneity	—	Used in a general sense to mean that the participants, interventions, and measurement of outcomes are similar across a set of studies. Used specifically to describe the effect estimates from a set of studies where they do not vary more than would be expected by chance.	https://training.cochrane.org/handbook

(*Continued*)

(Continued)

Terms	Acronym	Definition	Reference
I²	—	A measure of study heterogeneity; indicates the percentage of variance in a meta-analysis.	https://training.cochrane.org/handbook
Integrative medicine	—	Chinese herbal medicine combined with pharmacotherapy or other conventional therapy.	
Mean difference	MD	In meta-analysis: A method used to combine measures on continuous scales, where the mean, standard deviation and sample size in each group are known. The weight given to the difference in means from each study (e.g., how much influence each study has on the overall results of the meta-analysis) is determined by the precision of its estimate of effect, mathematically, this is equal to the inverse of the variance. This method assumes that all of the trials have measured the outcome on the same scale.	https://training.cochrane.org/handbook
Meta-analysis	—	The use of statistical techniques in a systematic review to integrate the results of included studies. Sometimes misused as a synonym for systematic reviews, where the review includes a meta-analysis.	—
Moxibustion	—	A therapeutic procedure involving ignited material (usually moxa) to apply heat to certain points or areas of the body surface for managing disease.	World Health Organization. Regional Office for the Western Pacific. (2007) WHO international

(Continued)

Terms	Acronym	Definition	Reference
			standard terminologies on traditional medicine in the Western Pacific Region. Manila: WHO Regional Office for the Western Pacific.
Non-controlled studies	—	Observations made on individuals, usually receiving the same intervention, before and after the intervention but with no control group.	https://training. cochrane.org/ handbook
Obese/obesity	—	An abnormal increase in the proportion of fat cells, mainly in the viscera and subcutaneous tissues of the body. Generally, an adult is regarded as medically obese if they have a body mass index of greater than or equal to 30 kg/m².	Harris P, Nagy S, Vardaxis N. (2019) *Mosby's Dictionary of Medicine, Nursing and Health Professions.* 3rd revised Australian and New Zealand edition. Elsevier, Australia
Other Chinese medicine therapies	—	Other Chinese medicine therapies include all traditional therapies except Chinese herbal medicine and acupuncture/moxibustion, such as *tai chi, qigong, tuina,* and cupping.	
Overweight		More than normal body weight; a body mass index of greater than or equal to 25 kg/m².	Harris P, Nagy S, Vardaxis N. (2019) *Mosby's dictionary of medicine, nursing and health professions.* 3rd revised Australian and New Zealand edition. Elsevier: Australia

(Continued)

(*Continued*)

Terms	Acronym	Definition	Reference
PubMed	PubMed	Bibliographic database.	http://www.ncbi.nlm. nih.gov/pubmed
Qigong 气功	—	Physical exercises and breathing techniques.	—
Randomised controlled trial	RCT	Clinical trial that uses a random method to allocate participants to treatment and control groups.	—
Risk of bias	—	Assessment of clinical trials to indicate if the results may overestimate or underestimate the true effect because of bias in study design or reporting.	https://training. cochrane.org/ handbook
Risk ratio (relative risk)	RR	The ratio of risks in two groups. In intervention studies, it is the ratio of the risk in the intervention group to the risk in the control group. A risk ratio of one indicates no difference between comparison groups. For undesirable outcomes, a risk ratio that is less than one indicates that the intervention was effective in reducing the risk of that outcome.	https://training. cochrane.org/ handbook
Standardised mean difference	SMD	In meta-analysis: A method used to combine results for continuous scales that measure the same outcome but measure it in different ways (e.g., with different scales). The results of studies are standardised to a uniform scale to allow data to be combined.	https://training. cochrane.org/ handbook

(*Continued*)

Terms	Acronym	Definition	Reference
Summary of findings	SoF	Presentation of results and rating the quality of evidence based on the GRADE approach.	http://www.gradeworkinggroup.org/
Tai chi (*taiji*) 太极	—	A Chinese martial art with health benefits.	—
Type 2 diabetes mellitus	—	A type of diabetes mellitus in which patients are not insulin-dependent or ketosis-prone, although they may use insulin for correction of symptomatic or persistent hyperglycaemia and they can develop ketosis under special circumstances such as infection or stress. Onset is usually after 40 years of age but can occur at any age.	Harris P, Nagy S, Vardaxis N. (2019) *Mosby's Dictionary of Medicine, Nursing and Health Professions*. 3rd revised Australian and New Zealand edition. Elsevier, Australia
Transcutaneous electrical nerve stimulation	TENS	Application of transdermal electrical current to acupuncture points via conducting pads.	—
Tuina 推拿	—	Chinese massage: Rubbing, kneading, or percussion of the soft tissues and joints of the body with the hands, usually performed by one person on another, especially to relieve tension or pain.	World Health Organization. Regional Office for the Western Pacific. (2007) WHO international standard terminologies on traditional medicine in the Western Pacific Region. Manila: WHO Regional Office for the Western Pacific.
Wanfang database	Wanfang	Chinese language bibliographic database.	http://www.wanfangdata.com/

(*Continued*)

(Continued)

Terms	Acronym	Definition	Reference
World Health Organisation	WHO	WHO is the directing and coordinating authority for health within the United Nations system. It is responsible for providing leadership on global health matters, shaping the health research agenda, setting norms and standards, articulating evidence-based policy options, providing technical support to countries, and monitoring and assessing health trends.	http://www.who.int/about/en/
Zhong Hua Yi Dian 中华医典	ZHYD	The Zhong Hua Yi Dian (ZHYD) "Encyclopaedia of Traditional Chinese Medicine" is a comprehensive series of electronic books on compact disc. The collection was put together by the Hunan electronic and audio-visual publishing house. It is the largest collection of Chinese electronic books and includes the major Chinese ancient works, many of which are from rare manuscripts and are the only existing copies. These books cover the period from ancient times up to the period of the Republic of China (1911–1948).	Hu R, ed. (2000) *Zhong Hua Yi Dian [Encyclopaedia of Traditional Chinese Medicine]*. 4th ed. Hunan Electronic and Audio-Visual Publishing House, Chengsha.
Zhong Yi Fang Ji Da Ci Dian 中医方剂大辞典	ZYFJDCD	Compendium of Chinese herbal formulae with over 96,592 entries derived from classical Chinese books. The Nanjing Chinese Medicine Institute compiled the ZYFJDCD and first published it in 1993.	Peng HR, ed. (1994) *Zhong Yi Fang Ji Da Ci Dian [Great Compendium of Chinese Medical Formulae]*, 1st ed. People's Medical Publishing House, Beijing.

Index

Evidence-based Clinical Chinese Medicine

(*Continued from page ii*)

Forthcoming